S0-BMS-927

The Auditory Brainstem Response

CONTRIBUTORS

Paul J. Abbas, PhD
The University of Iowa
Wendell Johnson Speech and
  Hearing Center
Iowa City, IA 52242

Steven J. Allen, MD
Department of Anesthesiology
University of Texas Medical School
  and Hermann Hospital
Houston, TX 77030

Grant A. Berry, MA
Speech and Hearing Center
Hospital of the University
  of Pennsylvania
Philadelphia, PA 19104

L. Clarke Cox, PhD
Department of Speech and Hearing
Cleveland State University
Cleveland, OH 44115

Terese Finitzo-Hieber, PhD
Callier Center for Communication
  Disorders
The University of Texas at Dallas
Dallas, TX 75080

Thomas J. Fria, PhD
Department of Otolaryngology
University of Pittsburgh
  School of Medicine; and
Division of Audiology
Children's Hospital of Pittsburgh
Pittsburgh, PA 15260

Sandy Friel-Patti, PhD
Callier Center for Communication
  Disorders
The University of Texas at Dallas
Dallas, TX 75080

Karen M. Gollegly, MA
Section of Otolaryngology and Audiology
Dartmouth-Hitchcock Medical Center
Hanover, NH 03755

Michael P. Gorga, PhD
The Boys Town National Institute
  for Communication Disorders in
  Children
Omaha, NE 68131

James W. Hall III, PhD
Department of Otolaryngology–Head
  and Neck Surgery
University of Texas Medical School
  and Hermann Hospital
Houston, TX 77030

Kurt Hecox, MD, PhD
Department of Neurology
University of Wisconsin–Madison
Madison, WI 53706

Martyn L. Hyde, PhD
Silverman Research Centre
Mount Sinai Hospital
Toronto, Ontario M5G 1X5
Canada

John T. Jacobson, PhD
Department of Communicative Disorders
Speech and Hearing Center
University of Mississippi
University, MS 38677

Peter J. Jannetta, MD
Department of Neurological Surgery
University of Pittsburgh
  School of Medicine
Pittsburgh, PA 15213

James Jerger, PhD
Department of Otorhinolaryngology
  and Communicative Sciences
Baylor College of Medicine
Texas Medical Center
Houston, TX 77030

Robert W. Keith, PhD
Department of Otolaryngology and
  Maxillofacial Surgery
Division of Audiology and
  Speech Pathology
University of Cincinnati Medical Center
Cincinnati, OH 45267

Paul Kileny, PhD
Departments of Audiology and
  Clinical Electrophysiology
Glenrose Rehabilitation Hospital
Edmonton, Alberta T5G 0B7
Canada

Nina Kraus, PhD
David T. Siegel Institute for
  Communicative Disorders
Michael Reese Medical Center; and
Department of Surgery (Otolaryngology)
Chicago, IL 60616

George E. Lynn, PhD
Departments of Audiology and
  Neurology
Wayne State University
  School of Medicine
Harper Grace Hospital
Detroit, MI 48201

Judy Mackey-Hargadine, MD
Division of Neurosurgery
University of Texas Medical School
  and Hermann Hospital
Houston, TX 77030

Thomas M. Mahoney, PhD
Bureau of Communicative Disorders
Utah Department of Health
Salt Lake City, UT 84113

John W. R. McIntyre, MD
Department of Anesthesiology
University of Alberta Hospital
Edmonton, Alberta T6G 2B7
Canada

Aage R. Møller, PhD
Department of Neurological Surgery
University of Pittsburgh
  School of Medicine; and
Presbyterian–University Hospital
Pittsburgh, PA 15213

Frank E. Musiek, PhD
Section of Otolaryngology and Audiology
Dartmouth-Hitchcock Medical Center
Hanover, NH 03755

Terrey Oliver, MS
Division of Audiology and
  Speech Pathology
Baylor College of Medicine
Texas Medical Center
Houston, TX 77030

Marilyn Pérez-Abalo, MD
Department of Neurophysiology
National Center for Scientific
  Investigation
Playa, Havana
Cuba

Terence W. Picton, MD, PhD
Department of Medicine
University of Ottawa
Ottawa General Hospital
Ottawa, Ontario K1H 8L6
Canada

Daniel Read, BA
Human Neurosciences Research Unit
University of Ottawa
Ottawa, Ontario K1H 8M5
Canada

Daniel M. Schwartz, PhD
Divison of Hearing and Speech Sciences
Vanderbilt University
  School of Medicine
Nashville, Tennessee 37232

Andrée Smith, PhD
Department of Audiology
Children's Hospital of Eastern Ontario
Ottawa, Ontario K1H 8L1
Canada

Brad Stach, MA
Division of Audiology and Speech
  Pathology
Baylor College of Medicine
Texas Medical Center
Houston, TX 77030

David R. Stapells, PhD
Department of Neurosciences
University of California–San Diego
  School of Medicine; and
Children's Hospital & Health Center
San Diego, CA 92123

Laszlo Stein, PhD
David T. Siegel Institute for
  Communicative Disorders
Michael Reese Medical Center; and
Department of Surgery (Otolaryngology)
University of Chicago
Chicago, IL 60616

Narayan P. Verma, MD
Department of Neurology
Wayne State University
  School of Medicine
Detroit, MI 48201

Bruce A. Weber, PhD
Center for Speech and Hearing Disorders
Duke University Medical Center
Durham, NC 27710

Don W. Worthington, PhD
The Boys Town National Institute
  for Communication Disorders in
  Children
Omaha, NE 68131

The Auditory Brainstem Response

Edited by John T. Jacobson, PhD

COLLEGE-HILL PRESS, San Diego, California

College-Hill Press, Inc.
4284 41st Street
San Diego, California 92105

Library of Congress Cataloging in Publication Data
Main entry under title:

The auditory brainstem response.

    Bibliography: p.
    Includes index.
    1. Audiometry, Evoked response.   2. Auditory evoked response. 3. Brainstem—Diseases—Diagnosis.   4. Hearing disorders—Diagnosis.   I. Jacobson, John T., 1943-
RF294.5E87A9   1984   617.8'86075   84-14253
ISBN 0-933014-15-5
    0–88744–268–4 (paper)

Dedication

To Claire, Vanessa, and Seth,
and for Marion, a source of constant inspiration

CONTENTS

PREFACE

The development of auditory brainstem response (ABR) measurement has changed our entire perspective on auditory and otoneurological assessment. Given that ABR has become an acceptable clinical procedure, intense demands have been placed on professionals to integrate the ABR methodology into the routine audiological test battery. Unfortunately, the advantages of ABR in the clinical setting are frequently offset by minimal academic exposure to auditory evoked potentials and limited clinical experience by the clinician. In an effort to meet clinical pressures, professionals and students alike have sought workshops, seminars and educational centers in an attempt to foster their knowledge and clinical expertise.

This textbook was conceived to fulfill two purposes: 1) to provide a literary source which focuses specifically on the role of ABR in a clinical setting; and 2) to offer a comprehensive description of the current state of knowledge in ABR measurement. This book is intended to serve as a graduate level text in audiology, otoneurology and other associated disciplines. With minor exception, this book will focus on clinical application and diagnostic assessment and therefore will be of interest to professionals and students in clinical and research facilities who are either currently involved or intend to develop auditory evoked potential laboratories. Throughout this textbook, emphasis has been directed toward a basic understanding and framework from which the clinician may expand and develop their knowledge base in ABR. Finally, this book has been designed to be used as a primary resource text in conjunction with original scientific research.

I would like to express my appreciation to each author who contributed to this textbook. For the many letters and phone calls they received requesting opinions, tapping their expertise and ultimately providing the clinical direction this book has taken, I am greatly indebted. To Jerry Northern who laid the groundwork and encouraged me to pursue such an undertaking as well as providing me with space and secretarial assistance during my sabbattical, a special thanks. To Barb Hansen who assisted me in manuscript preparation, personal correspondence and has done much to keep me afloat during those difficult times, a most appreciated thank you. A special acknowledgement to Aage Møller who allowed me to reproduce an illustration he submitted in his chapter and is found on the cover of this textbook. Finally, to my family whose patience and understanding made this book possible despite my idiosyncrasies, thanks for hanging in there.

John T. Jacobson

FOREWORD

The decade of the Eighties will be remembered by clinicians and scientists as the era of evoked potential measurement. The application of signal averaging techniques has influenced nearly every area of science. We can now examine miniscule periods of time to extract bioelectric information about the nervous system that in previous years was considered impossible. Signal averaging has opened untold avenues and created new vistas for examining the neural physiology of all sensory systems.

As a classic example of technology preceding application, clinicians and researchers are having a heyday developing procedures to make the most of this high-tech instrumentation. Seemingly, each current issue of every clinical journal contains new information on innovative applications of evoked potentials to basic science, identification and diagnosis of neurological problems, as well as the treatment and management of hearing impaired individuals.

The field of hearing and audition is no exception, and the use of auditory evoked potentials has had tremendous influence on all of us working with hearing-impaired patients or searching for the missing pieces in normal auditory physiology. In these past few years, with the development of auditory brainstem short-latency evoked potentials, our accuracy in detection of auditory pathway lesions has increased tremendously; confirmation of hearing loss in infants has become a practical reality leading to earlier intervention than ever before possible; auditory testing of difficult patients, such as multiply-handicapped children and functional hearing loss patients, has become routine in daily clinical activity. In short, the use of auditory brainstem responses has become a mandatory piece of the current audiologic test battery.

However, it is time to start documenting the uses of auditory brainstem responses in an orderly and complete treatise so that university training programs, as well as working clinicians and involved researchers, can go to a single source for a comprehensive review of the topic. John Jacobson has accepted and fulfilled that task by bringing together an outstanding group of experienced professionals to produce a very readable and worthy textbook. I have watched the initiation, development and completion of this textbook through the unwavering dedication of Dr. Jacobson, and I view the final result with satisfaction that this textbook fulfills his goals and purposes.

Dr. Jacobson has organized the material in this book into five major sections. Section I includes four introductory and basic chapters necessary for the understanding of the auditory brainstem response (ABR). The five chapters of Section II focus on auditory aspects while the five chapters of Section III emphasize neurologic aspects of ABR. Section IV features chapters describing pediatric clinical applications; and Section V has interesting chapters on special applications of auditory brainstem response measurements including hearing aid applications and presentation of illustrative case studies. All in all, the reader will find a well organized collection of materials dealing with all aspects of the auditory brainstem response.

My congratulations to all the contributors for achieving the utmost in their assignments which will help all of us understand better this exciting method of analyzing the auditory system.

Jerry L. Northern, Ph.D.
Professor of Otolaryngology
University of Colorado School of Medicine

SECTION I
FOUNDATIONS

Chapter 1

An Overview of the Auditory Brainstem Response

John T. Jacobson

Pity me not, but lend thy serious hearing to what I shall unfold

Hamlet
Wm. Shakespeare

INTRODUCTION

The clinical application of the auditory brainstem response (ABR) has provided a unique diagnostic dimension that has transcended interdisciplinary boundaries. The proliferation of the ABR technique has provided a mutual appreciation of the expertise and responsibilities of hearing specialists concerned with the needs of the auditorally and neurologically impaired. In the audiology community, no other test procedure has caused so much interest, generated such attention, and been so widely accepted. The wealth of information published on the ABR has for the most part been positive. Manufacturers have enthusiastically entered the competitive marketplace, producing an array of instrumentation and associated software. This latter contribution has done much to bring electrophysiological measures from the realm of experimental research to routine clinical use.

Today, with the ease of recording auditory evoked potentials (AEP) and the relatively inexpensive investment required, many clinical programs heretofore unable to provide such expertise and services have added the ABR to the clinical neurophysiological armamentarium. Too often, however, the introduction of ABR finds its way into the clinical setting due to administrative and professional pressures, not necessarily from a willingness to use it on the part of the clinician who is placed in the position of delivering responsible services.

In many instances, the scheduling and testing of patients may often occur before clinicians are adequately trained, have the opportunity to become "comfortable" with instrumentation and procedures, or have the time to establish the laboratory standards and norms so critical in the overall diagnostic process. Under these circumstances, misinterpretation is frequently inevitable, and unfortunately not entirely the fault of the clinician. When either technical, procedural, or interpretative errors occur, the credibility of the examiner and the electrophysiological test may come under seemingly justified criticism. This is of particular concern to those who have had previous clinical experience with the ABR. Regardless of one's level of expertise, anyone who has tested a patient experiences insecurity and frustration when, in a diagnostic assessment, replicable ABR tracings are unobtainable. Where does the fault lie? With the subject (pathology), the instrumentation (technical and/or procedural), or with the examiner (what have *I* done)? Nonetheless, despite these and other limitations addressed herein, the ABR has more than adequately proven itself as one of the leading clinical tools in the diagnosis of peripheral auditory dysfunction and neural brainstem integrity.

One reason the ABR has gained such rapid acceptance is its ability to objectively detect, localize, and monitor auditory and neurological deficits in difficult-to-test populations. This diverse clinical caseload includes any patient unable or unwilling to participate in traditional behavioral test protocol. Here, two caveats are in order. While no overt response is necessary from the patient, minimal cooperation is required. The adult patient must remain immobile, the baby should sleep. Another caveat is that a great deal of knowledge and experience is required to accurately identify and interpret abnormal ABR recordings. Subjectivity is inherent in every evaluation. And, as is the case in any subjective assessment, the key to resolution is the development of a substantial normative data base, personal hands-on experience, a consistent approach in the interpretative process, and a willingness to admit to an inconclusive outcome. It is hoped that this book will succeed in providing sufficient clinical information to answer many questions that the reader may have while simultaneously raising a number of queries for future study.

Finally, although this textbook concentrates primarily on only one latency epoch of the AEP, let us not forget the importance of the comprehensive test battery, which undoubtedly assists in the identification, diagnosis, and quantification of auditory and neurological disorders. As audiologists we must also open our clinical vistas and familiarize ourselves with other existing sensory evoked potentials (EPs) and their contribution to the overall diagnostic scheme. These potentials include the somatosensory and visual EPs. Many facilities, particularly those involved in neurological study, have successfully applied a multimodality EP approach. The integration of sensory EPs may prove to be the most powerful diagnostic entity in the clinical arena.

Historical Perspective

The monitoring of spontaneous bioelectric activity generated from the central nervous system (CNS) and recorded from the human scalp was first described by Berger (1929). These random electric events comprise the electroencephalogram (EEG). This pioneering effort was followed by the work of Loomis, Harvey, and Hobart (1938), who first reported alterations in human EEG patterns brought about by the introduction of sensory stimulation. This process of extracting stimulus-related bioelectric events from ongoing EEG activity set the stage for future clinical development in various aspects of evoked potential measurement.

In stimulus-related response measures, the spontaneous EEG voltage far exceeds that of the EP. As a consequence, throughout the history of EP development, various techniques have focused on means of eliminating unwanted physiological noise from response recordings. To this end, several attempts have been made to extract the EP from the EEG pattern (Dawson, 1951, 1954; Geisler, Frishkopf, & Rosenblith, 1958). Currently, the process of averaging has been the most successful in this pursuit. Clark (1958) and co-workers (1961) developed the principle of algebraic summation of bioelectric events elicited by stimulus synchronization (time-locked repetition). This operation functions through a process of analog-to-digital conversion whereby EEG voltage is converted and expressed as a numerical value (binary system). During the conversion process, information is maintained and the signal-to-noise ratio (SNR) remains constant so long as the sampling rate is adequate. Because the EP is predicated on event-related stimuli, it assumes a constant time relationship to the signal onset; in contrast, the ever-present unwanted noise is random. Theoretically, noise has no time relationship to stimulus onset and thus EPs can be extracted from the noise of the random EEG activity. Regardless of the process, however, the resulting response will always be contaminated to some degree by residual noise

(Picton, Liden, Hamel, & Maru, 1983). Hence, the necessity for further SNR reduction techniques (see Hyde, chapter 3).

Davis (1939) and Davis and colleagues (1939) initially described the results of a series of auditory evoked cortical potentials obtained from alert and sleeping humans. Their observations showed small but consistent changes in raw EEG tracings with the introduction of repeatable auditory stimuli. These AEPs were most robust when recorded from the vertex: hence, the commonly used designation, the "V" or vertex potential.

Following the discovery of the cortical AEPs from the human scalp, clinical interest was focused on the refinement of technical and procedural variables. During this era, two additional AEPs, the compound cochlear nerve action potential (AP) (Ruben, Sekula, Bordley, Knickerbocker, Nager, & Fisch, 1960) and what is currently referred to as the middle latency response (MLR) (Goldstein & Rodman, 1967) were being successfully explored. Each response has significantly contributed to the overall understanding of EPs; a historical summary of their development can be found in Davis (1976), Gibson (1978), Moore (1983), and Reneau and Hnatiow (1975).

The most recent electrophysiological procedure to dominate clinical auditory practice has been the ABR. In reviewing pertinent literature, the brainstem response should be considered an outgrowth of research activity conducted in the exploration of the cochlear microphonic (CM), the compound action-potential (AP), and the cortical response. Most of the early investigation monitoring the CM and AP involved the use of invasive techniques not readily available to the clinic setting. As a consequence, a good deal of attention was centered on alternative procedures to surgical recording methods. Among those investigating noninvasive electrode placement were Sohmer and Feinmesser (1967), who offered the first account of EPs generated from the brainstem. They reported a series of four wave components, the first two waves comprising the N_1–N_2 complex of the acoustic nerve AP. The latter two waves were of questionable origin and it was surmised that the responses were either repetitive firing of the acoustic nerve or neural discharge patterns from the brainstem pathway. While later confirmed (Sohmer & Feinmesser, 1973), it was the work of Jewett (1970) and colleagues (Jewett & Romano, 1972; Jewett, Romano, & Williston, 1970; Jewett & Williston, 1971) who definitively identified and described the origin of the far-field scalp-recorded ABR. In a light and revealing commentary, Jewett (1983) discusses his first encounter with the brainstem response while recording cortical activity in anesthetized animals. Convinced that these responses found "at the far left of the display screen" (p. xxv) were artifacts, investigative pursuits were restricted to informal seminars and discussions. After a relatively quiescent period, collaborative interest in the brainstem response was resumed and the result produced the now renowned series of publications by Jewett and co-workers previously cited. During this period, other investigators (Moore, 1971; Yoshie, 1968) also began to explore various aspects of the acoustic nerve AP using noninvasive procedures. Whether these researchers or others knowingly recorded brainstem potentials is a moot point. The evidence was now in.

Since the inception of the recorded brainstem potentials, two additional derivatives have been identified. They are the *following frequency response* (Moushegian, Rupert, & Stillman, 1973) and the *slow negative wave* occurring at about 10 ms (Davis & Hirsh, 1979). These potentials are recorded in response to frequency-related tonal stimuli. To date, the use of these two responses has had limited clinical success (see chapter 9).

It is not the intent of this writer to review in detail the historical events which have led to the current status of the ABR. That information may be found in each chapter of this text in a precise and sequential order. Suffice it to say that the ABR has come to embrace virtually every aspect and population associated in auditory and ontoneurological investigation. For a comprehensive review of the historical development of the ABR, the reader is encouraged to read Fria (1980) and Moore (1983).

Classification

Auditory evoked potentials comprise a series of neuroelectric responses generated at all levels of the auditory mechanism. Using scalp electrodes, as many as 15 AEPs have been identified within the first 500 ms poststimulus onset (Picton, Hillyard, Krauz, & Galambos, 1974; Picton, Woods, Baribeau-Braun, & Healey, 1977).

The stimulus-dependent responses used in clinical application take the form of either receptor or neurogenic potentials. Receptor potentials are generated from cochlear hair cells and consist of the CM and the summating potential (SP). The CM is considered a bioelectric analog of the auditory stimulus since it faithfully reproduces the signal input. The CM has no measurable latency delay to signal onset, represents basal region outer hair cell activity, and has no physiological threshold reducing its clinical value. The SP is seen as a negative DC voltage shift lasting the duration of the input signal. As in the CM, the SP is reflective of hair cell status and thus any pathology of the ear directly affects voltage amplitude; therefore, SP abnormality is restricted to end-organ disorders.

In contrast to receptor potential generation, neurogenic potentials originate from the acoustic nerve and other neural sites within the auditory CNS. They comprise action potential discharges and graded postsynaptic potentials and are of significant clinical interest. The following is a general classification of neurogenic AEPs.

In the absence of any formally adopted terminology, a number of classifications have been used interchangeably to describe AEPs. The two most familiar employed in clinical practice refer to the site of neural generation and the response latency. For example, the brainstem response and cortical or vertex potential reflect origins of neural activity.[1] These potentials and others are also described in terms of their latency. In Davis (1976) responses are described in order of their latency epoch and may be expressed as follows: "first" (cochlear microphonic, summating potential and acoustic nerve: 0–2 ms); "fast" (acoustic nerve and auditory brainstem response: 2–10 ms); "middle" (thalamus and auditory cortex: 8–50 ms); "slow" (primary and secondary areas of the cerebral cortex: 50–300 ms); and "late" (primary and association areas of cerebral cortex: 300+ ms).

The latency designations are used less frequently in favor of the generator descriptions. However, this does not always hold true; take for example the MLR, which may have cortical and thalamic origin. This response is almost exclusively referred to by its latency (MLR) found, in time, between the "fast" and "slow" response epochs. Other AEP classifications include stimulus–response relationship and electrode placement. A summary of receptor and neurogenic potentials is present in Table 1-1. For a detailed account of classification systems the reader is encouraged to review Davis, 1976; Jacobson and Hyde, in press, and Picton and Fitzgerald, 1983.

THE ABR

Description

The auditory brainstem response is considered a far-field recording by virtue of the fact that monitoring electrodes attached to the scalp are removed from the site of the electric field source. The ABR latency epoch consists of five to seven wave peaks measured within the first 10 ms. In the newborn and infant population, the response usually consists of only three wave

---

[1]The terminology used to reflect the neural response location may not be anatomically correct. The first and second waves of the auditory brainstem response do not originate from the brainstem but rather regions of the acoustic nerve (see Møller and Jannetta, chapter 2).

TABLE 1-1.
A Classification System of Auditory Evoked Potentials and their Descriptions

Common name	Physiological description	Anatomy source	Latency epoch	Latency range (ms)	Stimulus– response	Electrode– response
Cochlear microphonic (CM)	Receptor	Hair cells	First	0	Sustained	Near-field
Summating potential (SP)	Receptor	Hair cells	First	0	Sustained	Near-field
Action potential (AP) (N_1N_2) (ECochG)	Neurogenic	Auditory nerve	First	~2	Transient	Near and Far-field
Auditory brainstem response (ABR) (I–VII)	Neurogenic	Auditory nerve Brainstem	First Fast	<10	Transient	Far-field
Slow-negative (SN_{10})	Neurogenic	Brainstem	Fast	~10	Transient	Far-field
Frequency following response (FFR)	Neurogenic	Brainstem	Fast	Tone duration	Sustained	Far-field
Middle latency response (MLR) (N_0, P_0, N_a, P_a, N_b, P_b)	Neurogenic	Thalamus Auditory cortex	Middle	8–50	Transient	Far-field
Event-related potential (40 Hz)	Neurogenic	Brainstem–Thalamus Auditory cortex	Fast? Middle?	12–50	Transient? Sustained?	Far-field
Slow-vertex response (SVR) P_1, N_1, P_2, N_2	Neurogenic	Cerebral cortex (primary and association)	Slow	50–300	Transient	Far-field
Sustained cortical potential (SCP)	Neurogenic	Cerebral cortex (P & A)	Slow	Tone duration	Sustained	Far-field
Late positive component (P_{300})	Neurogenic	Cerebral cortex (P & A)	Late	250–350	Perceptual	Far-field
Cognitive negative variation (CNV)	Neurogenic	Cerebral cortex (association)	Late	300+	Perceptual	Far-field

NOTE: From Jacobson & Hyde, 1984

peaks (I, III, and V) whose latency and amplitude differ from adult values (Jacobson, Morehouse, & Johnson, 1982). The designated time interval of the brainstem response is usually based on the number of identifiable wave components, pathological considerations, and technical variables. For instance, lesions of the acoustic nerve and auditory brainstem (Section III) may diminish or totally eliminate wave amplitude, thereby altering the original number of waves and their component morphology. Technical aspects will also affect the latency epoch. These aspects include factors such as electrode placement, stimulus polarity, rate, filtering characteristics, and stimuli, all of which may influence the latency, amplitude, and morphology of the brainstem response. For example, transient stimuli are most often used in EP study because of their ability to initiate the neural synchronization of certain cell types whose onset discharge patterns are necessary in ABR production. These click stimuli elicit ABR wave components that have a relatively stable latency as a function of intensity (e.g., wave V = 5.8 ms at 60 dB nHL). However, even in a normal ear, a change in the auditory signal (e.g., low-frequency tone pip having a longer rise time) will prolong the wave V latency to 13–15 ms at low intensity levels.

Wave nomenclature. There are several methods of identifying wave peak ABR components. Throughout this book, the order-sequence described by Jewett and Williston (1971) has been adopted to identify individual waves. This nomenclature, which uses Roman numerals (I–VII) to designate wave peaks, is the one most commonly found in the literature and the least subject to misinterpretation.

Electrodes. Two additional forms of descriptive confusion involve the terms given to electrodes and their relationship with the visual appearance of the ABR tracing. In bipolar recordings used in ABR measures, three electrodes are usually applied to the scalp and commonly referred to as the "active," "reference," and "ground." These terms are misleading and do not accurately represent the underlying physiological events. ABR measures are based on neural synchronized discharges from subcortical levels. These electrical fields generated from caudal regions of the auditory mechanism are transmitted within a volume conductive medium of extracellular fluid and tissue. Thus, any electrode located on the scalp and remote from the electric field source will potentially register neural activity; therefore, the label "reference," suggesting a nonactive or indifferent electric site, is not applicable in such recording methodology.

Two sets of alternative electrode terms are gaining popularity. They are "positive" and "negative," related to electrode input at the preamplifier stage, and "noninverting" and "inverting," describing amplifier function. The third electrode, the "ground" or, more appropriately, the "common" electrode, serves as a reference electrode for the other two. The primary responsibility of the differential preamplifier is to amplify the resulting neural activity after a process of polarity reversal at the inverting electrode. The degree of internal noise cancellation is called the common-mode rejection ratio and is described fully in chapter 3.

Finally, a comment is necessary to explain the polarity direction of a brainstem response tracing. Most clinics in North America subscribe to a vertex/forehead-positive convention in an upward direction. In contrast, there is a tendency for European and Scandinavian facilities to reverse the sequence; that is, vertex-positive displayed downward. This direction in polarity is controlled by switching electrode input at the preamplifier stage. With the exceptions of chapters 2 and 9, all brainstem response tracings in this book follow the vertex-positive upward convention.

Validity

During the past decade and a half, there has been a dramatic increase in the efficiency of specialized audiological test procedures in otoneurological diagnoses. Today, individual tests are closely scrutinized in terms of their performance. The validity of a test, measured by the proportion of confirmed results, strongly influences its use and longevity. Improvements in technology and instrumentation, specific test selection in site-of-lesion analysis, and the incorporation of the test battery have all contributed to the overall improvement in accuracy of diagnostic prediction.

With the role of audiological services expanding to provide increased precision concerning peripheral and central deficits, the clinician can no longer be content with a test that simply provides a relatively high degree of sensitivity, that is, the ability of a test to correctly identify patients with auditory or otoneurological abnormalities. To improve diagnostic accuracy, a test must go beyond sensitivity as a measure of test validity. A test must also be accountable in terms of identifying patients with normal auditory function (i.e., specificity).

The test performance of the ABR in clinical practice has achieved a relatively high degree of validity. This is especially evident in the diagnosis of retrocochlear lesions where it is not unexpected to find hit rates of ABR abnormality exceeding 95%, whereas false positive rates are usually less than 10% (Eggermont, Don, & Brackman, 1980; Glasscock, Jackson, Josey, Dickins, & Wiet, 1979; Selters & Brackman, 1979; Terkildsen, Osterhammel, & Thomsen, 1981). An example of the illustrative accuracy of ABR in retrocochlear disorders has been reported by S. Jerger (1983). Analyzing data gathered by Musiek, Sachs, Geurkink, and Weider (1980), who reviewed the literature to discover 179 patients with acoustic tumors and a second group of 776 presumed cochlear-impaired subjects, Jerger found that the ABR produced sensitivity and specificity scores of 97 and 88%, respectively. In addition, test efficiency, an indicator of overall accuracy and measured by the total number of correctly identified patients, was 91%. In her analysis, the acoustic reflex measure had the next best rating, with a 78% efficiency.

The high-risk infant population is another group for which the ABR has proven itself in terms of test efficiency. Although there are a number of complicating issues in neonatal testing, such as middle ear effusion, transient neurological deficits, correct gestational age estimates, and appropriate follow-up services, the predictive rate of the ABR appears superior to all other newborn test procedures (see Fria, chapter 17, and Jacobson & Morehouse, 1984). The point to be gained here is that in special populations and in cases of retrocochlear disease, the ABR has established the best overall test performance used in audiological services.

Clinical Application

The ABR is the most recent electrophysiological procedure to be integrated into the audiological test battery. The development of the ABR has focused on two principal areas of application: (1) the evaluation and diagnosis of the peripheral auditory system and related pathology, and (2) the neural integrity of the acoustic nerve and caudal levels of the brainstem pathway (Hecox & Jacobson, 1984).

In the assessment of auditory sensitivity, one of the primary objectives of the ABR is to identify, as closely as possible, the patient's hearing status. This is normally accomplished in one of two ways. The first involves the monitoring of the response amplitude brought about by decreases in stimulus intensity until the presence of a brainstem response is no longer replicated. In ABR, the wave V component is used to estimate threshold and the resulting difference between the electrophysiological and behavioral thresholds. Threshold is dependent on pathological conditions and technical parameters used in ABR measurement. Due to these variables, the two thresholds are unlikely to be identical. The electrophysiological threshold is about 10 dB poorer in adults and approximately 20 dB elevated in the infant population when compared to psychophysical estimates.

The second method applies an input–output function as a means of assessing auditory sensitivity. In the case of the ABR, this usually describes the relationship between the stimulus intensity and the latency of the brainstem response. This is known as the latency–intensity function and involves a comparison of wave V latencies at several intensity levels to a norm. The result is a slope function measured in milli- or microseconds per decibel. While somewhat variable, the adult slope function is about 0.04 ms/dB with a range of 0.03 to 0.06 ms/dB (Galambos & Hecox, 1978). The advantage of the latency–intensity function is that it provides a standard by which site-of-lesion determination may be evaluated. Deviations of greater than 0.06 ms/dB are indicative of sensorineural pathology, whereas slope functions of 0.03 ms/dB or less suggest primarily high-frequency hearing loss (Hecox & Jacobson, 1984). For slope functions that parallel but are offset in latency, conductive pathology is suspect.

The second major application of the ABR and perhaps most significant in its role as a diagnostic tool is the identification of neurological abnormalities. As discussed, the sensitivity of the ABR to predict eighth nerve and brainstem lesions has been uncanny. This ability has not been exclusively limited to space-occupying lesions but also encompasses demyelinating and degenerative diseases and vascular lesions. The ABR is also being used in the examination of high-risk neurologically impaired newborns confined to the neonatal intensive care nursery. Finally, neurological application of the ABR is being used with growing interest as an intraoperative monitoring technique and in comatose and brain dead patients.

Implicit in neurological application is the understanding that any EP, including the ABR, will reveal only functional abnormality and not specific pathologic locus. The complexity of the brainstem pathway and the size, number, and impingment of the lesion will influence the resulting response. Second, it is important to recall that any peripheral abnormality will affect the interpretation of the neurological assessment. Therefore, it is imperative to know the condition of the peripheral mechanism and its influence on the brainstem response prior to judgmental inference about neurological status.

From this brief overview it can be seen that the ABR technique has become an integral part of audiological and neurological batteries. It must, however, be handled with great respect and only by knowledgeable professionals. Its variability, subjectivity, and sophisticated instrumentation do not lend themselves to use by the casual operator.

REFERENCES

Berger, H. (1929). Uber das elektroenkephalogram des menschen. *Archives fur Psychiatrie und Nervenkrankheiten, 87,* 527–570.

Clark, W. A., Jr. (1958). *Average response computer (ARC-1).* Quarterly Progress Report No. 49. Research Laboratory of Electronics, Massachusetts Institute of Technology. Cambridge, MA: MIT Press.

Clark, W. A., Jr., Goldstein, M. H., Jr., Brown, R. M., Molnar, C. E., O'Brien D. F., & Zieman, H. E. (1961). The average response computer (ARC): A digital device for computing averages and amplitudes and time histograms of electrophysiological responses. *Transactions of IRE, 8,* 46–51.

Davis, H., (1976). Principles of electric response audiometry. *Annals of Otology, Rhinology, and Laryngology, 85,* Supplement 28.

Davis, H., Davis, P. A., Loomis, A. L., Harvey, E. N., & Hobart, G. (1939). Electrical reactions of the human brain to auditory stimulation during sleep. *Journal of Neurophysiology, 2,* 500–514.

Davis, H., & Hirsh, S. K. (1979). A slow brainstem response for low-frequency audiometry. *Audiology, 18,* 445–461.

Davis, P. A. (1939). Effects of acoustic stimuli on the waking human brain. *Journal of Neurophysiology, 2,* 494–499.

Dawson, G. D. (1951). A summation technique for detecting small signals in a large, irregular background. *Journal of Physiology, 115,* 2P-3P.

Dawson, G. D. (1954). A summation technique for the detection of small evoked potentials. *Electroencephalography and Clinical Neurophysiology, 6,* 65-84.

Eggermont, J., Don, M., & Brackman, D. (1980). Electrocochleography and auditory brainstem electric responses in patients with pontine angle tumors. *Annals of Otology, Rhinology, and Laryngology,* Supplement 75.

Fria, T. J. (1980). The auditory brainstem response: Background and clinical applications. *Maico Monographs in Contemporary Audiology, 2,* 1-44.

Galambos, R., & Hecox, K. (1978). Clinical application of the auditory brainstem response. *Otolaryngologic Clinics of North America, 11,* 709-722.

Geisler, C. D.,. Frishkopf, L. S., & Rosenblith, W. A. (1958). Extracranial responses to acoustic clicks in man. *Science, 128,* 1210-1211.

Gibson, W. P. R. (1978). *Essentials of clinical evoked response audiometry.* New York: Churchill Livingstone.

Glasscock, M., Jackson, C., Josey, A., Dickins, J., & Wiet, R. (1979). Brainstem evoked response audiometry in clinical practice. *Laryngoscope, 89,* 1021-1034.

Goldstein, R., & Redman, L. B. (1967). Early components of averaged evoked responses to rapidly repeated auditory stimuli. *Journal of Speech and Hearing Research, 10,* 697-705.

Hecox, K., & Jacobson, J. T. (1984). Auditory evoked potentials. In J. L. Northern (Ed.), *Hearing disorders.* Boston: Little, Brown.

Jacobson, J. T., & Hyde, M. (in press). An introduction to auditory evoked potentials. In J. Katz (Ed.), *Handbook of clinical audiology.* Baltimore: Williams & Wilkins.

Jacobson, J. T., & Morehouse, C. R. (1984). A comparison of auditory brainstem response and behavioral screening in high risk and normal newborn infants. *Ear and Hearing, 5,* 247-253.

Jacobson, J. T., Morehouse, C. R., & Johnson, M. J. (1982). Strategies for infant auditory brainstem response assessment. *Ear and Hearing, 3,* 263-270.

Jerger, S. (1983). Decision matrix and information theory analyses in the evaluation of neuroaudiologic tests. *Seminars in Hearing: The Neuroaudiologic Evaluation, 4,* 121-132.

Jewett, D. L. (1970). Volume conducted potentials in response to auditory stimuli as detected by averaging in the cat. *Electroencephalography and Clinical Neurophysiology, 28,* 609-618.

Jewett, D. L. (1983). Introduction. In E. Moore (Ed.), *Bases of auditory brain-stem evoked responses.* New York: Grune & Stratton.

Jewett, D. L., & Romano, M. N. (1972). Neonatal development of auditory system potentials from the scalp of rat and cat. *Brain Research, 36,* 101-115.

Jewett, D. L., Romano, M. N., & Williston, J. S. (1970). Human auditory evoked potentials: Possible brain stem components detected on scalp. *Science, 167,* 1517-1518.

Jewett, D. L., & Williston, J. S. (1971). Auditory evoked far fields averaged from the scalp of humans. *Brain, 94,* 681-696.

Loomis, A., Harvey, E., & Hobart, G. (1938). Disturbances of patterns in sleep. *Journal of Neurophysiology, 1,* 413-430

Moore, E. (1971). *Human cochlear microphonics and auditory nerve action potentials from surface electrodes.* Unpublished PhD dissertation, University of Wisconsin, Madison.

Moore, E. (Ed.), (1983). *Bases of auditory brain-stem evoked responses.* New York: Grune & Stratton.

Moushegian, G., Rupert, A. L., & Stillman, R. D. (1973). Scalp-recorded early response in man to frequencies in the speech range. *Electroencephalography and Clinical Neurophysiology, 35,* 665-667.

Musiek, F., Sachs, E., Geurkink, N., & Weider, D. (1980). Auditory brainstem response and eighth nerve lesions: A review and presentation of cases. *Ear and Hearing, 1,* 297-301.

Picton, T. W., & Fitzgerald, P. G. (1983). A general discription of the human auditory evoked potentials. In E. J. Moore (Ed.), *Basis of auditory brainstem evoked responses (pp. 141-156). New York, Greene & Stratton.*

Picton, T. W., Hillyard, S. H., Krauz, H. J., & Galambos, R. (1974). Human auditory evoked potentials. I. Evaluation components. *Electroencephalography and Clinical Neurophysiology, 36,* 179-190.

Picton, T. W., Linden, R. D., Hamel, G., & Maru, J. T. (1983). Aspects of averaging. *Seminars in Hearing, 4,* 327-340.

Picton, T. W., Woods, D. L., Baribeau-Braun, J., & Healey, T. (1977). Evoked potentials audiometry. *Journal of Otolaryngology, 6,* 90-118.

Reneau, J. P., & Hnatiow, G. Z. (1975). *Evoked response audiometry: A topical and historical review.* Baltimore: University Park Press.

Ruben, R. J., Sekula, J., Bordley, J. E., Knickerbocker, G. G., Nager, G. T., & Fisch, U. (1960). Human cochlear responses to sound stimuli. *Annals of Otology, Rhinology, and Laryngology, 69,* 459-476.

Selters, W., & Brackman, D. (1979). Brainstem electric response audiometry acoustic tumor detection. In W. House & C. Luetje (Eds.), *Acoustic tumors.* Baltimore: University Park Press.

Sohmer, H., & Feinmesser, M. (1967). Cochlear action potentials recorded from the external ear in man. *Annals of Otology, Rhinology, and Laryngology, 76,* 427-438.

Sohmer, H., & Feinmesser, M. (1973). Routine use of electrocochleography (cochlear audiometry) in human subjects. *Audiology, 12,* 167-173.

Terkildsen, K., Osterhammel, P., & Thomsen, J. (1981). The ABR and MLR in patients with acoustic neuromas. *Scandinavian Audiology,* Supplement *13,* 103-108.

Yoshie, N. (1968). Auditory nerve action potential responses to clicks in man. *Laryngoscope, 78,* 198-215.

Chapter 2

Neural Generators of the Auditory Brainstem Response

Aage R. Møller
Peter J. Jannetta

INTRODUCTION

The usefulness of auditory brainstem responses (ABRs) in making otoneurological diagnoses depends upon knowing the anatomical origin of the various components of the ABR that can be identified and upon knowing how various pathologies change these potentials. It is generally accepted that the ABR recorded from electrodes placed on the scalp represent the far field of the potentials generated by the fiber tracts and nuclei of the ascending auditory pathway.

Throughout the first decade that ABRs were used to make otoneurological diagnoses the origins of the potentials were determined on the basis of results of animal experiments (Achor & Starr, 1980a, b; Britt & Rossi, 1980; Buchwald & Huang, 1975; Huang & Buchwald, 1977; Rossi & Britt, 1980). Although one may accept the hypothesis that the ascending auditory pathway in such commonly used experimental animals as cats, rats, and monkeys is similar in its organization to that of man, there is certainly one difference, namely, that the auditory nerve in man is much longer than it is in the small animals usually used in auditory research: the auditory nerve in small animals such as cats, rats, and guinea pigs is 0.3 to 0.5 cm long, while it is about 2.5 cm long in man (Lang, 1981). Since the auditory nerve is composed of relatively slow-conducting fibers, this means that the conduction time in man is also longer than in small animals: about 1 ms versus 0.1 to 0.2 ms. In addition, while peak I in the ABR in man and small animals is generated by the distal end of the auditory nerve, the remaining peaks originate in different loci in man and in small animals. This fact complicates any hypotheses regarding the origin of the different components of the ABR in man that are based on the results of experiments in animals such as the cat.

Recent studies in which a comparison has been made between the ABR and the potentials recorded directly from different structures of the ascending auditory pathway in man have provided new insights into the neural generators of the human ABR (Møller & Jannetta, 1981, 1982a, b, 1983b, c, 1984; Møller, Jannetta, Bennett, & Møller, 1981; Møller, Jannetta, & Møller, 1981). In other studies abnormalities in the ABR patterns of patients with confirmed lesions in the ascending auditory pathway were examined to gain insight into the origins of the ABR. By correlating the location of the lesion with changes in the ABR, information about the origin of the different components of the ABR was obtained (Sohmer, Feinmesser, & Szabo, 1974; Starr & Achor, 1975; Starr & Hamilton, 1976; Stockard & Rossiter, 1977).

Even more difficult to determine than the origins of components of the ABR is the relationship between the type of anatomical changes observed during intracranial surgical procedures and the changes in the ABR. At present this problem is being studied primarily by creating specific lesions in animals and then analyzing the changes which occur in the recorded far-field potentials (Achor & Starr, 1980b). However, in these studies the differences between the auditory nervous systems of animals and man must also be considered.

The interpretation of ABRs is complicated by the complexity of the ascending auditory pathway: the auditory system is more complex than other sensory systems and there are several connections between the left and right sides. The main nerve tracts and nuclei of the auditory system are outlined on a schematic diagram (Figure 2-1): there are four main relay nuclei between the ear and the auditory cortex. The auditory nerve terminates in the cochlear nucleus complex, which mainly contains second-order neurons, but also contains neurons of higher order. Three fiber tracts connect the hemispheres: nuclei of the most dorsal, the stria of Monakow, mainly terminate in the nucleus of the contralateral-lateral lemniscus and the inferior colliculus; the other two tracts are the medial stria (stria of Held) and the ventral stria (trapezoidal body). All three striae make connections with the numerous subnuclei of the superior olivary complex. Some fibers leaving the cochlear nucleus reach the nucleus of the ipsilateral lateral lemniscus. The superior olivary complex contains mainly third-order neurons and serves as the first relay nucleus that receives input from both ears. From the superior olivary complex connections are made to the inferior colliculus via the lateral lemniscus, mostly by neurons that receive their input from the opposite ear. Fibers leaving the inferior colliculus reach the thalamic auditory relay nucleus (medial geniculate body) via the brachium of the inferior colliculus. The primary auditory cortex receives its input from this nucleus. It is generally assumed that ABRs represent electrical events generated in subcortical structures.

Potentials recorded from the auditory nervous system at a point distant to the generators (far-field potentials) are thought to be of two kinds, namely, summations of the neural discharges of many fibers or nerve cells and potentials generated by dendrites. Potentials of the first type are dependent upon the locking of discharges to the time pattern of the stimulus sound, and are characterized by sharp peaks. The latter type of potentials are slow potentials that are much less dependent on synchrony of firing and are thus less dependent on the transient nature of the stimulus.

We shall in the following sections discuss the different potentials that can be recorded from the cochlea, the auditory nerve, and the nuclei and nerve tracts of the ascending auditory pathway.

NEURAL GENERATORS

Electrical Potentials of the Ear and the Auditory Nerve

Several different sound-evoked potentials can be recorded from the cochlea: the cochlear microphonic (CM), the summating potential (SP), and the compound action potential (CAP) (see, e.g., Dallos, 1973). These potentials can be recorded from an electrode placed on the round window or from various types of electrodes placed inside the cochlea. Different types of sounds may evoke all three potentials but each potential is most clearly elicited in response to a particular type of sound. Thus, the CM is best seen in response to pure tones of relatively low frequency, the SP is best elicited by bursts of high-frequency tones, and the CAP is seen best in response to transient sounds. In small animals such as cats, guinea pigs, and rats the CAP that can be recorded from the cochlea shows two negative peaks (N_1 and N_2), the earliest one (N_1) representing the synchronization in many nerve fibers of the auditory nerve and the latter one (N_2) representing the discharges of nerve cells in the cochlear nucleus (Fisch & Ruben, 1962; Møller, 1983a; Ruben, Hudson, & Chiong, 1982).

The potential recorded intracranially from the auditory nerve in man has a triphasic shape: the earliest potential is a small positive deflection, which is followed by a large negative peak, which in turn is followed by a smaller positive deflection (Møller & Jannetta, 1981) (Figure

FIGURE 2–1.
Schematic drawing of the ascending auditory pathway. VCN: ventral cochlear nucleus; DCN: dorsal cochlear nucleus; SO: superior olivary complex; TB: trapezodial body; SM: stria of Monakow (dorsal stria); SH: stria of Held (intermediate stria); LL: lateral lemniscus; IC: inferior colliculus; MG: medial geniculate body (from Møller, 1983b).

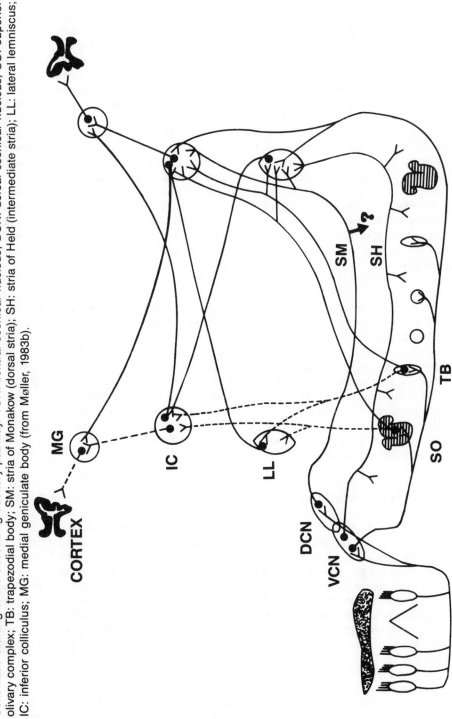

2-2). This type of response is to be expected when recording from a long nerve with a field potential which is the second derivative of the action potential (Lorente de No, 1947).

Figure 2-2 also shows how the potentials recorded from the intracranial portion of the auditory nerve change as a function of stimulus intensity (given in decibel equivalents above normal hearing threshold). The two curves in each graph were recorded from two different locations on the nerve. More distal responses have shorter latencies than do those recorded more proximally. The latency of the negative peak varies with the sound intensity. It is slightly more than 3 ms in response to short bursts of a 2000-Hz tone at 100 dB equivalent above normal hearing threshold (Møller, Jannetta, Bennett, & Møller, 1981; Møller & Jannetta, 1981), a time which is much longer than the latencies recorded from small animals and about 1 ms longer than the N_1 that can be recorded from the round window of the human cochlea (Eggermont, 1974; Elberling 1976). This additional delay in N_1 is due to the greater length of the auditory nerve in man, which leads to a rather slow conduction time (20 m/s) (Engstrom & Rexed, 1940; Lazorthes, Lacomme, Ganbert, & Planel, 1961). This may also explain why there is no clear evidence of an N_2 potential when recording from the promontorium in man (Eggermont, 1974; Elberling, 1976; Spoor, Eggermont, & Odenthal, 1976). In small animals the N_2 has been shown to originate in the cochlear nucleus and is conducted well to the recording site (round window) because the distance is short. The much longer distance between the cochlea and the cochlear nucleus in man compared to that in small animals leads to poor conduction of the evoked potentials of the cochlear nucleus to the recording site (promontorium). Examples of compound action potentials (CAPs) recorded from the round window in a rat and from the promontorium in man are seen in Figure 2-3.

A comparison of the potential recorded directly from the eighth nerve and the ABR recorded differentially from electrodes placed on the vertex and just above the pinna shows that the potential recorded from the proximal end of the auditory nerve appears with the same latency as does peak II of the ABR (Figure 2-4) (Møller, Jannetta, Bennett, & Møller, 1981; Møller, Jannetta, & Møller, 1981, 1982; Møller & Jannetta, 1983c; Spire, Dohrmann, & Prieto, 1982). The recordings shown in Figure 2-4 were obtained in patients undergoing neurosurgical operations to treat cranial nerve dysfunctions; in most cases microvascular decompression was performed to relieve hemifacial spasm or trigeminal neuralgia (Jannetta, 1977; Jannetta, 1981a, b). The results of analyzing these recordings led us to revise earlier interpretations of the origins of the ABRs in man that assumed that the second peak was generated by secondary neurons located in the cochlear nucleus.

Potentials Generated by the Cochlear Nucleus and Superior Olivary Complex

When a recording electrode on the eighth nerve is moved from a location near the porus acusticus to a location that is close to the brainstem, the amplitude of the potential decreases and the shape of the potential changes (Figure 2-5A, B). The potentials recorded from the eighth nerve near the porus acusticus have shorter latencies than do those recorded from the nerve at a location near the brainstem. In addition, when responses are recorded near the brainstem a slow negative potential is seen to follow the sharp negative peak (Figure 2-5B) and a second negative peak is seen about 1 ms after the first negative peak. This second negative peak is most likely generated by second-order auditory neurons located in the cochlear nucleus, while the slow potential is probably generated by dendrites in the cochlear nucleus (Møller & Jannetta, 1982a).

The cochlear nucleus in small animals dominates the brainstem and is located near the entrance of the eighth nerve, but in man it is a comparatively small part of the brainstem and is pushed backwards by the larger inferior cerebellar peduncle. It is, therefore, difficult to gain direct access to the cochlear nucleus of man in a lateral approach. Thus our conclusion that

FIGURE 2–2.

Recordings made from the auditory nerve of a patient undergoing a neurosurgical operation in which the eighth nerve was exposed. The results obtained at different stimulus intensities are shown in decibels above normal human hearing threshold. The sound stimuli were 2,000-Hz tone bursts of 5-ms duration presented through an insert earphone. The solid lines represent responses from a location slightly more distal on the nerve than the responses represented by dashed lines (From Møller & Jannetta, 1981). Negativity is upward in this and all subsequent figures except where specified.

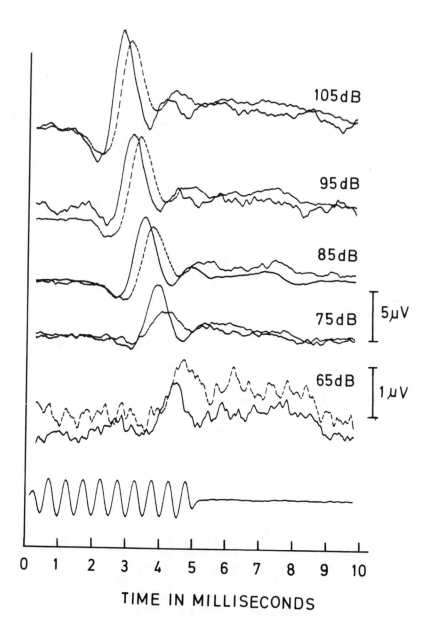

TIME IN MILLISECONDS

FIGURE 2–3.
Compound action potentials recorded from the round window of a rat (from Møller, unpublished) (top) and from the promontorium of a human subject with normal hearing (bottom) (from Eggermont et al., 1976).

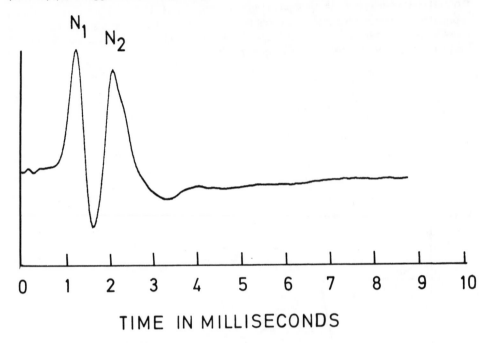

TIME IN MILLISECONDS

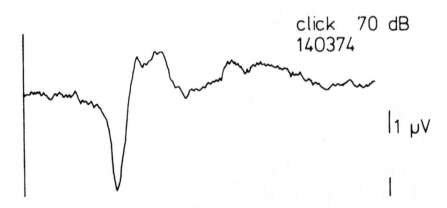

click   70 dB
140374

$1 \mu V$

the second negative peak in the CAP recorded from the eighth nerve near the brainstem is generated in the cochlear nucleus was reached by comparing recordings made at different locations on the eighth nerve. The latency of the first negative peak increases as the electrode is moved along the nerve from the porus acusticus toward its entrance into the brainstem. This result indicates that this peak is generated by propagated activity in a nerve trunk. The latency of the second peak, however, remains unchanged while its amplitude increases (Figure 2-5A, B) as the recording site is moved toward the brainstem indicating that the source of this

FIGURE 2–4.

Comparison between potentials recorded from the intracranial portion of the eighth nerve and those recorded differentially from electrodes placed on the scalp at the vertex and at a position just above the ipsilateral pinna. Both potentials were recorded at the same time during the operation and both were subjected to the same digital filtering. (A) and (B) show results from two different patients. Lower curves are consecutive averages of the potentials recorded from the scalp to show replicability. The sound stimuli were 5-ms-long tone bursts with an intensity of about 90 dB above normal hearing threshold (From Møller & Jannetta, 1983c).

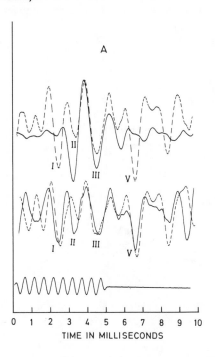
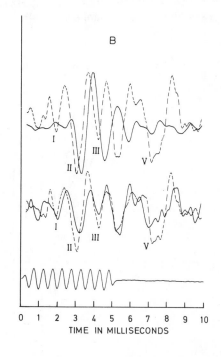

second peak is located in the brainstem and not in the nerve trunk along which the electrode is moved (Møller & Jannetta, 1982a, 1983a). When these intracranial recordings are compared to the ABRs recorded simultaneously from scalp electrodes, this peak is seen to appear with the same latency as does peak III of the ABR (Figure 2-5D).

In a patient who was operated upon for a tumor of the fourth ventricle it was possible to obtain direct access to the medial side of the cerebellar peduncle and thus the cochlear nucleus or its vicinity (Møller & Jannetta, 1983b). Recordings from this location showed a potential with a large negative peak (Figure 2-6), the latency of which was similar to this second negative peak in the recording from the root entry zone (REZ) of the eighth nerve mentioned above (Figure 2-5B). The initial positive deflection seen in the recording in Figure 2-6B is assumed to have originated in the proximal portion of the auditory nerve, where it enters the cochlear nucleus. It may therefore be assumed that this second peak is generated by secondary auditory neurons located in the cochlear nucleus. This lends strong support to the hypothesis that peak III is generated mainly in the cochlear nucleus. Originally, it was thought that peak III originated in the superior olivary complex, but the facts that an additional delay occurs in the auditory nerve and that peak III has a much larger amplitude than peak II support the hypothesis that peak III is generated by a relatively large nucleus, such as the cochlear nucleus.

FIGURE 2–5.
Comparison between potentials recorded at different locations on the auditory nerve and brainstem from a patient undergoing microvascular decompression operations for hemifacial spasm. (A) Recording from the eighth nerve near the porus acusticus. (B) Similar recording made near the entrance of the eighth nerve into the brainstem. (C) Recording made from a location on the brainstem about 4 mm medial and rostral to the entrance of the eighth nerve that is assumed to overlie the superior olivary complex. (D) ABR recorded simultaneously from scalp electrodes. The stimuli were 2,000-Hz tone bursts of 5-ms duration presented with an interstimulus interval of 150 ms. The recording bandpass for the potentials recorded intracranially was 3 to 3,000 Hz and the ABR was digitally filtered to enhance the peaks (from Møller & Jannetta, 1984).

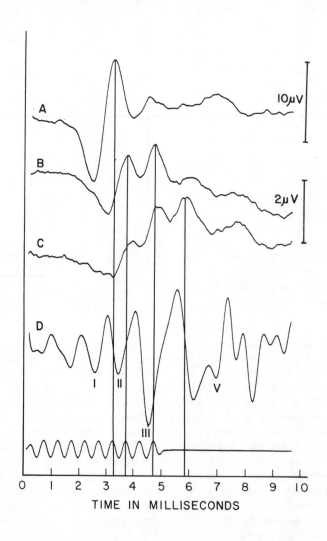

While it is relatively easy to record the evoked potentials from the superior olivary complex in animals, it is difficult to record from this nucleus in man due to the relatively small size of these nuclei, which necessitate a very precise placement of the recording electrode, and the fact that the nuclei are located below the lateral surface of the brainstem. Figure 2-5C shows recordings made from a location on the brainstem that is presumed to overlie the superior olivary complex. This recording is dominated by a negative peak, the latency of which is about 1 ms longer than that of the second negative peak in the recording made near the brainstem (the response from the cochlear nucleus). A peak with the same latency but with a much smaller amplitude can be seen in the recording from the REZ (Figure 2-5B). When the recording electrode is moved from the REZ to a location on the brainstem that is presumed to be over the superior olivary complex, this third peak rose in amplitude, indicating that this latter location is closer to the source of this third peak than was the entrance to the brainstem. The latency of this third peak is about 1 ms longer than that of the second negative peak, indicating that its source is third-order auditory neurons. Third-order auditory neurons are known to be located mainly in the superior olivary complex, although presumably there are a number of third-order neurons also in the cochlear nucleus of man, as has been shown to be the case in animals. Although this third peak has a latency that is close to that of peak IV in the ABR recorded simultaneously (Figure 2-5D), determination of the generators of peak IV is complicated by the fact that the major parts of the ascending auditory pathway cross the midline at this level while some parts continue uncrossed toward higher auditory centers.

The conclusions that can be drawn from the results of this work are that peak I originates exclusively from the distal part of the eighth nerve; that peak II originates mainly from the proximal part of the eighth nerve, although there may be some small contribution from other more distal parts of the auditory nerve; that peak III is mainly generated by the neurons in the cochlear nucleus but may receive some small contribution from nerve fibers entering the cochlear nucleus; and that the neural generator of peak IV is third-order neurons, mostly those located in the superior olivary complex but also those in the cochlear nucleus and probably also in the nucleus of the lateral lemniscus. Although other studies of the neural generators of ABRs in man based on intracranial recordings have obtained essentially similar results (Hashimoto, Ishiyama, Yoshimoto, & Nemoto, 1981; Spire et al., 1982), this interpretation, particularly regarding peaks III and IV, should be taken as a simplification. There is no doubt that other sources in addition to these two nuclei also contribute to peaks III and IV of the ABR.

In comparing potentials recorded intracranially to the ABRs recorded in the traditional way (the difference between responses from electrodes placed on the vertex and the ipsilateral mastoid) we found that the intracranial potentials did not always occur precisely with the same latencies as did peaks in the ABRs (Møller, 1983a). There was thus not always an exact match in time between potentials recorded intracranially and those recorded extracranially. A similar observation was made by Hashimoto et al. (1981). We ascribe that occasional lack of an exact match between the peaks of potentials recorded intracranially and those recorded extracranially to the way ABRs are traditionally recorded: namely, differentially between electrodes placed at the vertex and the ipsilateral mastoid. Since both of the recording electrodes are located at sites that are electrically active (vertex and mastoid), the resulting potential will be the difference between the potentials recorded at these two locations. If the peaks of the potentials recorded at these two sites do not occur at precisely the same time, the resulting difference potential (and thus the ABR) will have peaks that occur with latencies that are different from those of the peaks in the potentials occurring at either of the two electrode locations (Terkildsen, Osterhammel, & Huis in't Veld, 1974). This difference is illustrated in Figure 2-7, which shows potentials recorded intracranially from the eighth nerve and from two locations on the scalp using a noncephalic reference, namely, the vertex and a location just above the pinna. The bottom tracings show the intracranial potentials and the potential that is the difference between the

FIGURE 2–6.
Recordings from the vicinity of the cochlear nucleus made in a patient undergoing an operation for a tumor located in the fourth ventricle. (A) Recordings made from the cerebellar peduncle at a location medial to the cochlear nucleus and near the floor of the fourth ventricle. (B) The same recording after digital filtering. (C) Simultaneous recording from an electrode placed on the vertex (with a noncephalic reference). The stimuli were 2,000-Hz tone bursts of 5-ms duration presented at 95 dB to the ipsilateral ear (From Møller & Jannetta, 1983b).

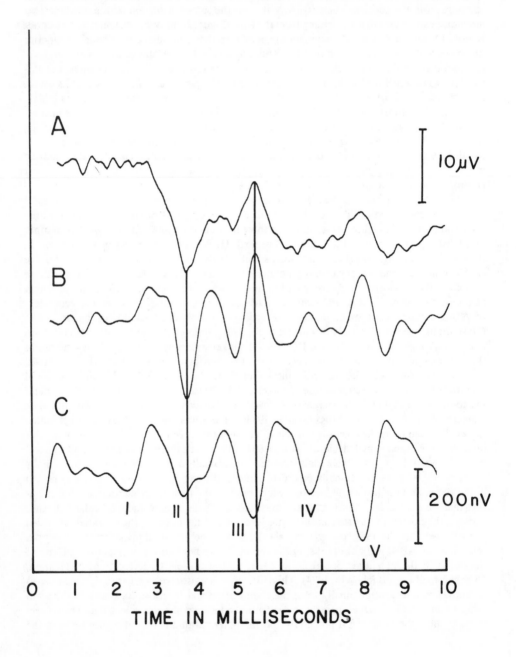

FIGURE 2–7.
Comparison between recordings made intracranially from the eighth nerve (solid lines) and those made simultaneously from the vertex and from a position immediately above the pinna ("mastoid") using a noncephalic reference (dashed lines). In the upper and middle tracings negativity is shown as an upward deflection for the intracranial response as well as for the scalp response. The bottom tracing also shows the difference between the scalp (vertex-mastoid) recording (shown with vertex-negativity upward) and the intracranial recording, but the intracranial recording is shown inverted (negativity is a downward deflection). The recording from the nerve was done at a location medial to the porus acusticus. All curves were subjected to digital filtering to attenuate the slow components. The stimuli were 1-ms-long tone bursts at 100 dB presented at intervals of 120 ms. The amplitude scale was the same in the recording from the scalp where noncephalic reference electrodes were used (two upper tracings) (from Møller & Jannetta, 1984).

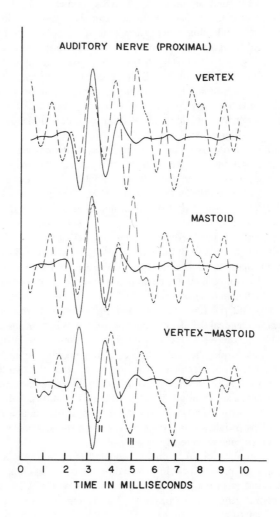

two scalp locations (the latter representative of the ABR recorded traditionally). The responses were obtained in a patient in whom a retromastoid craniectomy was performed. It is evident that the peaks of the intracranial recordings match the peaks of the scalp recordings more exactly when recordings made independently from the two sites using a noncephalic reference are compared rather than when potentials recorded intracranially are compared to the difference between the potentials recorded at these two sites (conventional ABRs). In the example shown in Figure 2-7, the vertex electrode recorded early, high-amplitude components of the ABR. More often, earlier components of recordings from the vertex have smaller amplitudes and peaks V, VI, and VII are more evident. In recordings from the mastoid the first three or four peaks usually have the largest amplitudes while peaks V, VI, and VII have relatively low amplitudes.

Potentials Recorded from the Inferior Colliculus

It has generally been assumed that peak V in the ABR is generated by the inferior colliculus. While this is most likely true in the small experimental animals usually used in auditory research, recordings from the inferior colliculus in man show that this is unlikely to be the case in man. Typical potentials recorded from the inferior colliculus in man in response to contralateral sound stimulation are shown in Figure 2-8. In this figure the earliest potential is a positive peak occurring with a latency equal to that of peak V in the ABR recorded from the scalp (Møller & Jannetta, 1982b). This positive peak is followed by a large negative deflection on which several smaller peaks are riding. This sharp positive potential is most likely generated by the lateral lemniscus as it enters the inferior colliculus, while the slow negative potential following this is likely a dendritic potential of the inferior colliculus.

When the potentials recorded from the inferior colliculus are compared to the ABR, both being recorded in such a way that low frequencies are preserved (Figure 2-9A), it is seen that the negative peak in the response from the inferior colliculus has about the same latency as does the vertex negative potential (Møller & Jannetta, 1982b, 1983c), usually known as the SN_{10} (Davis & Hirsh, 1976). This indicates that the main neural generator of this potential is most likely the inferior colliculus.

When the slow potential is removed by filtering, a series of two to three peaks is seen to follow the initial positive peak, as shown in Figure 2-9B. These sharp peaks probably represent synchronized firing of neurons in the inferior colliculus. When the potentials recorded intracranially from the inferior colliculus are compared to those recorded from the vertex using a noncephalic reference, the latencies of peaks V, VI, and VII of the potentials recorded from the scalp (Figure 2-9B) and the first, second, and third peaks of the potentials recorded intracranially look nearly identical (Møller & Jannetta, 1983c). When the intracranially recorded potentials are compared to the ABRs recorded in the traditional way, differentially between a mastoid and a vertex electrode, the match between the peaks in the intracranial and scalp recordings is less perfect. This discrepancy is due to the fact that the two locations (mastoid and vertex) from which the ABRs are recorded differentially from the scalp are both active and the latencies of the peaks are slightly different for the two locations. A differential recording from these two locations consequently differs from the recordings made from either of the two locations alone. (This problem was addressed earlier in this chapter when the potentials recorded from the auditory nerve were discussed.)

A schematic conceptualization of the neural generators of the ABR in man is shown in Figure 2-10. This illustration represents a simplified diagram of the main part of the ascending auditory pathway and indicates the main neural generators of the ABR. It is important to emphasize that the neural generators of peaks IV, V, VI, and VII are complex in that more than one anatomical structure contributes to each peak and that each anatomical structure contributes to more than one peak.

FIGURE 2-8.

Recordings from the inferior colliculus obtained in patients undergoing neurosurgical operations. The stimuli were 2,000-Hz tone bursts of 5-ms duration presented to the contralateral ear.

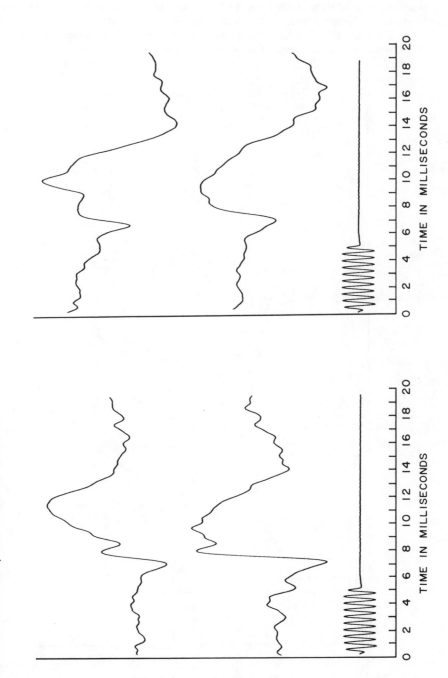

FIGURE 2–9.
Recordings from the inferior colliculus (solid lines) compared to recordings made simultaneously from the vertex using a noncephalic reference (dashed lines). (A) Recording bandwith 3 to 3,000 Hz; response was digitally lowpass filtered with a triangular weighting function 0.8-ms wide. (B) Same data as in (A) but after attenuating the low-frequency components by digital filtering (from Møller & Jannetta, 1984).

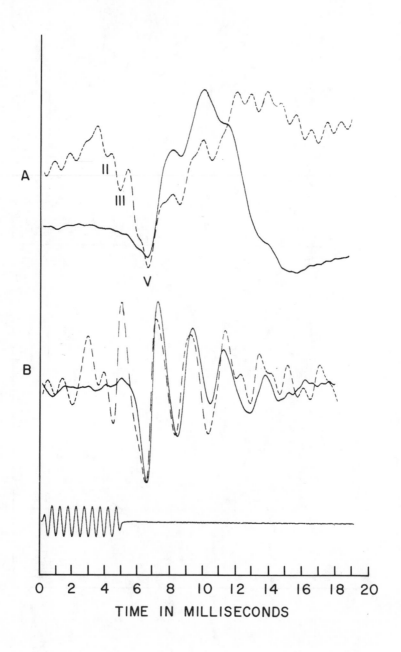

FIGURE 2-10.
Schematic illustration of the neural generators of the ABR in man.

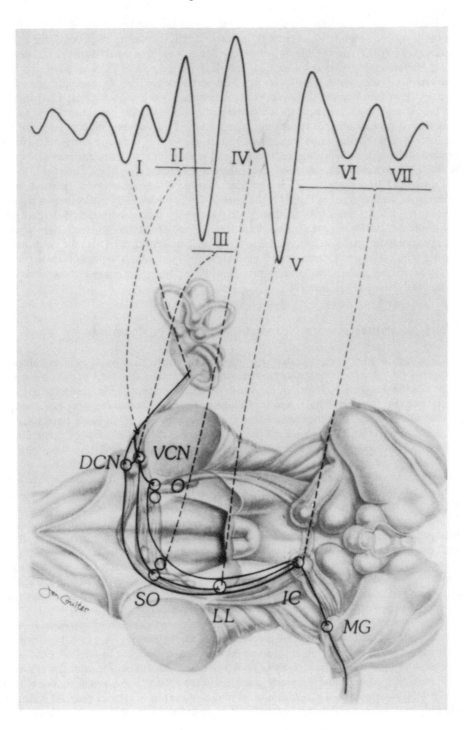

Differences Between Results Obtained in Man and Those Obtained in Experimental Animals

From studying recordings from cats it appears that the auditory nerve is the generator of peak I, the cochlear nucleus of peak II, the superior olivary nucleus of peak III, the lateral lemniscus of peak IV, and the inferior colliculus of peak V in this animal (Buchwald & Huang, 1975). However, as previously discussed, the data from small animals upon which this interpretation of the origins of ABRs are based cannot be used to identify the neural generators of the ABR in man because the auditory nerve in man is much longer (Lang, 1981) than it is in the cat as a natural consequence of the fact that man has a larger head than the cat. Also, while there is no evidence that the general organization of the human auditory system differs qualitatively from that of these small animals, it is known that there are certain differences between primates and carnivores in the nuclei of the ascending auditory pathway (Moore & Moore, 1971). Whether these differences are sufficient to cause significant differences in the ABRs recorded from these species is not clear. Another difference between man and small experimental animals such as the cat is the smaller size of the auditory nuclei in man relative to head size; that is, the volume of the cochlear nucleus in man is not much different from that in the cat, but because the human head is larger and the auditory nerve longer in man these structures are smaller in man relative to head size. This fact, together with the much longer distance from the recording electrode to the neural generators in man, is responsible for the much smaller amplitude of the potentials recorded from human subjects compared to those that can be recorded from small animals.

Effects of Pathologies on Near-field and Far-field Potentials

To understand the changes in the far-field potentials (ABRs) that result from pathological changes in the nerves it is necessary to understand the changes that such pathologies cause in the near-field potentials. However, the effects of various pathologies on the potentials that can be recorded from nerve tracts and nuclei have not been studied to the same extent as has the normal response. Thus, the changes that can be expected as a result of certain insults are largely unknown. Clinical experience, however, has shown that various types of pathologies result in a prolongation of the latencies of the various peaks in the ABR.

The effects of pathologies such as tumors on the far-field potentials (ABR) have been studied extensively in patients whose site of lesion is known. In animal experiments nuclei have been compressed and aspirated or nerve tracts have been severed to simulate the pathology caused by a tumor; the changes noted in the evoked potentials after such insults have been related to the location of the injury and the degree of damage inflicted, although generally it has been difficult to correlate the site or degree of damage inflicted with specific changes in the recorded ABR. Studies of patients with acoustic neuromas have been the most useful in correlating specific changes in the latencies of the peaks in the ABR to the particular lesion involved. ABRs are generally assumed to be among the more important data obtained in otoneurological testing of patients with intracranial lesions. For a more detailed account of the effects of neurological disorders on the ABR, see Section III of this book.

The uncertainty as to just what the neural generators of elements of the ABR are has, however, made it difficult to determine exactly which of the changes seen in ABRs are most specifically correlated with certain diseases. For instance, an increase in the latency of wave V of the ABR had generally been regarded as being indicative of an acoustic neuroma. However, when more information about the neural generators of the ABR was obtained, it became evident that in most patients who had acoustic nerve tumors a shift in latency of peak III occurred, a finding which agreed with previous findings that peaks I and II are generated by the auditory nerve and that peak III is generated by the cochlear nucleus (Møller & Møller, in press). The amplitudes of the potentials and their waveform morphology also change as a result of injury, but the two latter parameters are not as well utilized in clinical diagnosis as is the change in latency.

There are several factors that may change the amplitude of the evoked potentials, one of which is insult to the nerve. When recordings are made from the auditory nerve, cochlear nucleus, and probably also from more centrally located structures, the degree of synchrony (phase locking) of discharges is a large factor in determining the amplitude and the shape of the potential. If synchrony is impaired, the amplitude will change but the latency may be relatively unchanged.

It is more difficult to obtain accurate and reproducible measures of the amplitudes of evoked potentials than of their latencies. This is true of near-field as well as far-field potentials. Thus, the amplitudes of near-field potentials may be greatly affected by such factors as the exact placement of the recording electrode or shunting of fluid, while these same factors do not affect latency to any noticeable extent. This is one important reason why examining changes in latency has been preferred over studying changes in amplitude to detect various abnormalities. Nevertheless, there is no doubt that the amplitude and the waveform of the evoked potentials carry much information that can be of value in the diagnosis of disorders of the auditory nervous system. This is shown, for instance, in the discovery that putting traction on the auditory nerve in patients undergoing operations for cranial nerve dysfunction produces a number of changes in the shape of the CAP that can be recorded directly from the nerve, as well as causing an increase in the latency of the ABR (Møller & Jannetta, 1983a).

Another reason for studying characteristics of ABRs other than their latencies is that non-neural factors can affect latency. Notable among these is hearing loss resulting from defects in the conduction of sound to the inner ear (middle ear disorders) or from damage to hair cells in the inner ear. These factors prolong the latency of impulse conduction, and if not taken into account may lead to a mistaken interpretation of the ABR. When click sounds with broad spectra are used as stimuli, it is mainly the high-frequency part of the spectrum that is the effective stimulus in people with normal hearing. Since high-frequency sounds only travel a short distance on the basilar membrane, this travel time contributes only slightly to the latency of the ABR in people with normal hearing. However, in people who have lost their high-frequency hair cells (commonly the elderly or people who have noise-induced hearing losses) the lower-frequency components constitute the effective stimulus; since these components travel a longer distance on the basilar membrane there is an additional delay which adds to the latency time of all the peaks. If not taken into account, this latency increase may be confused with an increased neural conduction time. There are several ways of compensating for this possibility in testing for neural conduction deficits. One way is not to use absolute latency values but instead to use the interwave latencies between waves I and III or waves I and V; another way is to test the responses to tonebursts rather than click sounds. The latter method works because the location of maximal deflection of the basilar membrane in response to tones is independent of the sensorineural hearing loss, which in turn means that the time it takes for the traveling wave to reach the location of maximal response of a pure tone is independent of the population of sensory hair cells. Consequently, the latency of the response to tone bursts is relatively independent of the size of the hair cell population, as long as there are some hair cells present. For this reason the latency of the response to low-frequency tone bursts (of, e.g., 2,000 Hz) is less dependent on degree of cochlear hearing loss than are the latencies of the responses to click sounds. The relationship between frequency specificity and brief tones is discussed later in this book, in chapter 9.

REFERENCES

Achor, L., & Starr, A. (1980a). Auditory brain stem responses in the cat. I. Intracranial and extracranial recordings. *Electroencephalography & Clinical Neurophysiology, 48,* 154–173.

Achor, L., & Starr, A. (1980b). Auditory brain stem responses in the cat. II. Effects of lesions. *Electroencephalography & Clinical Neurophysiology, 48,* 174–190.

Britt, R., & Rossi, G. (1980). Neural generators of brain stem auditory evoked responses. Part I. Lesion studies. *Neuroscience Abstracts, 6,* 594.

Buchwald, J., & Huang, Ch. (1975). Far-field acoustic response: Origins in the cat. *Science, 189,* 382–384.

Dallos, P. (1973). *The auditory periphery.* New York: Academic Press.

Davis, H., & Hirsh, S. (1976). The audiometric utility of brain stem responses to low-frequency sounds. *Audiology, 15,* 181–195.

Eggermont, J. J. (1974). Basic principles of electrocochleography. *Acta Otolaryngologica (Stockh.), 316* (Supplement).

Eggermont, J. J., Spoor, A., & Odenthal, D. W. (1976). Frequency specificity of tone-burst electrocochleography. In R. J. Ruben, C. Elberling, & G. Salomon (Eds.), *Electrocochleography.* Baltimore: University Park Press.

Elberling, C. (1976). Simulation of cochlear action potentials recorded from the ear canal in man. In R. J. Ruben, C. Eberling, & G. Salomon (Eds.), *Electrocochleography.* Baltimore: University Park Press.

Engstrom, H., & Rexed, B. (1940). Uber die Kaliber Verhaltnisse der Nerven Fasern im N. Statoacusticus des Menchen. *Zeitschrift Mikroskopisch-Anatomische Forschung (Leipzig), 47,* 448–455.

Fisch, U. P., & Ruben, R. J. (1962). Electrical acoustical response to click stimulation after section of the eighth nerve. *Acta Otolaryngologica (Stockh.), 54,* 532–542.

Hashimoto, I., Ishiyama, Y., Yoshimoto, T., & Nemoto, S. (1981) Brainstem auditory evoked potentials recorded directly from human brain-stem and thalamus. *Brain, 104,* 841–859.

Huang, Ch., & Buchwald, J. (1977). Interpretation of the vertex short-latency acoustic response: A study of single neurons in the brain. *Brain Research, 137,* 291–303.

Jannetta, P. J. (1977). Etiology and definitive microsurgical treatment of hemifacial spasm. *Journal of Neurosurgery, 47,* 321–328.

Jannetta, P. J. (1981a). Hemifacial spasm. In M. Samii & P. J. Jannetta (Eds.), *The cranial nerves.* New York: Springer-Verlag.

Jannetta, P. J. (1981b). Vascular decompression in trigeminal neuralgia. In M. Samii & P. J. Jannetta (Eds.), *The cranial nerves.* New York: Springer-Verlag.

Lang, J. (1981). Facial and vestibulocochlear nerve, topographic anatomy and variations. In M. Samii & P. J. Jannetta (Eds.), *The cranial nerves.* New York: Springer-Verlag.

Lazorthes, G., Lacomme, Y., Ganbert, J., & Planel, H. (1961). La constitution du nerf auditif. *La Presse Medicale, 69,* 1067–1068.

Lorente, de No, R. (1947). Analysis of the distribution of action currents of nerve in volume conductors. *Studies of the Rockefeller Institute of Medical Research, 132,* 384–482.

Møller, A. R. (1983a). On the origin of the compound action potentials (N_1, N_2) of the cochlea of the rat. *Experimental Neurology, 80,* 633–644.

Møller, A. R. (1983b). *Auditory physiology.* New York: Academic Press.

Møller, A. R., & Jannetta, P. J. (1981). Compound action potentials recorded intracranially from the auditory nerve in man. *Experimental Neurology, 74,* 862–874.

Møller, A. R., & Jannetta, P. J. (1982a). Auditory evoked potentials recorded intracranially from the brainstem in man. *Experimental Neurology, 78,* 144–157.

Møller, A. R., & Jannetta, P. J. (1982b). Evoked potentials from the inferior colliculus in man. *Electroencephalography & Clinical Neurophysiology, 53,* 612–620.

Møller, A. R., & Jannetta, P. J. (1983a). Monitoring auditory functions during cranial nerve microvascular decompression operations by direct recording from the eighth nerve. *Journal of Neurosurgery, 59,* 493–499.

Møller, A. R., & Jannetta, P. J. (1983b). Auditory evoked potentials recorded from the cochlear nucleus and its vicinity in man. *Journal of Neurosurgery, 59.*

Møller, A. R., & Jannetta, P. J. (1983c). Interpretation of brainstem auditory evoked potentials: Results from intracranial recordings in humans. *Scandinavian Audiology (Stockh.), 12,* 125–133.

Møller, A. R., & Jannetta, P. J. (1984). Neural generators of the brainstem auditory evoked potentials (BAEP). In *Proceedings of the Second International Evoked Potentials Symposium,* Cleveland, Ohio (October 18–20, 1982), Wolburn, MA: Butterworth.

Møller, A. R., Jannetta, P. J., Bennett, M., & Møller, M. B. (1981). Intracranially recorded responses from human auditory nerve: New insights into the origin of brain stem evoked potentials. *Electroencephalography & Clinical Neurophysiology, 52,* 18–27.

Møller, A. R., Jannetta, P. J., & Møller, M. B. (1981). Neural generators of the brain stem evoked responses: Results from human intracranial recordings. *Annals of Otology, Rhinology, & Laryngology, 90,* 591–596.

Møller, A. R., Jannetta, P. J., & Møller, M. B. (1982). Intracranially recorded auditory nerve response in man: New interpretations of BSER. *Archives of Otolaryngology, 108,* 77–82.

Møller, M. B., & Møller, A. R. (in press). Auditory brainstem evoked responses (ABR) in diagnosis of eighth nerve and brainstem lesions. In M. L. Pinheiro & F. E. Musiek (Eds.), *Assessment of central auditory dysfunction: Its foundations and clinical correlates.* Baltimore: Williams & Wilkins.

Moore, J. K., & Moore, R. Y. (1971). A comparative study of the superior olivary complex in the primate brain. *Folia Primatology (Basel), 16,* 35–51.

Rossi, G., & Britt, R. (1980). Neural generators of brainstem evoked responses. Part II. Electrode recording studies. *Neuroscience Abstracts, 6,* 595.

Ruben, R. J., Hudson, W., & Chiong, A. (1982). Anatomical and physiological effects of chronic section of the eighth nerve in cat. *Acta Otolaryngologica (Stockh.), 55,* 473–484.

Sohmer, H., Feinmesser, M., & Szabo, G. (1974). Sources of electrocochleographic response as studied in patients with brain damage. *Electroencephalography & Clinical Neurophysiology, 37,* 663–669.

Spire, J. P., Dohrmann, G. J., & Prieto, P. S. (1982). Correlation of brainstem evoked response with direct acoustic nerve potential. In J. Courjon, F. Manguiere, & M. Reval (Eds.), *Advances in neurology: Clinical applications of evoked potentials in neurology* (Vol. 32). New York: Raven Press.

Spoor, A., Eggermont, J. J., & Odenthal, D. W. (1976). Comparison of human and animal data concerning adaptation and masking of eighth nerve compound action potentials. In R. J. Ruben, C. Elberling, & G. Salomon (Eds.), *Electrocochleography.* Baltimore: University Park Press.

Starr, A., & Achor, L. (1975). Auditory brain stem responses in neurological disease. *Archives of Neurology, 32,* 761–768.

Starr, A., & Hamilton, A. (1976). Correlation between confirmed sites of neurological lesions of farfield auditory brain stem responses. *Electroencephalography & Clinical Neurophysiology, 41,* 595–608.

Stockard, J., & Rossiter, V. (1977). Clinical and pathological correlates of brain stem auditory response abnormalities. *Neurology, 27,* 316–325.

Terkildsen, K., Osterhammel, P., & Huis in't Veld, F. (1974). Far field electrocochleography, electrode positions. *Scandinavian Audiology (Stockh.), 3,* 123–129.

Chapter 3

Instrumentation and Signal Processing

Martyn L. Hyde

Introduction

The term "signal processing" is very broad, covering almost any manipulation of data; usually, the data are in the form of a voltage which changes over time, obtained by probing the activity of some biological or physical system. This chapter deals with some of the principles of signal processing which underlie ABR methods and instrumentation. The emphasis is not upon specific instrumentation systems, but upon the *functions* performed using common system components. For both background and more detailed information, see the sources cited in the References. Matters relating to stimuli are covered in depth in the chapter by Gorga et al. (chapter 4 of this volume).

Although the physiologic and electrodynamic bases of the auditory brainstem response (ABR) waveform are not well understood, it is clear that we can record minute changes in potential on the head that are associated with synchronized patterns of neural activity deep within the brain. The overriding problem is that these potentials are obscured by concurrent potentials from many other sources, both physiologic and nonphysiologic. Denoting the total measured potential as the *activity,* the ABR as the *signal,* and all other potentials as *noise,* the activity at any point on the head is usually assumed to be the algebraic sum of the signal and noise components. This assumption requires that the various components of activity are independent of each other, and in particular that the presence of a signal has no effect on the concurrent noise; this is reasonable for the ABR, but not necessarily true for all evoked potentials (EP).

Some common components of activity are listed in Table 3-1. The accurate detection and estimation (quantitative measurement) of the ABR in the face of so many noise components is the major technical issue that governs test methodology, instrumentation, and clinical utility of the ABR.

Differential Recording and Amplification

If we were restricted to recording from a single point on the head, with reference to an absolute potential ground, we would probably not be aware of the ABR, because many of the noise components are several orders of magnitude larger. We are obliged, therefore, to measure not absolute potentials but potential *differences* between two or more points on the head. This is called differential recording, and it improves the signal-to-noise ratio (SNR) because many of the noise components, such as radio-induced potentials and cardiac potentials, are similar at all points on the head. By taking differences, these noise components are at least partially cancelled.

TABLE 3–1.
Some common components of the electrical activity recorded from the head.

Physiologic	Nonphysiologic
ABR	Electromagnetic potentials:
Other evoked potentials	— radio signals
Spontaneous EEG	— power line radiation
Electromyogenic potentials	— stimulus transducer radiation
Cardiac potentials	Electrostatic potentials
Electro-ocular potentials	Internal noise of instrumentation
Electrodermal potentials	

The effect of differential recording, and the importance of recording electrode position, can be appreciated by visualizing the overall distribution of potential over the head as a contour map, analogous to geographical survey maps depicting height above sea level. The overall pattern is termed the topography of potential; each and every signal and noise component will have its own topographic distribution, which will evolve over time. The key to improving the SNR is to place the electrodes at sites where the signal differs, but the noise is similar. Note that if the ABR were to radiate from the brainstem in such a way that the potential at any time were the same over the head, then differential recording would not work. It is very important to remember that in the measurement and interpretation of the ABR, we are dealing not with the actual potential at any single site, but with differences.

Since the ABR is extremely small, it must be amplified to a convenient size for further electronic manipulation. The differential recording and amplification functions are combined in the differential preamplifier. For a single differential recording channel, three electrodes are required: the noninverting (positive), inverting (negative), and common (ground) electrodes. The more old-fashioned terms such as "active" and "reference" are not really appropriate; often, the noninverting and inverting electrode sites are both highly "active," in the sense that there is significant signal at both sites. The terminology used here is more cumbersome, but helps to remind us what is really going on.

Usually, the noninverting electrode is placed on the scalp vertex, or high on the forehead, in the midline. The inverting electrode is in the periauricular region of the ear being stimulated (stimulation is usually monaural, by headphone). The common electrode is in the contralateral periauricular region, most often on the mastoid or earlobe. This electrode montage allows registration of all the common waves in the ABR, but is not necessarily optimal for any specific ABR component. It is immaterial whether the noninverting and inverting electrodes are reversed; all that will happen is that the recorded waveform will be inverted. Debates about which way up the ABR should be recorded are interminable and sterile; what matters is that we know which way is up, which is not always the case!

Effectively, the differential preamplifier subtracts the activity at the inverting electrode from that at the noninverting electrode, and multiplies the difference by the gain factor, typically 100,000. The common electrode is required as an electrical reference point for the amplifier, though the activity at the common site does not contribute significantly to the amplifier output. A measure of the amplifier's ability to reject similar activity at both inputs is the *common-mode rejection ratio,* or CMRR. This is the ratio of amplifier output when a signal is presented to only one input, relative to the output when the same signal is presented to both inputs. Typical values for CMRR exceed 80 dB; in voltage terms, this means that the output for the common-mode activity will be more than 10,000 times smaller than for the single-input condition.

The CMRR varies with frequency and is often tuned to be maximal for the most problematic noise source, for instance, 60 Hz power line interference. Periodic readjustment is required to maintain optimal values (see Gorga et al., chapter 4). A 10 dB loss in CMRR is equivalent to tripling the common-mode noise level at the preamplifier output, an increase which could have a drastic effect on the precision of ABR measurements.

The electrical impedance of each electrode/skin interface is typically in the range of 1–10, and because the preamplifier input impedance is of the order of megaohms or higher, there will be very little loss of voltage across the interface. Thus, the interface impedance has a negligible effect on the ABR waveform itself. The impedance is important for two reasons: impedances may all be very good in absolute terms, that is less than 2, but if one electrode is 1500 ohms and the other 500 ohms, the CMRR will be reduced. Second, the absolute impedance affects the size of the voltage developed at the amplifier input by any electrical current source (such as electromagnetically induced noise current) in a proportional manner, so high impedances degrade recording not by affecting the signal, but by increasing the input noise level.

Differential amplification, in spite of being an essential step in rendering the ABR detectable, is by no means sufficient. The main reason for this is that much of the physiologic noise that obscures the ABR is not identical at the noninverting and inverting electrodes; in fact, it is largely uncorrelated noise and its ability to obscure the signal is almost unaffected by the differential action.

In practice, the dominant noise source affecting ABR measurements is electromyogenic noise. Its effects on the SNR are profound. In infants, for example, the root-mean-square (RMS) noise level can change by more than an order of magnitude, depending on whether the infant is deeply asleep or awake and fretting. While the scalp topography of the ABR is quite well documented, at least for normal adult subjects, there is little information about myogenic noise topography. It is conceivable that such studies would lead to changes in electrode placement to give superior SNRs, but it seems unlikely that the gains would be substantial.

All electrical components in the recording instrumentation generate some internal noise, which is added to the noise picked up by the electrodes. The only point in the system where this matters is the input stages of the preamplifier, where the noise is magnified by the very high gain. Amplifier noise is typically equivalent to about 1 μV RMS at the scalp, so usually the other noise components are much more important. However, when recording from sleeping infants or from anesthetized patients, amplifier noise is a substantial proportion of the total effective input noise.

Differential recording is a major step in improving the SNR, but it must be stressed that it can have profound and complex effects on the ABR waveform; this fact is all too often forgotten. A given wave component will appear at the preamplifier output only to the extent that it is different at the electrode sites. Also, a potential which is truly scalp-positive, for example, may be either positive or negative at the preamplifier output, depending on whether it appeared predominantly at the noninverting or inverting electrode.

Filtering the Differential Preamplifier Output

Filtering is a further step in the effort to improve SNR. The general objective is to preferentially suppress those frequency components of the activity containing particularly high amounts of noise energy. Often, filters are included in the amplifier, but it is frequently necessary to use additional filters for increased flexibility.

Filters are described as analog or digital; an analog filter manipulates the input activity as a continuous *voltage–time* process which can take any real value. A digital filter operates on a series of discrete numbers, which are obtained by sampling the activity sequentially. At present, most filters used in ABR work are analog devices. Digital filters can be made to simulate

Figure 3–1.
A to *D*: Some ideal (solid) and realizable (dotted) filter moduli. *E*: Moduli for 12, 24, and 48 dB/octave Butterworth filters. Note the linear roll-off on log-log axes, and the common −3dB point. The abscissa is f/f_c for a low-pass filter, and f_c/f for a high-pass filter, where f_c is the cutoff frequency. *F*: The phase function for a Butterworth filter. The left-hand ordinate indicates positive phase shift (phase lead) for a high-pass filter; the right-hand ordinate indicates negative phase shift (phase lag) for a low-pass filter. Full scale is 180°, 360°, or 720°, for 12, 24, and 48 dB/octave filters, respectively. The abscissa is f/f_c for all cases.

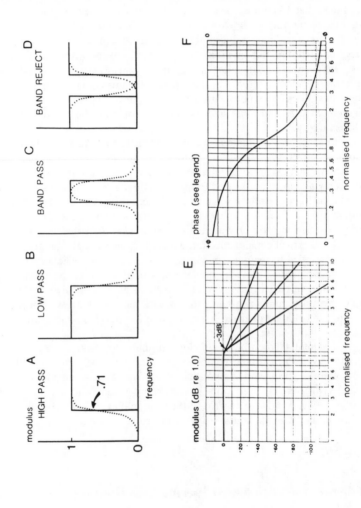

analog filter properties, but the reverse is not always true. For example, consider a digital filter in which a section of the digitized activity is stored, prior to manipulation by some numerical algorithm. It is possible, in such a filter that has memory, to essentially run the stored activity backwards through the algorithm, to reverse time. This is obviously not possible in a simple analog filter, which processes the input data as they occur. For many reasons, the power and flexibility of digital filters are much greater than those of analog filters.

Any filter can be expressed in terms of its effect on the frequency distribution of the energy at its input, that is, on the energy density spectrum of the input signal. A general formula for the filter action is

$$M (\omega) \exp [-j\o(\omega)]$$

where $M(\omega)$ is the modulus at frequency ω, and $\o(\omega)$ is the phase shift at the corresponding ω. If the modulus is unity at some particular ω, then the size of that input frequency component is unaltered by the filter; in the regions of ω where the modulus is less than unity, the filter suppresses input energy.

A useful concept is that of the ideal filter, which passes some input frequency components unchanged, but totally suppresses others. Common types of ideal filter moduli are shown in Figure 3-1. In practice, such moduli can only be approximated by real filters, whether analog or digital; examples of this are also shown in the figure. There are many ways of designing filters; some common designs are designated Butterworth, Bessel, Chebychev, and so on, which terms relate to the underlying mathematical formula used in the design. These common types differ in the extent to which they approximate the ideal modulus functions, and in the amount of phase shift. The Butterworth design is the most common.

A consequence of these approximations in real filters, which are often quite limited, is that the actual amount of attenuation achieved outside the filter passband is small. For example, a 12 dB/octave high-pass filter with a cutoff frequency of 100 Hz will only attenuate 60 Hz activity by a factor of about three, whereas a 24 db/octave filter with the same cutoff frequency will attenuate 60 Hz by a factor of about eight.

The extent to which filtering will improve the SNR depends on the amount of overlap of the signal and noise spectra. If these are identical, the filter will not alter the SNR at all. If, on the other hand, there is no overlap, an ideal filter would completely eliminate the noise and a real filter might also perform quite well, depending on its slope and the amount of overlap. For the ABR, the signal and noise spectra overlap strongly, and so the SNR enhancement achievable by filtering is modest. This issue is actually very complex and has not been studied in any real depth, so it is difficult to say exactly how effective a particular filter will be, or to specify filters that will be optimal for various recording conditions and clinical applications.

One of the consequences of filtering signal and noise components that have overlapping spectra is that the filter alters the signal. It does this by two mechanisms: first, by attenuating some signal frequency components, and second, by altering the phase of the various frequency components, even those which are not significantly attenuated. This latter effect, known as phase distortion, usually dominates the changes in ABR waveform. Whether this distortion matters or not depends entirely on what use is being made of particular ABR features. If the goal of the measurement is merely to detect the ABR, which is often the case when estimating audiometric thresholds, the distortion may not matter or may even improve response detectability. For making inferences about the presence or absence of a retrocochlear lesion, on the other hand, ABR detection may be secondary to precise calculations involving absolute, interaural, or interpeak latencies; here, the filter effects must be considered more carefully.

Some generalizations can be made about the distortions introduced by the high-pass and low-pass components of a bandpass filter. The low-pass filter will smooth out the high-frequency components, and will introduce a time lag in each frequency component, equal to $d\o(\omega)/d\omega$.

If this rate of change of the phase shift depends on ω, that is, if the phase shift is not zero or linear over ω (in which case the time lag is either zero or a constant), then it follows that signal energy components at different frequencies will be delayed by different amounts; this is the mechanism of ABR phase distortion.

A high-pass filter will introduce time lead (i.e., negative delay) by the same argument, and, because high-pass filters tend to encroach on regions of significant response energy, their effects on signal waveform are often more profound than those of commonly used low-pass filters. In general, high-pass filtering will depress the amplitude of any given peak in the wide-band ABR, and will introduce an artifactual succeeding peak of opposite polarity. More severe filtering may abolish the wide-band peak, depress the succeeding peak, and induce a later artifactual peak of the same polarity as the original peak. An example is shown in Figure 3-2. Such artifacts may be quite useful clinically, but it is pointless to speculate about their physiologic sources. These distortions can occur for all peaks in the ABR sequence, and their summed effect can be quite complex, in terms of relating peaks in the filtered waveform to those in the wide-band waveform.

It was mentioned earlier that the degree to which filters will improve the SNR depends upon the spectra of the signal and noise components. With standard filter designs we are quite restricted in terms of tailoring the filter to spectra that occur; usually, only the cut-off frequency is adjustable. It is possible that more advanced filters, which would take account of the spectral details, might be beneficial, but this is an area for much further research. The difficulty is that what we really want the filter to do is optimize either response detectability or the precision with which we can measure specific waveform features. This is quite a complex problem which draws on sophisticated statistical and pattern recognition concepts. A further complication is that so many factors affect the signal and noise conditions which will be encountered, such as the stimulus parameters, the state of the patient, the presence of pathology, and so forth. Certainly, no single filter will be best for all conditions.

It is to be expected that digital filters will become increasingly common in ABR systems. They are more flexible, can be applied nondestructively in many ways to stored ABR data, and can easily be structured to avoid phase distortion. More advanced formulations which take spectral details into account, such as the Wiener filter, have yet to be proven useful.

The use of narrow-band filters, which focus upon a frequency region where the signal and noise energy ratio is relatively favorable, has been proposed for many EPs, including the ABR. The disadvantage of such filters is that they render all input activity, whether signal or noise, into a sinusoidal form with a frequency which is approximately that of the filter passband center. This can degrade the recognizability of response, relative to wide-band recordings, by suppressing morphological cues.

Special filters designed to suppress specific noise components, notably 60 Hz power line pickup, are available in several ABR systems. These are often called *notch* filters, a special case of the bandstop type. The trouble with notch filters is that they usually cause considerable phase distortion, and should be used only as a last resort in very adverse recording situations, such as in the operating room or in the field. It is far better to solve nonphysiologic noise problems at the source than to try and compensate by signal processing tricks.

Analog to Digital Conversion (ADC)

Following differential amplification and filtering, the next steps in SNR enhancement require that the activity be converted to digital form. This is a process of sampling the activity and generating an integer (whole number) that approximates the value of the activity at the instant of sampling. This is done rapidly, at regular intervals. The result is a sequence of digits (a time series) that represents the activity.

The two relevant features of ADC are the sampling rate and the resolution of the convertor. The Nyquist sampling theorem states that if the total information content of the activity is to be preserved, the activity must be sampled at a rate at least twice that of its highest frequency component. Thus, if the activity contains energy up to 5000 Hz, the sampling rate must be 10,000 Hz or greater to avoid irrevocable loss of information. Since there is not usually a frequency at which the input energy spectrum suddenly goes to zero, it is customary to sample at a rate at least 2.5 times the cutoff frequency of the low-pass filter which precedes the ADC. In practice, this is rarely an issue for the ABR because we require the activity to be digitized at a sufficiently high rate that the time series closely resembles the waveform of the activity itself, for purposes of visual inspection; this practice leads to rates substantially higher than the Nyquist rate. For example, to produce a time series that adequately defines an ABR peak in response to a click stimulus of moderate intensity, a sampling rate of at least 10,000 Hz is required, yet there is little response energy above 2000 Hz.

The consequence of sampling at an insufficient rate is an inability to visually assess the waveform; in particular, peak locations may be altered, and peak amplitudes underestimated. If the rate actually satisfies the Nyquist theorem, it is possible to recover the true waveform by a mathematical transformation of the time series, but this procedure is tedious and almost never done. If the rate actually fails the Nyquist criterion, then the true activity is not recoverable, and certainly not visually interpretable. Signal energy at frequencies above the sampling rate will be represented in the time series as low-frequency distortions, a phenomenon known as aliasing.

The only common occasion when attention to sampling rate might be necessary is when multichannel ABR recordings are required. If a basic sampling rate for a single data channel of 20,000 Hz were used, multiplexing this into four data channels would give a rate of 5000 Hz per channel, which is not usually adequate.

The ADC resolution is usually expressed as a number of binary digits (bits); for example, an 8-bit conversion can produce 2^8 (256) distinct output integers. Thus, the entire continuous input voltage range is mapped onto 256 output values; this is called quantization, and the resulting errors are quantization errors. If the input range were equivalent to, say, 50 μV at the patient's head, the maximum quantization error would be about 200 nV. This error could be significant if it were necessary to inspect the ADC output directly, but in fact this output is passed to a further manipulation (summation or averaging), which has the effect of increasing the effective resolution dramatically. For example, if each of two quantities can take values from zero to 256, then their sum can take values from zero to 512. Thus, an 8-bit ADC is perfectly adequate for ABR work; in fact, quite reasonable results can be obtained with only a 1-bit conversion, which is equivalent to capturing only the sign of the input data. In practice, the ADC operations in ABR instrumentation have no significant effect on the SNR.

Summation or Averaging

The operation of summation or averaging of the digitized activity has a massive effect on the SNR, and is a critical step in making the ABR detectable and measurable. The reader may be familiar with the basic concepts, so the following development is a little more formal than usual. Some knowledge of simple statistical principles is required. Suppose the section of the time series containing the response to a single stimulus is termed an elementary record. The ABR will not be visible in any such record, so further SNR enhancement is required. Let n such elementary records be collected, following delivery of n identical stimuli, with each record

Figure 3–2.

Effects of high-pass filtering on the ABR. The top waveforms in each column are a typical response from a young normal infant to 500 Hz 40 dB nHL tone pips in band-reject masking noise. The window length is 25.6 ms, and the recording bandwidth was 1–1500 Hz; a small amount of digital smoothing was applied. This is the true, essentially unfiltered, response waveform; only a broad vertex-positive wave V peak is visible. The left-hand column shows the effect of increasing high-pass cutoff frequency for a regular 24 dB/octave Butterworth filter. Note the depression of wave V, development of a succeeding negative wave (SN_{10}), and a later positive wave, and the peak latency changes. The right-hand column shows the results for the same filter moduli, but with phase distortion removed digitally. Comparison of the two columns shows the distortions introduced by the modulus alone (right side) and the modulus plus phase effects (left side).

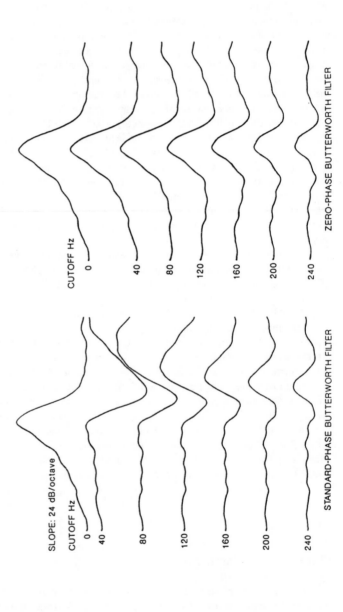

being exactly synchronized to the corresponding stimulus event. The elementary record is modeled as the sum of a signal (the ABR) and a noise (everything else) process. This can be written as:

$$x(t) = s(t) + n(t),$$

where $x(t)$ is the activity, and $s(t)$ and $n(t)$ are the signal and noise components, respectively. In terms of digitized sequences, this can be written as:

$$x(j) = s(j) + n(j),$$

where j is an integer in the range 1 to m, and represents the successive samples in each elementary record. If n such records are collected, a matrix of n rows and m columns is developed, and any data point in the matrix can be represented as:

$$x(ij) = s(ij) + n(ij),$$

where the index i goes from 1 to n, and denotes the successive records.

If the signal part is identical for each of the n records, then the index i can be dropped because $s(ij)$ depends only upon j, the position of the sample point in each record, thus:

$$x(ij) = s(j) + n(ij).$$

The i index is retained for the noise components, which are random and therefore may differ in each record, as will the overall activity x.

The secret of summation or averaging lies precisely in this difference between the signal and the noise; the signal is assumed to be deterministic (nonrandom) and identical for all stimulus repetitions, whereas the noise is random. The argument is as follows:

The SNR for any elementary record is some ratio of the *size* of the signal and the noise. The signal changes with time, that is, with j, so we need the concept of SNR at any particular value of j. We might choose a j which corresponds to the latency of wave V, for example. The SNR is more formally the RMS ratio, and the RMS of a constant quantity is the quantity itself, so the RMS of $s(j)$ is $s(j)$. The noise $n(ij)$ is usually assumed to be taken from a population of values that is normally distributed (Gaussian) with mean zero and variance σ^2. This is true for any i and j, in which case the statistics of the noise do not change over time, and the noise is said to be stationary. The RMS value of $n(ij)$ equals its standard deviation σ, if the process has zero mean value.

At any j, therefore, the SNR in the elementary record is simply $s(j)/\sigma$.

Suppose we now add up all n values of $x(ij)$ for each value of j individually. This will produce an array of sums, denoted by $X(j)$, where:

$$X(j) = x(1j) + x(2j) + \ldots + x(nj),$$

that is, we merely sum each column of the data matrix $[x(ij)]$. What is the SNR in this sum array? At any j, the size of the signal component is simply n times the value in each record, because the signal is identical at any j in all records. Thus the signal RMS becomes $n.s(j)$. With regard to the noise, statistical theory tells us that the variance of the sum of n independently and identically distributed random variables is the sum of their individual variances, so the variance of the noise component at any j in the sum is $n.\sigma^2$. The noise RMS is the standard deviation, which is the square root of the variance, so the noise RMS is $\sigma.n^{1/2}$. It follows that the SNR in the sum record is $n.s(j)/\sigma.n^{1/2}$, which equals $n^{1/2}.s(j)/\sigma$; thus the SNR in the sum is $n^{1/2}$ times the SNR in the elementary record. If the initial SNR were 0.1, say, then the SNR in the sum of 1000 records would be about 3.2.

Many commercial ABR systems merely sum the records, but some of them actually divide the sum by the number of records, in other words, they produce an array which is the true average of the accumulated records. This procedure produces exactly the same improvement in SNR, but the underlying statistical arguments change slightly. Here, the SNR of the signal component in the average is $s(j)$, at any j, because the average value of a constant is that constant. The variance of the average of n independently and identically distributed random variables is the sum of the individual variances divided by n^2, that is, the variance of the average is $n.\sigma^2/n^2$, which equals σ^2/n, so the RMS value is $\sigma/n^{1/2}$. It follows that the SNR in the average record is $n^{1/2}.s(j)/\sigma$, which is the same result as for summation alone. The only real difference between the two procedures lies in the visual appearance of the displayed result as the procedure progresses. For summation, the response will appear to grow steadily relative to a noise background which also grows, though not as rapidly. For averaging, there is no impression of growth, but rather one of gradual convergence to a response-like waveform, as the noise variance in the average decreases.

Since summation or averaging takes up most of the time in any ABR measurement session, and since the output SNR governs the reliability of interpretive decisions, it is of interest to consider exactly how much averaging is required. In practice, the choice of n is often based on popular consensus rather than on quantitative rationale, and it is common to encounter published recommendations lacking any formal rationale. Informal views of experienced workers are probably useful, but it is better to have a quantitative argument. The difficulty is that the specification of n is a very complicated statistical problem which requires the definition of an explicit measurement goal; such goals have not yet been well formulated. However, as technology and automation impact more heavily on evoked potential techniques, some quantitative arguments will inevitably be required.

A basic ball-park figure for n can be derived easily. The bottom line on, say, an ABR determination for audiometric purposes is a reliable decision about the presence or absence of response in a given summed record. Of course, the summed or averaged record may still contain a lot of noise—it may even be entirely noise—so that decisions based on such records will be statistical ones having finite probability of error. It appears that human observers looking at averaged records are comfortable making response detection decisions that have fairly low rates of false-positive detection; they require SNRs of about 2 or more before deciding with confidence that the ABR is present. This means that the putative response peak in the average must be about twice the size of the visually estimated standard deviation of the noise fluctuations in the rest of the record. If the SNR in the average must be at least 2, and the typical SNR in the elementary record is about 0.05, which we know by comparing the typical ABR amplitude to the RMS EEG noise level, then about $(2/0.05)^2$, or 1600, records must be summed. This can be contrasted with the case for the cortical slow vertex response, where the typical elementary SNR is about 0.3, so that $(2/0.3)^2$, or roughly 50, records must be summed to achieve the required output SNR.

Attempting to be more precise than this is where the going gets tough. Suppose that one subject has on average twice the noise RMS of another, but that the ABRs are about the same size. To achieve similar levels of accuracy in detection decisions for the two subjects requires that the n be changed to compensate for the noise differences, about four times as many records being needed for the subject with the higher noise levels. The severity of the problem is readily appreciated if one considers that in a situation of fairly low EEG noise levels, averages of 2000 records are common practice. If a patient is encountered whose noise level is twice as large, the continued use of 2000 records per average is equivalent to the use of only 500 records per average in the well-behaved case; few would consider that number to be adequate.

Of course, one cannot continue averaging indefinitely; there is an upper bound to the test time. The bottom line is that if the source data are of poor quality and test time is constant, something has to give; no amount of data processing will make a silk purse out of a sow's ear. It is better to spend the available time getting fewer decisions which are reliable rather than many decisions which are not. The only real way to solve the problem of poor-quality activity is either to do more work, or to remove the problem at the source.

The use of large n, say up to 10,000, is not as daunting as it appears because many ABR applications rely primarily on wave V, and this wave is quite robust against increasing stimulus repetition rate. The use of high rates permits large n in reasonable test times, and an important concept which governs the choice of rate is the ratio of response amplitude to the RMS noise in the averaged record. This has been called efficiency (Picton, Linden, Hamel & Maru, 1983). The loss in amplitude of a response component as stimulus rate increases is offset by the reduction in noise level in the average, resulting from the use of larger n in a given test time. The compromise that maximizes the efficiency is likely to be a desirable test protocol. When only wave V is important, rates greater than 35/s are more efficient; even when it is required to detect or measure wave I, rates greater than about 20/s are more efficient.

These arguments concerning the required n, and the test efficiency, are often not taken into account in clinical ABR testing. By far the most common practice is to use a constant and somewhat arbitrary n for all subjects, in which case accuracy will vary drastically with noise levels. It seems more reasonable to strive for a consistent accuracy, rather than merely to set a dial to a convenient number which ignores activity characteristics.

Unfortunately, current instrumentation rarely provides adequate information on which to base a quantitative strategy for selecting n. As systems become more sophisticated, it is to be hoped that data characteristics such as noise RMS will be extracted automatically, and either displayed in a helpful way to the tester or used in automatic control paradigms that guide the averaging to achieve consistent and known levels of accuracy, both for response detection decisions and for waveform description.

It is worth noting that if the amount of time to be expended on averaging for a given stimulus condition allows the acquisition of, say, 8000 records, then this could be done as a single average or as two independent averages of 4000 records each. Which is preferable? If the noise really conformed to the normally distributed stationary model mentioned earlier, then the single average is the most efficient procedure. In fact, the noise is often quite nonstationary; in many ways it behaves like what is termed a *contaminated* normal process, a mixture of one low-variance process which is normal and stationary and another process which has higher variance and may be nonstationary. The primary source of the high-variance contaminant, in ABR measurements, is electromyogenic activity. In such a case, it is useful to split the total data set into two subsets of 4000 records, and to require that for any waveform to be considered a response, it must be present and fairly consistent in both subsets.

Often, the result of averaging still contains a lot of noise, and the decisions about detection or measurement are quite difficult, even with two averages to compare. The use of no-stimulus averages as a way of describing the noise alone, and therefore as a guide to reliable response detection decisions, has a superficial appeal but little analytical foundation. It is nonstationary noise that is the source of most ABR measurement problems, and there is no guarantee whatsoever that the noise estimates gained in a control average will be representative of the test averages. The major role of control recordings in ABR work lies in ruling out the presence of nonrandom, nonphysiologic noise components, such as power line artifacts.

There are two simple procedures which do provide some insight into noise processes; the first is simply to delay the stimulus so that a reasonable amount of prestimulus summated activity can be visually compared with the region containing the putative response. Such prestimulus activity is in principle a much better reference condition than an independent control average, because the actual noise conditions in the test material are well represented. A problem with this procedure is that, because the ABR is only the beginning of a much more lengthy response series, especially including the middle-latency response (MLR) and possibly the postauricular myogenic response, the prestimulus epoch may contain these responses from previous stimuli, and be misleading. This is a problem especially with wide-band ABR recordings at high-stimulus repetition rates. Also, for high stimulus intensities the presence of a large stimulus artifact within the elementary record can trigger automatic artifact rejection systems (see below).

The second method is the so-called plus/minus reference, in which a second average is simultaneously accumulated, but with the sign of the data reversed for half the records. Any deflection present in both the regular average and the reference average cannot be response, according to the data model developed above. Note that if the reference is accumulated with sign alternation of every other record in the sequence, this will defeat the alternation of stimulus polarity as a device for reducing stimulus artifact. Also, the reference average will contain better approximations of nonstationary noise events contaminating the regular average if the sign change is done only once, rather than every other record. The plus/minus reference is a useful tool, which is underutilized in current ABR systems.

Locking to Phase-Coherent Noise Components

It is assumed in the averaging model that the noise is a random process. This is true for most of the physiologic noise contaminants, but is clearly untrue for such noise components as 60 Hz power line interference, and associated harmonics or periodic transients, which can arise from exposed power lines and fluorescent lighting, for example. Averaging goes hand in hand with stimulus repetition, and the rates of repetition can determine the extent to which averaging will suppress these noise components. For example, averaging at 60 records per second, or at any repetition rate which is an integer submultiple of 60, such as 30, 20, or 10, will cause the power line noise to be locked in phase with the averaging sequence; the noise, then, will be enhanced by the same factor as the response. In fact, running a no-stimulus average at 60/s is an excellent test for the presence of noise related to the power line.

All that is required to avoid this phase locking is to adjust the repetition rate so that it is not an exact submultiple of 60. However, the pattern of artifact that can result from any given repetition rate can be quite complex, and the precise rates to be used in clinical or research measurements must be carefully and periodically checked for absence of nonphysiologic noise.

The stimulus sequence itself can induce physiologic "noise" (unwanted activity) which is synchronized to the averaging cycle, and which can seriously distort the ABR, especially at stimulus repetition rates above about 35/s. The postauricular myogenic response and the MLR are the main offenders; the latter phenomenon is precisely what underlies the recording conditions for the so-called 40-Hz event-related potential, which can be a significant source of ABR distortion. Its effects can be reduced by raising the high-pass filter cutoff frequency to 100 Hz or so, which will abolish much of the MLR. This is fine for otoneurologic ABR work, with high-intensity click stimuli, but does not solve the problem when near-threshold tone pip stimuli are used, for ABR audiometry. Here, the ABR energy distribution shifts to low frequencies which are not much higher than those where the MLR is concentrated, and any filter which suppresses the MLR will then also affect the ABR quite strongly.

Editing or Artifact Rejection

The SNR increase due to averaging was based on the common assumption of normally distributed stationary noise. It is the assumption of stationarity that is strictly necessary, for averaging to work; the data need not be normally distributed. It is important to realize that the SNR enhancement by the square root of n in summation or averaging is based upon arguments of long-term expectation; in fact, the enhancement actually achieved in any single average is itself a random variable with an expectation of root n. One of the factors that contribute to unreliable outcomes of individual averages is the occurrence of extreme data values, that is, large voltage deflections in individual elementary records. A single isolated artifact of size $100 \mu V$ will have a value of 100 nV in an average of 1000 records, and may simulate or abolish a genuine response of similar size. Such extremes commonly arise from myogenic activity, and it is sound practice to reduce their incidence in the average by rejecting those records which contain them.

Artifact rejection systems are important and common components of ABR instrumentation. The problem lies in the available amount of control of the voltage level at which rejection will occur, and in how to use it. In some systems, data rejection occurs on both positive and negative extremes, when the ADC registers either limiting value. Yet, it is the effective size of the rejection voltage level at the patient's head which matters. If 1V of activity at the ADC triggers the rejection, then, if the gain of the preceding preamplifier is 50,000, say, the effective rejection level at the preamplifier input is $20 \mu V$. If the only way of controlling this level is by adjusting the preamplifier gain, then a situation can arise in which the choices of effective rejection level at the head are too restricted by virtue of switched, as opposed to continuous, gain control. More flexible systems permit the rejection levels to be set at almost any value, for example, as a percentage of the full-scale data display.

The management of artifact rejection levels is not a simple matter, and can have quite strong effects on the quality of averages. The most common error is insufficient use of rejection, that is, setting the rejection levels too large, relative to the general amount of fluctuation in recorded activity. In making the decision, the major drawback of using low rejection levels, ones that give many rejections, is that the time taken to acquire a given number of records is increased.

If the noise were really stationary, the mean (or sum) array without any artifact rejection is the most powerful estimator of the true signal waveform. Any deletion or alteration of any value in the sample can result only in loss of information. Thus, artifact rejection never improves the quality of well-behaved data; what it does do, however, is tend to produce average records that are relatively well behaved even when the source data are littered with nonstationary artifactual extreme values. The cost is acquisition time; we do not get something for nothing.

In practice, the recorded activity rarely contains isolated extreme values. It is far more common to see lengthy periods of well-behaved, low-variance activity, interspersed with bursts of high-variance activity resulting from episodic electromyogenic noise. A sensible course is to set the artifact rejection limits so that little of the well-behaved activity is rejected, but all of the high-variance activity is. This can be done by "tuning" the rejection level while observing the displayed activity, so that about 5–10% of the "good" activity is rejected. If the patient goes into a myogenic episode, then almost all of the bad activity will be rejected. This also avoids having to manually interrupt and resume the averaging.

In the event that the activity from a given patient does not show these periods of low and high variance, the task is more difficult. If the absolute voltage level is sustained and higher than usual, the cause is probably a steady level of myogenic disturbance, often seen in patients who are tense and anxious. Here, there is no clear distinction between good and bad activity; it is all fairly bad, and there are three possible courses of action. By far the best course is to improve the quality of the source data, perhaps by calming and reassuring the patient, or by medication. The next best course is to set the rejection level to give about 10% rejection, and increase the amount of averaging in an attempt to compensate for the increased noise variance. The least desirable course is to ignore the poor quality of the data, and suffer the ensuing loss of accuracy in response detection or estimation.

It is worth noting here that there are obvious and simple ways in which ABR data acquisition might be improved. For example, the role of a filter is to preferentially suppress noise, yet the most effective artifact rejection strategy would require accurate and sensitive detection of significant noise events. Thus, the artifact rejection system would operate more effectively if its input were not the actual data to be averaged, but rather some other parallel data stream which had been filtered or otherwise manipulated so as to optimize the detection of noise events. It might even be desirable to employ different electrode derivations for the express purpose of artifact detection.

The Validity of ABR Data Models

There is a subtle, but considerable, gap between the rationale for averaging developed above and the operations actually performed in practical ABR measurements. The model for averaging dealt exclusively with the amplitude of activity *at arbitrary poststimulus times,* whereas it is amplitudes and latencies of *observed peaks* in the average record which dominate many ABR applications. Do the laws of averaging, and all the attendant protocol manipulations based upon those laws, actually apply to these important, clinically utilized response features? This is a hard question to answer; a peak in an averaged record is a maximum (or minimum) of a time series which has substantial correlation between neighboring points; the statistical distributions of such quantities are quite difficult to derive analytically. The real problem here is that we do not know in advance the points that will be selected as probable response features; rather, we select them after looking at the averaged record. The properties of data that are selected a posteriori are very different from those defined prior to data collection. For example, the voltage at precisely 6 ms after stimulus delivery may well be normally distributed with zero mean, in the absence of a response. The theory of averaging will be correct, for the amplitude of activity at that point. By contrast, the voltage which is most likely to be measured as a response peak is actually chosen because it is the largest excursion in a certain range of latency where the response is expected to lie. Even if there is no genuine response, some peak will probably exist in the target latency range, and so the actual amplitude selected will never be zero or negative; thus, it is certainly not distributed in the same way as the amplitude at the point selected a priori.

The behavior of ABR peak latency estimates is even more difficult to describe analytically. The latency of an observed maximum or minimum in an averaged record is quite a complicated function of the amplitude distribution throughout the record; it is by no means obvious that latencies will be normally distributed, even if the amplitude distribution of the activity is. Nor is it clear that latencies will conform exactly to the SNR enhancement laws of averaging derived above.

The other important assumptions of the averaging model are that the ABR and the noise are statistically independent, and that the ABR is constant for all elementary records. Neither of these assumptions is verified satisfactorily, and both are extremely difficult to validate. A common flaw in published studies in this area is to equate the failure to detect a phenomenon with absence of the phenomenon, even though the methods used were not at all sensitive.

In summary, the statistical models for ABR data are speculative but plausible. The effects of signal processing operations such as averaging are superficially predictable, given reasonable but unproven assumptions. Some simple considerations can guide the choice of instrumentation and protocols, but current procedures are largely intuitive and qualitative. Much further research is required to validate data models and to understand fully the effects of signal processing operations on clinically useful response measures. Technical advances should not blind us to the importance of source data quality; sometimes, 5 minutes spent reassuring a patient or checking an electrode will be more useful than hours of exotic data massage.

After Averaging

Having accumulated one or more average records, the usual goals are either to make a decision about response presence or absence, or to measure specific features of the response. Most ABR systems provide simple helpful facilities to achieve these goals. Some systems permit inspection and manipulation of records concurrently with acquisition of new averages, which saves time. Usually, several averages can be displayed simultaneously, vertical scaling can be adjusted, and vertical shifting so that records can be superimposed is helpful in identifying consistent features between records. There is often a data smoothing function, which is a form of digital low-pass filtering helpful in removing unwanted high-frequency components. Many systems have the facility to add and subtract entire averages, a feature which is often useful when response identification is difficult, and is essential if any of the "derived response" techniques are to be used. Interactive cursor management for picking peaks and getting numerical readout of amplitude and latency are standard, as are plotting facilities. Disk storage of records is widely available, as are interfaces to general purpose microcomputers, for further manipulation or storage.

Future Trends

There are many ways in which the clinical value of ABR measurements could be improved, and many of these are highly technical; a few areas have already been mentioned. Rapid advances can be expected in the extent to which the instrumentation system will evaluate and control data acquisition, as well as aid in interpretation. In estimating the ABR threshold, for example, we can expect future systems not only to implement simple procedures such as the plus/minus reference automatically, but also to control the number of records averaged, adjust artifact rejection criteria, quantify noise conditions, apply optimal digital filters, indicate how long it will take to achieve a specified detection accuracy, implement statistical tests for response detection, change the stimulus conditions, and so on. Some of these areas are extremely complex, but are being intensively investigated and implemented on systems connected to powerful general purpose computers. Ultimately, these procedures will be incorporated in packaged clinical systems.

In otoneurologic applications, similar progress can be expected. In particular, systems will incorporate automatic response feature detection and measurement, and will include decision-making algorithms for response evaluation and diagnostic classification. Here, recent advances in collection and display of multichannel ABR data are especially promising. It must be recognized that while the vast majority of ABR measurements and reports to date deal with single-channel recordings, such methods give a very narrow and possibly quite misleading view of the true, three-dimensional pattern of activity in the auditory system. The problem with multichannel recording is the sheer volume of data generated, and it is necessary to integrate and display the data so that they can be appreciated by the investigator. Recent advances indicate that multichannel recording may offer new insight into the neurophysiological basis of the ABR, and opportunities for radical improvement in breadth and quality of clinical applications.

In spite of the technical advances behind present-day ABR techniques, it is no exaggeration to say that we have only scratched the surface. There is enormous scope for technical and concomitant clinical advance, but progress will require the pooling of diverse skills. The task of integrating multichannel recording, advanced signal processing and pattern recognition techniques, high-speed interactive computer graphics, and even adaptive decision-making systems from the area of artificial intelligence research is a most challenging and potentially rewarding one.

REFERENCES

Arlinger, S. (1981). Technical aspects on stimulation, recording and signal processing. In T. Lundborg (Ed.), Scandinavian Symposium on Brain Stem Response (ABR). *Scandinavian Audiology (Stockholm),* Supplement 13.

Beagley, H. A. (Ed.) 1979). *Auditory investigation. The scientific and technical basis.* New York: Oxford University Press.

Beauchamp, K., & Yuen, C. (1979). *Digital methods for signal analysis.* London: Allen & Unwin.

Bendat, J., & Piersol, A. (1966). *Measurement and analysis of random data.* New York: Wiley.

Coats, A. C. (1983). Instrumentation. In E. J. Moore (Ed.), *Bases of auditory brain-stem evoked responses.* New York: Grune & Stratton.

Doyle, D. J., & Hyde, M. L. (1981). Analogue and digital filtering of auditory brainstem potentials. *Scandinavian Audiology (Stockholm), 10,* 81-89.

Glaser, E. M., & Ruchkin, D. S. (1976). *Principles of neurobiological signal analysis.* New York: Academic Press.

Hamming, R. W. (1983). *Digital filters.* Englewood Cliffs, NJ: Prentice-Hall.

Picton, T. W., Linden, R. D., Hamel, G., & Maru, J. T. (1983). Aspects of averaging. *Seminars in hearing, 4,* 327-341.

Chapter 4

Stimulus Calibration in ABR Measurements

Michael P. Gorga
Paul J. Abbas
Don W. Worthington

INTRODUCTION

In both psychophysical and physiological studies of hearing, we are concerned with the relation between stimulus and response. To understand this relation, it is essential that we describe the stimulus that we are delivering to the ear to elicit the response. This need exists for clinical and experimental studies alike. In this chapter, we list some stimulus characteristics that are particularly pertinent to auditory brainstem response (ABR) measurements. In addition, we attempt to provide brief descriptions of how these stimulus features can be measured. In the interest of conserving space, we do not engage in a detailed description of the physics of sound and we assume some basic knowledge on the part of the reader. Other references are available that provide more general acoustical descriptions (Backus, 1969; Durrant, 1983; Green, 1976; Pickles, 1982; Small, 1973; Yost & Nielsen, 1977). Herein, we present calibration procedures appropriate for the description of stimulus intensity, rate, duration, phase (polarity), temporal waveform, and amplitude spectrum.

STIMULUS INTENSITY

The stimuli that are used to elicit ABRs present special problems for stimulus intensity measurements. The duration of these stimuli is often short relative to the response of a sound level meter (SLM). While SLMs are available which are capable of responding with sufficient speed,[1] often these devices are not found in clinical settings. In the absence of such devices, a variety of physical and biological calibration procedures have been substituted, some of which are reviewed below.

Tone Bursts

There is some confusion in the literature regarding the terminology used for frequency-specific stimuli. As an example, both short-duration pure tones (≤ 10 ms) and filtered clicks have been referred to as tone pips. The "logon," described by Davis (1976), is derived by gating a

[1]The Bruel and Kjaer sound level meter (Type 2209), having a time constant of 10 μs for its peak detector, is an example of one instrument that can follow relatively short-duration stimuli.

sinusoid with Gaussian envelopes. We consider sine waves of any duration as members of the class of stimuli referred to as *tone bursts*. For these stimuli, calibration of amplitude is straightforward. We simply increase the duration of the tone burst until it is long relative to the response time of the SLM, and then measure the sound pressure level. In this way, we can specify intensity in dB SPL (re: 20 μPa) by measuring the sound pressure level of a continuous stimulus which has the same amplitude as the peak amplitude of the tone burst. In the procedures to follow, we use SLMs for sound pressure measurements, but such devices are more a convenience than a necessity. One easily could use a coupler with a microphone, attenuators, one or more amplifiers, and a voltmeter to do the same thing. For both approaches, the devices must be calibrated using a known source such as that provided by a pistonphone.

Clicks or Unidirectional Voltage Pulses

Clicks are probably the single most commonly used stimulus in ABR measurements. They are unidirectional rectangular voltage pulses with (theoretically) instantaneous rise and fall times. The duration of these clicks may vary but is seldom less than 40 μs or greater than 500 μs. Most SLMs cannot follow such rapid voltage changes. Even though the response of an earphone (which transduces electrical energy to acoustical energy) will not be as rapid as the voltage pulse, it will still be fast relative to the response of many SLMs. SLMs exist which are capable of "capturing" such short-duration events (see footnote 1). These meters will have the capability of both responding with a relatively short time constant and maintaining the reading on the meter face until it is reset manually. With a calibrated SLM, therefore, it is possible to make direct measurements of the peak dB SPL for an impulsive sound such as a click or short-duration pure tone.

Many SLMs, however, cannot capture these transient pressure changes. One approach to measuring the SPL in these circumstances is to route the AC (alternating current) output of the SLM to an oscilloscope. Oscilloscopes, which plot voltage as a function of time (i.e., the temporal waveform), are capable of extremely fast response. Thus, these devices can follow the rapid pressure changes caused by click stimuli. In this procedure, the amplitude of the acoustic click is measured with the oscilloscope. Subsequently, a long-duration sine wave is used as the signal and its peak (or peak-to-peak) voltage is adjusted so that its amplitude equals that of the previously measured click. Peak voltage for a click is defined between the baseline and its maximum amplitude, whereas peak-to-peak voltage is defined between the maximum positive and negative peaks of the click, which probably are not equal. In estimates of peak equivalent sound pressure level (peSPL), the amplitudes of the click and the comparative sinusoidal waveforms should be measured using similar approaches.

A SLM is used to measure the sound pressure of the sine wave. The response of the SLM is short relative to the duration of either a long-duration or steady-state sine wave. The frequency of the sine wave should be selected so that it is within the flat or maximum portion of the earphone response (e.g., 2000 Hz for a TDH49 earphone). The amplitude of the click is designated, then, in terms of its peak equivalent SPL when compared to the pure tone. The actual estimate of equivalent SPL will depend upon whether comparisons are made between peak or peak-to-peak voltages. The reason for this is that a sinusoid is symmetrical around zero (i.e., the negative and positive sides of the waveform are identical), whereas clicks are often asymmetrical pressure changes. The extent of the differences between peak and peak-to-peak equivalent estimates will depend upon the degree of asymmetry in the click (Arlinger, 1982; Campbell, Picton, Wolfe, Maru, Baribeau-Braun, & Braun, 1981; Stapells, Picton, & Smith, 1982). Although it is true that, once an operational definition is established, either approach will lead to repeatable estimates of stimulus amplitude, there is no uniformly used definition of peak equivalent.

An alternative approach to the physical measurements outlined above uses a behavioral threshold reference, often referred to as "dB $_n$HL". In this approach, behavioral thresholds for the clicks (or tone bursts) are measured in a group of normal-hearing young adults. The mean behavioral threshold for this group becomes 0 dB $_n$HL for auditory evoked potential measurements. All other intensities are referred to this reference. Thus, 80 dB $_n$HL refers to a stimulus that is 80 dB above the level of the behavioral threshold for a group of normal-hearing listeners for that specific stimulus.

It is essential that these behavioral measurements be made in a sound-treated environment if the ABR data are to be used to estimate hearing sensitivity. In threshold applications, the ambient room noise can be sufficiently intense to elevate thresholds. It is not advisable to measure normal behavioral thresholds in these nonstandard environments in order to set a reference. The thresholds for normal-hearing subjects may be elevated, whereas the thresholds for hearing-impaired persons may not be, depending upon both the level and spectrum of the noise and the magnitude and configuration of the hearing loss. It is for these same reasons that we recommend that ABR threshold assessments be performed only in sound-treated environments. One situation where this is particularly relevant is when ABRs are used to assess hearing sensitivity in patients from an intensive care nursery (ICN). Noise levels in an ICN are quite variable and often will be sufficient to shift thresholds in normal-hearing subjects. In this application, the test should be performed when it is safe to transport the child to a sound-treated environment, which is usually at a time just prior to discharge.

If ABR measurements have to be made in the ICN and a behavioral threshold reference must be used, then it probably is better to obtain both behavioral and electrophysiological measurements in the same sound environment. Infants with mild-to-moderate hearing losses may be missed by this approach, but infants with severe-to-profound losses should be identified. This procedure, of course, will work only if the behavioral and electrophysiological data are collected in the same sound environment and this environment remains constant. Unfortunately, this is seldom the case in an ICN. Using behavioral threshold references established for a sound-treated environment may be tried, but this could lead to an intolerably high false-positive rate if the passing criterion is the same as the one used in a controlled, sound-treated environment.

Interpretation of ABR data based on behavioral threshold references is complicated by other factors. The ABR is thought to derive only from the synchronous onset discharges of a group of neurons. The observation that ABR threshold is independent of stimulus duration supports this hypothesis (Gorga, Beauchaine, Reiland, Worthington, & Javel, 1982; Hecox, Squires, & Galambos, 1976). On the other hand, behavioral thresholds will depend upon stimulus duration (Plomp & Bouman, 1959; Watson & Gengel, 1969; Zwislocki, Hellman, & Verrillo, 1962). The use of a behavioral reference, therefore, may not be appropriate since the reference response is altered by duration, whereas the electrophysiological response is not. In fact, this reference may result in errors in threshold estimates for hearing-impaired listeners (Gorga et al., 1982).

A related problem stems from the decisions which need to be made about the rate of stimulus presentation at which the behavioral thresholds are estimated. It has long been recognized that behavioral threshold will decrease as repetition rate increases, again due to integration of energy (Garner, 1947; Thurlow & Bowman, 1957). Yet ABRs tend to be observed less easily for high stimulation rates, presumably as a result of adaptation. If behavioral threshold references are to be used, it probably is wisest to determine behavioral thresholds with the highest repetition rate that does not affect ABR thresholds. This approach may result in the most sensitive (or lowest) behavioral threshold while avoiding adaptation effects in the ABR. We would note that recent evidence indicates that adaptation may not be evident in ABR threshold measurements for repetition rates as high as 50/s (Thornton & Sprague, 1983).

Finally, such factors as the psychophysical technique and the number of subjects may affect the accuracy of behavioral threshold references. These are some of the reasons why comparison between evoked potential and behavioral measurements may be difficult. Unfortunately, these are precisely the comparisons we hope to make. We are not yet ready to discard behavioral references but the clinician should be aware of the many pitfalls when such comparisons are attempted.

TEMPORAL CHARACTERISTICS

There are a variety of temporal characteristics of concern in ABR measurements. These include the temporal waveform, stimulus rate, duration, rise/fall time, and polarity (or phase). Some of these features can affect the ABR we measure. As a result, we need to describe the temporal parameters of ABR eliciting stimuli.

Temporal Waveforms

The temporal waveform of the acoustic click can be evaluated by taking the AC output of the SLM and routing to an oscilloscope whose trace is triggered by the click. The acoustic properties of the click will be determined by the stimulus-delivery system. The properties of any system can be estimated from its temporal response to a click. This is often referred to as the impulse response. This temporal waveform may be used as the "signature" of the earphone. For a given earphone, the temporal response to a click is measured and recorded at the initial calibration. This waveform is stored for future reference. Any changes in the waveform at subsequent calibration measurements alert the clinician to the possibility that the earphone response has changed. Although a variety of other techniques could be used to alert the clinician to changes in earphone response, this simple approach can be performed as a convenient screening measure for the earphone.

Stimulus Rate

Calibration of stimulus rate is simple and straightforward. Two approaches are suggested here. Using an oscilloscope, one could measure the time interval (Δt) between comparable positions of successive clicks (or tone bursts). This interval may be related to frequency (or rate) by the simple equation

$$\text{Frequency} = 1/\Delta t$$

Rate, therefore, can be estimated using the above rule. As an example, if clicks are presented with an interval between them of 100 ms (i.e., $\Delta t = 100$ ms or 0.1 s), then rate = 10 per second (rate = $1/\Delta t = 1/0.1 = 10$).

Alternatively, devices are available that count events per unit time. One can simply route the signal to these counters and measure the rate directly. Such measurements are more accurate than those derived from the oscilloscope. We point out that the timing circuits accompanying most commercially available systems are quite stable. Still, periodic checks of stimulus rate are simple enough that they should be part of a routine calibration procedure.

Stimulus Duration

The simplest technique for measuring stimulus duration also uses an oscilloscope, since these measurements can be made from the plot of voltage as a function of time. We can use this approach for measurements of both the electrical and acoustical waveforms. Electrical waveforms are measured from the stimulus generation equipment, whereas acoustical waveforms are produced by the earphone and can be measured with a SLM. Simply apply either the AC output of the SLM or the voltage at the back of the earphone to the input of the oscilloscope, adjust the sensitivity and time base so that the entire signal can be viewed, and then measure its duration, using the calibrated time base. The duration of tone bursts can be measured either electrically or acoustically. It is often difficult, however, to define stimulus duration for clicks acoustically since the response of the earphone will cause the click to be less well defined temporally. For this reason, click duration is usually measured from the electrical signal. (Nonetheless, the response of the earphone is critical and will be discussed in a later section.)

There are a variety of operational definitions that are used for stimulus duration. The duration of the plateau section of the waveform can be used for clicks. Of course, if the click changes amplitude instantaneously at onset and offset, this estimate will be the same regardless of the points used along the voltage waveform (i.e., 0 to 0 voltage points should equal 50% up — 50% down points of the maximum amplitude which, in turn, should equal the duration of the plateau or steady-state portion of the click).

Alternate approaches are possible for tone burst stimuli. Most investigators define stimulus duration between half-voltage points on the rise and fall envelopes of the waveform. Other approaches are to define duration between the two zero-amplitude points or to use the length of the steady-state or plateau portion of the waveform. If rise/fall time, rise/fall envelopes, and duration are described explicitly (regardless of the operational definition), one can convert data from one of the above sets of rules to another.

Stimulus Rise/Fall Time

Rise/fall time describes how rapidly a stimulus is turned on and off. This temporal parameter is of interest mainly for tone burst stimuli. There are a variety of common definitions for rise/fall time. In one approach, rise/fall time is defined as the interval between zero amplitude and maximum amplitude (0–100%). In another, rise/fall time is defined as the interval between 10 and 90% maximum amplitude of the voltage waveform. Finally, this interval may be defined in terms of the number of cycles of a sine wave. For example, a rise/fall time of 2 cycles would equal 4 ms at 500 Hz but would equal 0.5 ms at 4000 Hz.

Regardless of how rise/fall time is defined, these intervals can be measured from the voltage waveform. Using an oscilloscope, the waveform should be displayed from onset to offset. It may be necessary to use relatively short stimuli in order to allow a view of the entire stimulus. The oscilloscope trace should be triggered by the stimulus for ease of examination. Also, it may be wise to use an extremely high-frequency signal. Recall that we are trying to estimate the time interval for a stimulus either to rise or fall from maximum amplitude. As a result, we will be measuring the envelope of the stimulus at onset or offset. The envelope can be viewed most easily for higher frequencies where individual cycles are packed more densely.

Once the stimulus waveform envelope is displayed on the oscilloscope, rise/fall times can be measured in much the same way as duration, using the calibrated time base. This procedure should work regardless of how rise/fall time is defined.

STIMULUS POLARITY

The calibration of stimulus polarity (rarefaction or condensation) often presents problems for the practicing clinician. These extremely important calibrations, however, can be performed with relative ease. Three related techniques will be given below, starting with the most difficult approach.

The question we are addressing is what direction the earphone diaphragm moves, given a particular rectangular voltage input. This is not a trivial question because earphones are not wired in any uniform manner. Furthermore, the ABR response can be quite different depending upon stimulus polarity. Thus, this calibration needs to be completed before any ABR measurements are made.

One approach, recommended by Cann and Knott (1979), is to disassemble the earphone so that access to the diaphragm is possible. The earphone itself is firmly mounted and the piston of a micrometer is gently brought into contact with the diaphragm. A known DC voltage (such as that provided by a battery) is attached to the earphone and the direction of diaphragm motion is noted on the micrometer. In this way, the true positive and negative terminals can be known.

An alternate technique is to apply the same voltage to the back of the earphone and examine diaphragm motion through direct observation with a microscope. (These movements can be quite small and are often not detectable by the unaided human eye.) Again, positive and negative terminals can be identified.

A simpler technique which can be performed routinely uses standard calibration equipment. In this case, the DC (direct current) output of a SLM is routed to an oscilloscope. The SLM is fitted with a coupler and a microphone. The earphone then is placed atop the coupler. The oscilloscope should show a flat line at zero voltage. One should gently press against the back of the earphone (thus creating a positive pressure or condensation) and note the direction of the DC shift on the oscilloscope. This direction of voltage change would correspond to the condensation phase of the click, since it results from an increased pressure in the acoustic coupler. Next, connect the AC output of the SLM to the oscilloscope and present clicks to the earphone. Note the direction of the initial change in voltage on the face of the oscilloscope. If the shift is in the same direction as in the previous measurement, these are condensation clicks. If the shift is in the opposite direction of the "reference shift," the clicks are rarefaction pulses. Although it is true that the earphones are not wired in standard ways and that phase (polarity) shifts are possible through almost any measuring device, this method will define the acoustic waveform polarity produced by the particular earphone under test.

In contrast to clicks, sinusoids and tone bursts are symmetrical around zero voltage, having both positive and negative components. As a result, we are usually concerned with stimulus polarity at a fixed point in time (i.e., stimulus onset). In clinical evaluations using tone burst stimuli, it is often necessary to invert starting phase (or polarity) of the tone. This need arises due to problems with either stimulus artifact or cochlear microphonic potential. The stimulus artifact results from the electromagnetic force that is driving the diaphragm of the earphone and is directly proportional to the stimulus. The cochlear microphonic (CM) is an AC receptor potential (generated by the hair cells) which mimics the stimulus waveform. Both of these "potentials" may be recorded for the entire duration of the stimulus and could obscure the neural responses that are measured during ABR evaluations. By inverting stimulus polarity on alternate presentations, however, both stimulus artifact and CM can be canceled in the averaged

response while the neural potential remains. The calibration procedure is similar to the one used for clicks. Again, after calibrating the measurement system, view the temporal waveform on an oscilloscope. The direction of the initial voltage change (i.e., positive or negative) will be used to measure stimulus onset phase. Finally, for tone bursts with alternating phase, it should be possible to view the sine wave flip-flopping on the face of the oscilloscope.

AMPLITUDE SPECTRUM

In these calibrations, we are concerned with the amplitude as a function of frequency. From an audiological standpoint, we are continually concerned with measures that provide information relative to some response (e.g., threshold) as a function of frequency. The pure tone audiogram is one such measure. In this chapter, we do not discuss the problems or issues related to frequency-specific ABR measurements. We have discussed these issues previously (Gorga & Worthington, 1983) and these issues are also presented in chapter 9 of this volume. Rather, we concern ourselves only with measurements of the power or amplitude spectrum for the stimuli commonly used in ABR evaluations, and not with the interactions between stimuli and cochlear responses. Measurements of amplitude spectrum, although relatively simple, do require somewhat more elaborate equipment, including devices such as wave analyzers, spectrum analyzers, and plotters. In general, the filter sections of SLMs (having resolution bandwidths that usually are not less than one-third octave in width) are insufficient for these measurements. Unfortunately, the more sophisticated equipment is not available in all clinics. Of course, the importance of spectral information remains, regardless of available instrumentation.

Clicks

For all stimuli, there is a relation between the temporal waveforms and the amplitude spectrum. This relation will become somewhat more apparent as we discuss tone burst stimuli. One simple relation is that zeros (no energy) will occur in the amplitude spectrum at frequencies equivalent to integral multiples of ± 1 divided by duration. For example, an electrical click of 100 μs duration will have zeros at 10,000 Hz, 20,000 Hz, and so on (1/100 μs or 1/0.0001 = 10,000). A somewhat different spectrum may be measured for stimuli after they are transduced by an earphone. The earphone response will alter the temporal waveform (and therefore the amplitude spectrum) of the signal.

Figure 4-1 depicts the temporal waveform and amplitude spectrum of a 100-μs click, measured from the electrical signal applied to the back of an earphone. Note that the electrical click is a rectangular voltage pulse that is sharply defined in time (top panel). Its amplitude spectrum (bottom panel) indicates that this is a broad-band signal with zeros occurring at 10,000-Hz intervals.

Figure 4-2 depicts the same signal after transduction by a Beyer DT 48 dynamic earphone. These measurements were made with a sound level meter and a 1-inch microphone (Bruel & Kjaer, 4144). The acoustical waveform (top panel) is not as well defined as the electrical signal that is driving the earphone. This difference reflects the fact that the diaphragm of an earphone has inertia and cannot respond instantaneously. The amplitude spectrum (bottom panel) reflects this shaping as well. Note that the energy rolls off above 2500 Hz, although the zero at 10,000 Hz remains evident. While the 1-inch measuring microphone has its own frequency response which rolls off above 10,000 Hz, its response is constant for frequencies below 10,000 Hz. Thus, the differences for frequencies below 10,000 Hz between the bottom panels of Figures 4-1 and 4-2 reflect how the click has been altered by the earphone.

FIGURE 4-1.
Temporal waveform and amplitude spectrum of a 100-μs click measured electrically.

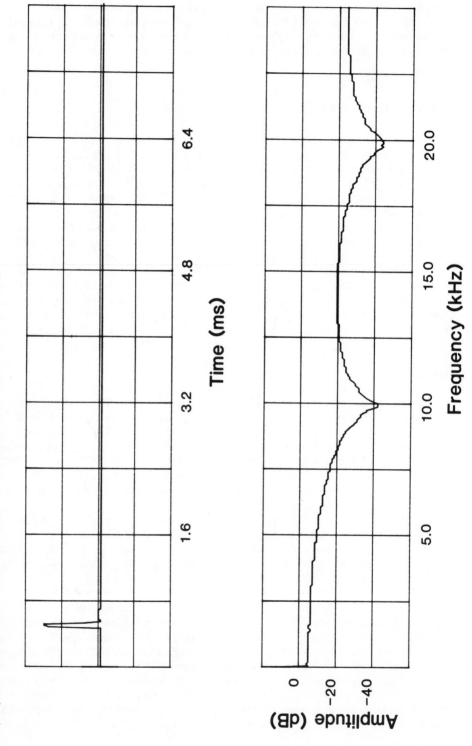

FIGURE 4–2.
Temporal waveform and amplitude spectrum of a 100-μs click measured acoustically (Beyer DT 48 earphone).

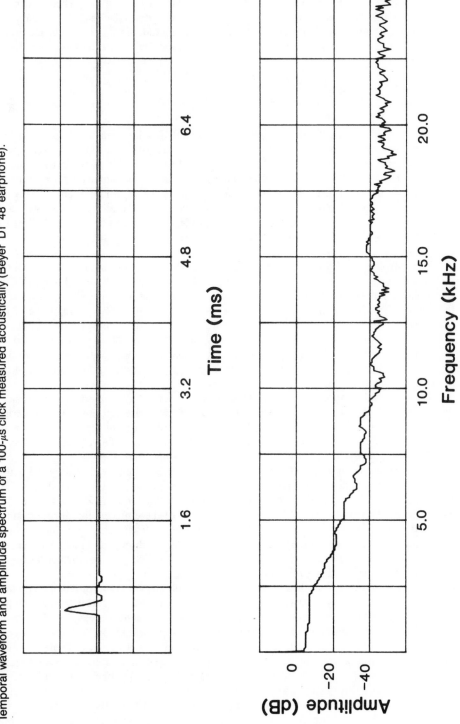

These measurements are made by routing the signal (either electrical or acoustical) to some device capable of measuring amplitude at individual components (or frequencies) within a complex stimulus. Wave analyzers or spectrum analyzers are useful devices for these analyses. If measurements are made for the electrical signal, the amplitude spectrum must be multiplied by the frequency response of the earphone in order to accurately estimate the stimulus delivered to the ear.

Tone Bursts

As stated previously, the short-duration, unidirectional voltage pulse (click) results in a basically broad-band stimulus. When tone burst stimuli are used, the general objective is to excite a narrow region along the cochlear partition. To achieve this goal, narrow-band or frequency-specific stimuli are used. Unfortunately, the stimulus requirements for eliciting an ABR often result in significant energy splatter to frequencies distant from the nominal or center frequency of the tone burst. Furthermore, the underlying response of the cochlea will itself limit the extent to which responses from specific cochlear regions can be measured (Gorga & Worthington, 1983). Prior to considering these physiological factors, however, stimulus considerations must be addressed.

Typically, the amplitude spectrum calculated over the entire duration of a tone burst has a main lobe of energy surrounded by side lobes at lower energy levels. The duration of the signal can affect the spacing between these side lobes. The gating function, which refers to the envelope by which a stimulus is turned on and off, affect the relative amplitude of the side lobes. Several examples of 2000-Hz tone, which is gated by different functions, are shown in Figure 4-3. Figures 4-3a and b plot amplitude spectra for 2 and 10-ms duration envelopes, respectively. Each sinusoid was gated with a cosine-squared envelope with rise and fall of 2 ms. Note that the spacing of the side lobes decreases with increased duration while the energy in the main lobe is increased.

The shape and duration of the rise and fall gating function are also important in determining the spectrum. Figures 4-3a to 3c show spectra of signals with rise/fall times of 2 and 5 ms, respectively. The longer the rise/fall time, the greater the amplitude difference between the main lobe and side lobes. Thus, a stimulus with 5-ms rise/fall times has relatively less energy away from the center frequency than a stimulus of 2-ms rise/fall time.

Finally, the relations between center and side lobe energy can be altered by the gating function used to turn signals on and off. For example, linear envelopes (or rise/fall times) will have greater side lobe amplitude than cosine^2 envelopes for equivalent rise/fall time. A comparison of Figures 4-3a and 3d illustrates the effects of these two gating functions on the amplitude spectra. Rise/fall times equal 2 ms for each panel. The cosine^2 function results in a more sharply defined amplitude spectra. For a more complete discussion of tone burst energy spectra, the reader is referred to Wightman (1971). Harris (1978) provides further details on the effects of different gating functions.

Having loosely described the kinds of effects rise/fall time and duration can have on tone burst spectra, let us briefly describe how these spectra can be measured. As with any stimulus, these measurements can be made from either the electrical or acoustical signal. If we know both the electrical spectra and the frequency response of our transducer (earphone), we can predict what we are delivering to the ear. It is a relatively simple exercise to measure the acoustical spectra directly, a measurement which will include the frequency response of the earphone. To accomplish this, take the AC output of the SLM and route it to either a wave analyzer or spectrum analyzer. Wave analyzers operate as a voltmeter with a very narrow input filter , so that energy within a limited frequency range (e.g., 6 Hz) is measured. By sweeping across the frequency range of interest (e.g., 20–20,000 Hz), one can estimate stimulus amplitude as a function

FIGURE 4–3.
Electrical spectra of a 2000-Hz tone burst; (a) the amplitude spectrum for a 2-ms cosine^2 gating function and 2-ms duration; (b) the amplitude spectrum of a 2-ms cosine^2 gating function with 10-ms duration; (c) same as Figure 4-3a, only with a 5-ms cosine^2 gating function; (d) same as Figure 4–3a, only with a 2-ms linear gating function.

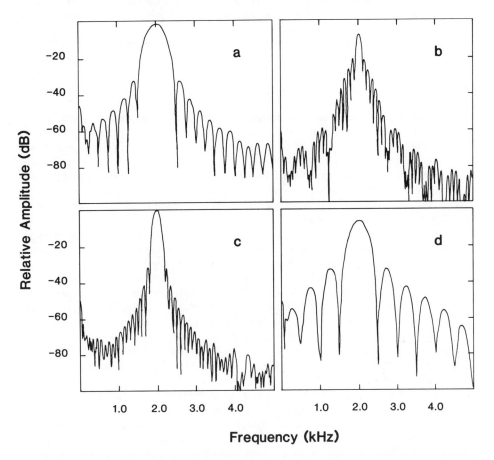

Frequency (kHz)

of frequency. The stimulus should be repeated at a relatively high rate while the wave analyzer sweeps across frequency slowly in order to obtain the most accurate estimate of the amplitude spectrum. Some spectrum analyzers are capable of capturing a short-duration stimulus on which they perform a Fourier analysis. Fourier analysis takes any simple or complex waveform and breaks it down into its individual sinusoidal parts. Any waveform can be described by this analysis because it provides a description of the relations between frequency, amplitude, and phase for all components within the stimulus. As output, these analyzers can provide plots of amplitude as a function of frequency (amplitude spectrum) and phase as a function of frequency (phase spectrum).

As a final note on frequency-specific stimuli, a variety of other approaches have been used. One approach has been to pass (broad-band) clicks through bandpass filters to create stimuli that are more sharply defined in the frequency domain. Of course, both the temporal waveform and the amplitude spectrum will be changed. These stimuli sometimes are referred to as filtered clicks or tone pips, although there is no universally accepted definition. Others will define tone pips as stimuli having rise and fall times equivalent to one cycle of the sine wave (without any plateau). The motivation for defining stimulus temporal parameters (rise/fall times and/or durations) in such a way is related to the fact that frequency is organized geometrically along the cochlear partition. Stimuli of different frequencies whose temporal characteristics are fixed in terms of the number of cycles of a sine wave will have uniform energy splatter in logarithmic frequency, thus presumably exciting equivalent areas along the cochlea. In contrast, stimuli with temporal characteristics fixed in time (regardless of frequency) will be characterized by uniform energy splatter on linear-frequency coordinates. As a consequence, high-frequency stimuli will excite more narrow regions than stimuli with lower center frequencies.

Noise

We often present noise during ABR evaluations. This noise may be presented contralaterally to eliminate the response of the non-test ear or ipsilaterally in order to restrict the portions of the cochlear partition responding to a given stimulus. Broad-band noise is commonly used as the contralateral masker for click-evoked ABRs. Its spectrum is determined principally by the frequency response of the earphone. This will make its spectrum similar to that of clicks with durations of 200 μs or less. (The one exception to this rule occurs for transducers with extended high-frequency responses, where the zeros in the click spectrum may occur at frequencies within the passband of the earphone.)

High-pass or notched noises are usually presented to the ipsilateral or stimulated ear in order to mask the responses from specific regions along the basilar membrane. For example, high-pass noise may be presented to eliminate or mask basal, high-frequency regions of the cochlea, ensuring that the measured response is generated by lower-frequency regions.

To describe these masking stimuli, we need to know cutoff frequency (or frequencies for notched noise), rejection rate, and noise floor. Cutoff frequencies are defined as those frequencies for which the power is one-half of the power in the passband. Thus, it is sometimes referred to as the half-power point or 3-dB down point. Rejection rate describes the slope of the function relating amplitude to frequency beyond the cutoff frequency. It is usually specified in decibels/octave. For example, if a high-pass noise has 2000 Hz as its 3-dB down point and the energy is 48 dB less at 1000 Hz, the rejection rate would be 48 dB/octave. Finally, noise floor measurements are concerned with how far the rejection of energy continues. In the above example, it is unlikely that, at 250 Hz, the energy would be 144 dB down from the passband. In fact, the energy probably would not be reduced nearly that much. This phenomenon is due to limitations imposed by the system noise floor. The noise floor (or, more accurately, the signal-to-noise ratio) is important to evaluate since it places a limit on how intense we can make the masking stimulus without causing direct masking in frequency regions of interest (i.e., regions distant from the main energy in the noise).

The noise floor may be determined by such devices as filters and amplifiers but could possibly be affected by distortion within the earphone. If the noise floor limits are imposed by the filter and/or amplifier, and if these devices precede the attenuator, then the signal-to-noise ratio should remain constant. On the other hand, the noise floor may be level dependent if the earphone is generating distortion products.

All of these measurements could be made with either a wave analyzer or spectrum analyzer. Again, it is a simple procedure to make these measurements of the acoustic spectrum since such measurements will include the frequency response of the earphone. This is particularly important for high-pass noise since most clinical earphones have reduced output for frequencies at or above 6000 Hz.

SUMMARY

We have tried to provide the reader with a list of stimulus characteristics that should be considered in ABR measurements. In addition, we have offered various approaches to the description of these characteristics. We reiterate that in order to understand any response, we must understand the stimulus that we are using to elicit that response.

REFERENCES

Arlinger, S. (1982). Comments on calibration of clicks for use in ABR. *ERA Newsletter, 80,* April.

Backus, J. (1969). *The acoustical properties of music.* New York: Norton.

Campbell, K. B., Picton, T. W., Wolfe, R. G., Maru, J., Baribeau-Braun, J., & Braun, C. (1981). Auditory potentials. *SENSUS, 1,* 21–31.

Cann, J., & Knott, J. (1979). Polarity of acoustic click stimuli for eliciting brainstem auditory evoked responses: A proposed standard. *American Journal of EEG Technology, 19,* 125–132.

Davis, H. (1976). Principles of electric response audiometry. *Annals of Otology, Rhinology, and Laryngology, 85,* Supplement 28.

Durrant, J. D. (1983). Fundamentals of sound generation. In E. J. Moore (Ed.), *Bases of auditory brain-stem evoked responses.* New York: Grune & Stratton.

Garner, W. R. (1947). The effect of frequency spectrum on temporal integration of energy in the ear. *Journal of the Acoustical Society of America, 19,* 808–815.

Gorga, M. P., Beauchaine, K. A., Reiland, J. K., Worthington, D. W., & Javel, E. (1982). The effects of stimulus duration on ABR and behavioral thresholds. Presented at the American Speech and Hearing Association Convention, Toronto.

Gorga, M. P., & Worthington, D. W. (1983). Some issues relevant to the measurement of frequency-specific auditory-brainstem responses. *Seminars in Hearing, 4,* 353–362.

Green, D. M. (1976). *An introduction to hearing.* Hillsdale, NJ: Lawrence Erlbaum Associates.

Harris, F. J. (1978). One the use of windows for harmonic analysis with the discrete Fourier transform. *Proceedings of the IEEE, 66,* 51–83.

Hecox, K., Squires, N., & Galambos, R. (1976). Brainstem auditory evoked responses in man. I. Effect of stimulus rise-fall time and duration. *Journal of the Acoustical Society of America, 60,* 1187–1192.

Pickles, J. O. (1982). *An introduction to the physiology of hearing.* London: Academic Press.

Plomp, R., & Bouman, M. A. (1959). Relation between hearing threshold and duration for tone pulses. *Journal of the Acoustical Society of America, 31,* 749–758.

Small, A. M. (1973). In F. D. Minifie, T. J. Hixon, & F. Williams (Eds.), *Normal aspects of speech, hearing and language.* Englewood Cliffs, NJ: Prentice-Hall.

Stapells, D. R., Picton, T. W., & Smith, A. D. (1982). Normal hearing thresholds for clicks. *Journal of the Acoustical Society of America, 72,* 74–79.

Thornton, A. R., & Sprague, B. H. (1983). Hearing threshold sensitivity estimation by evoked response audiometry. Presented at the American Speech and Hearing Association Convention, Cincinnati.

Thurlow, W. R., & Bowman, R. (1957). Threshold for thermal noise as a function of duration and interruption rate. *Journal of the Acoustical Society of America, 29,* 281–283.

Watson, C. S., & Gengel, R. W. (1969). Signal duration and signal frequency in relation to auditory sensitivity. *Journal of the Acoustical Society of America, 46,* 989–997.

Wightman, F. L. (1971). Detection of binaural tones as a function of masker bandwidth. *Journal of the Acoustical Society of America, 50,* 623–636.

Yost, W. A., & Nielsen, D. W. (1977). *Fundamentals of hearing: An introduction.* New York: Holt, Rinehart, and Winston.

Zwislocki, J., Hellman, R. P., & Verrillo, R. T. (1962). Threshold of audibility for short pulses. *Journal of the Acoustical Society of America, 34,* 1648–1652.

SECTION II
AUDITORY ASPECTS

Chapter 5

Normative Aspects of the ABR

Daniel M. Schwartz
Grant A. Berry

INTRODUCTION

Since the initial description of a procedure to record auditory evoked far-field electrical potentials from the human scalp (Jewett, Romano, & Williston, 1970; Jewett & Williston, 1971) the measurement of auditory brainstem responses (ABR) has had a major impact on the disciplines of audiology, otology, and neurology. Application of the ABR has been directed toward the identification and estimation of degree of hearing loss in patients with whom routine behavioral audiologic procedures are inappropriate (e.g., infants and difficult-to-test patients) and as the primary test of choice in neuroaudiologic diagnosis.

While the stability and robustness of the ABR are remarkably reliable and the normal variance of the peak latencies is acceptably small, it is critical to the measurement that normative data be collected within the individual laboratory or clinic. Several investigators have reported on the myriad of variables that can potentially alter one or more of the important parameters of the ABR and hence, lead to misinterpretation. Despite this knowledge, many clinicians in each of the aforementioned disciplines are recording and interpreting the ABR with little or no regard to normative data for their particular test system and measurement protocol. In fact, some distributors of auditory evoked potential instrumentation have gone so far as to suggest that one could utilize published normative data, thus permitting immediate initiation of the test procedure into clinical practice. Clearly, the lack of uniformity in ABR measurement variables among investigators precludes such a practice.

This chapter reviews the effects of the many recording variables that can influence the underlying response. It is hoped that review of this chapter will enlighten the clinician regarding the large variations in response latency, amplitude, and morphology that are produced by relatively minor manipulations in the controlling variables, and will underscore the need for the collection of normative data prior to using this powerful audiologic technique for assessing the neurologic integrity of the central auditory nervous system.

PHYSICAL CHARACTERISTICS OF THE ABR

The criteria for ABR interpretation are based, in general, on the (1) latency (in milliseconds) of individual waveforms, (2) latency differences between primary peak components (interpeak latency), (3) peak amplitude (in microvolts), (4) I–V amplitude ratio, and (5) waveform morphology. Since some of these parameters (e.g., latency and amplitude) lend themselves more to quantitative interpretation, diagnostic decisions are often based on alterations in one or more of these response parameters. Consequently, individual patient responses must be compared

---

© College-Hill Press, Inc. All rights, including that of translation, reserved. No part of this publication may be reproduced without the written permission of the publisher.

FIGURE 5–1.
Example of a normal ABR for an adult male. Shown is the Jewett scheme for peak labeling (vertex-positive up) and the measurement of absolute and interpeak latency and peak-to-trough amplitude.

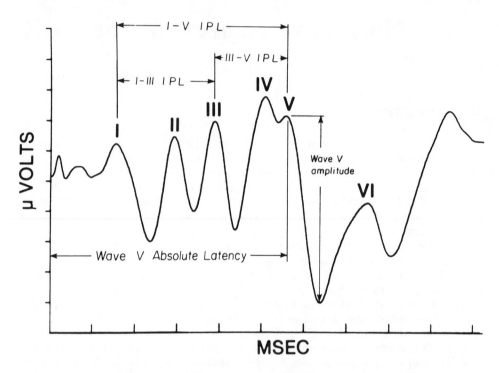

to a normative referent to determine if any of the response parameters falls outside of a prespecified range of normalcy.

Absolute Latency

The absolute latency of a given waveform can be defined as the time period (in milliseconds) between the onset of the acoustic stimulus (e.g., rectangular wave click) and the peak of the averaged response. Figure 5-1 illustrates the concept of measuring the absolute and interpeak latencies of the ABR. While no standard exists as to the exact point on the waveform for calculating absolute latency, prevailing opinion suggests that latency is measured at a point representing the beginning of the down-slope of a given peak component, as shown in Figure 5-1. This measurement convention is of particular value when a waveform does not present with a clearly defined peak, but rather shows a merging of two separate waveforms, as is often encountered in the IV/V complex, or has minor glitches at the peak of the response.

Clearly, the absolute latency of waveform V, the rostral component of the ABR, has received the most widespread clinical attention in differential diagnosis of otoneurologic disorders, as well as for deriving estimates of hearing sensitivity. The importance of wave V relates to its robust character and reliability under varying measurement conditions; as stimulus intensity decreases, wave V latency increases proportionally and by a predictable amount. This effect of increased latency with decreased stimulus intensity is common to all neural systems; that is, neural firing becomes less rapid as stimulus intensity decreases in magnitude. The effect is a more slowly rising postsynaptic potential with a resultant prolonged latency of synaptic transmission (Picton, Woods, Baribeau-Braun, & Healey, 1977). Alternatively, the earlier primary wave components I and III become unstable as intensity is reduced much below 50 dB normal hearing level (nHL).

Critical to the differential diagnosis of space-occupying lesions, either intrinsic or extrinsic to the brainstem, and the disruption of neuroelectric activity secondary to demyelinating disease, is the time difference between two primary peaks (I, III, and V) often described as the interpeak latency (IPL) or interwave interval (IWI). This time interval reflects, in part, neural conduction time and has been called a "central transmission" or "brainstem transmission" time measure (Fabiani, Sohmer, Tait, Garni, & Kinarti, 1979).

Table 5-1 summarizes the absolute and IPLs of responses recorded from normal hearers as reported by 10 different investigators. In general, stimulus intensity ranged between 60 and 70 dB SL, whereas stimulus repetition rate was usually 10/s. Although filter settings among studies typically spanned the frequency range 100–3000 Hz, filter slope was not uniform. Remarkably (perhaps fortuitously), despite differences in recording technique, the data presented in Table 5-1 show quite favorable interlaboratory agreement for individual waveform and IPL measures. On the average, the latency for wave I was 1.7 ms, with each subsequent wave thereafter occurring approximately 1.0 ms later in time. Moreover, between-laboratory standard deviations of all measures provide excellent support for the stability and reliability of the ABR at moderately high intensity levels. A review of the IPLs among published reports suggests an approximately 2.0-ms difference between peaks I–III and III–V and about a 4.0-ms I–V IPL in normal hearers.

Waveform Amplitude

In dissonance to the general agreement among researchers and clinicians regarding response latencies, measures of response amplitude (in microvolts) have not met with a great deal of clinical success, owing partly to the variability of the measure. Amplitude values do not appear to be normally distributed (Rowe, 1981), are highly susceptible to myogenic activity and noise level, are difficult to replicate, and are easily influenced by minor alterations in recording technique. Consequently, the measurement of absolute waveform amplitude does not enjoy the stability and reliability of its latency counterpart. This is true whether amplitude is measured from the peak of the wave component to its following trough or between peaks of contiguous components.

One technique for controlling the variability of the amplitude measure was proffered by Thornton (1975-1976). His approach was to plot normative data on coordinates that represented response amplitude on the ordinate and latency on the abscissa. Individual data points for each wave component are subsequently grouped within ellipses corresponding to a prespecified range of normal values (e.g., confidence intervals), thereby reflecting the variability of the measure.

An alternative to the absolute amplitude measure that has achieved increased clinical acceptance in recent years is the calculation of the relative I–V ratio. In normal patients, wave V is usually greater in amplitude than wave I, resulting in an amplitude ratio > 1.00 (Chiappa, Gladstone, & Young, 1979; Rowe, 1978; Starr & Achor, 1975). Hence, a I-V amplitude ratio of < 1.00 is considered abnormal and indicative of retrocochlear pathology (Musiek, Kibbe, Rackliffe, & Weider, 1984). To date, however, there remains a dearth of well-documented literature concerning the I-V amplitude ratio in a large pathologic population. Considerably more research is needed relative to the confounding effects of such variables as stimulus polarity, repetition rate, filter characteristics, and electrode sites prior to the general use of this relative amplitude

TABLE 5–1.
Normative ABR latency data across 10 laboratories

Laboratory	Stimulus intensity (dB SL)	Stimulus polarity	Repetition rate (cps)	Filter settings (Hz)	Wave latency (ms)									
					I	II	III	IV	V	I-III	III-V	I-V
Jewett and Williston (1971)	60–75	?	?	10–10,000	1.5	2.6	3.5	4.3	5.1	—	—	—
Lev and Sohmer (1972)	65	?	?	250–5000	1.5	2.5	3.5		5.0	—	—	—
Picton et al. (1974)	60	?	10	10–3000	1.5	2.6	3.8	5.0	5.8			
Starr and Achor (1975)	65	alt.	10	100–3000	1.6	2.8	3.8	4.8	5.5	—	—	—
Stockard and Rossiter (1977)	60	rar.	10	100–3000	1.9	3.0	4.1	5.2	5.9	2.1	1.9	4.0
Rosenhamer et al. (1978)	60	?	16.6	180–4500	1.7	2.9	3.9	5.2	5.9	2.26	2.0	4.27
Row (1978)	60	?	10	100–3000	1.9	2.9	3.8	5.1	5.8	1.97	1.97	3.94
Gilroy and Lynn (1978)	75	?	11	150–3000	1.55	2.67	3.60	4.69	5.40	2.05	1.9	3.83
Beagley and Sheldrake (1978)	70	?	10	250–3200	2.1	3.3	4.3	5.3	6.1	2.2	1.8	4.0
Chiappa et al. (1979)	60	alt.	10	100–3000	1.7	2.8	3.9	5.1	5.7	2.1	1.9	4.0
Own Data	75 dB (nHL)	rar.	11.1	75–1500	1.65	2.85	3.8	4.99	5.66	2.05	1.85	4.00

measure in clinical practice. If clinicians elect to employ the I–V amplitude ratio in the clinical decision-making process, it behooves them to establish their own normative data for this measure.

Waveform Morphology

The final response parameter used for interpreting the ABR is that of wave morphology. Morphology refers to the visual appearance or actual shape of the averaged response. Unlike latency and amplitude measures, however, interpretation of the ABR based on the clarity of the response is entirely subjective and is, at best, a qualitative descriptor.

Over the years a variety of nomenclature has been used to describe and label the various waveforms of the ABR. Jewett and Williston (1971) advocated the use of Roman numerals to label the seven distinct and sequential series of waves that occurred within the first 9 ms following the introduction of an acoustic transient. This nomenclature has, in general, become the convention. In contrast, other investigators have elected to describe individual peak components on the basis of wave latency, resulting in such designations as p6 (Davis, 1976); FFP7 (Terkildsen, Osterhammel, & Huis in't Veld, 1977). Still others label peaks chronologically (Thornton, 1975). Undoubtedly, our inability to adopt a standard nomenclature for peak identification has led to considerable confusion among those involved in ABR recording. Add to this the observation that many European investigators display their waveforms with a vertex-positive downward reference, in contrast to the North American convention of vertex-positive upward deflection, and the result becomes a quagmire of nomenclature similar to that experienced in the early days of acoustic immittance testing.

As noted previously, the clinical interpretation of ABR on the basis of wave morphology rests on the intuition of the individual examiner. While much of the early descriptions of the ABR led us to believe that these auditory far-field potentials were displayed as a distinct series of five to seven individual waveforms connected in time, clinical experience over the past decade has shown sufficient variability in response morphology among normal subjects to warrant the recommendation of studying a large series of normal records prior to using this technique in clinical evaluation. Figure 5-2, for example, exemplifies the morphologic variations that one can obtain on normal subjects. Observe that the well-known IV/V complex is not always apparent. At times, wave V seems to ride just below the crest of peaks IV (5-2A) or there may be a total fusion of waves IV and V into one broad peak (5-2H). Similarly, it is not uncommon to show bifurcation of waves I and/or III (2G, 2H) thus making it difficult to measure latency if one uses a peak reference point. Of particular importance is that response morphology can be affected by age, pathology, and measurement-related variables. In essence, therefore, alterations in wave morphology represent "soft" clinical signs of neuroauditory pathology.

To summarize, accurate and reliable interpretation of the ABR is based on the quantitative and qualitative assessment of waveform latency, amplitude, and morphology. Of these, the measurement of absolute and IPLs has met with the greatest clinical success for assessing the integrity of the auditory nervous system. Unquestionably, it is comforting to know that the latency of the individual components that make up the ABR remains relatively stable and within acceptable limits of statistical variation across what has now become hundreds of laboratories and clinics throughout the world. While some investigators continue to measure response amplitude both in its absolute and relative forms, considerably more research to identify all of the sources of normal variability is needed prior to formal adoption of this measure in differential diagnosis. Finally, alterations in waveform morphology can provide insight into rather insidious lesions in the retrocochlear and central auditory systems; however, interpretation of pathologic recordings based on waveform morphology is entirely subjective and should not be performed by the inexperienced or naive clinician.

FIGURE 5-2.
Normal variations in the ABR. (A) wave V is riding on the down-shoulder of wave IV; (B) wave IV is riding on the up-shoulder of wave V; (C) waves IV and V appear as a broad undulation (M configuration) with wave V amplitude less than IV; (D) wave V amplitude is greatly reduced from peak IV; (E) the classic IV/V complex; (F) waves I and II amplitude greater than IV/V; (G) bifid wave III; (H) bifid wave I and fused IV/V.

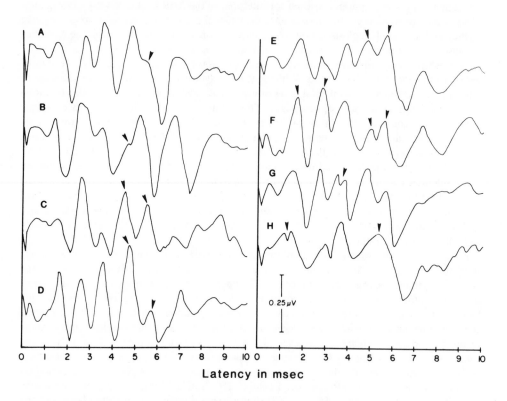

Latency in msec

FACTORS INFLUENCING THE NORMAL ABR

Due to the absence of standards to specify recording parameters and methods used to measure the ABR, it is imperative that each individual clinical facility establish its own normative data. Differences in electrical and electromagnetic field variation between clinical sites, as well as heterogeneity in stimulus recording and analysis parameters, electrode placement, and transducer type, all lead to small but significant differences in wave latency, amplitude, and morphology which together can cloud ABR interpretation.

Filter Characteristics

As with most bioelectric potentials, the ABR is embedded in a background of competing electrical activity (EMG). In fact, amplitudes of the electromyographic events often achieve voltage levels 100 times greater than those of the ABR. Obviously, then, the morphology of the averaged evoked potential will lose considerable resolution unless the frequency response of the recording system is set to reject the maximal amount of electrical interference.

One method of optimizing response clarity by reducing the signal-to-noise ratio is that of bandpass filtering. Investigators have applied various bandpass filter settings to record the ABR, as exemplified in Table 5-2. Undoubtedly, the heterogeneity of filter settings across laboratories and clinics may explain, in part, variations in normative values for the component waveforms of the ABR.

The choice of filter settings should be predicated on the frequency composition of the desired bioelectric potential, as well as on the interfering myogenic noise. In recent years, several investigators have indicated that the constituent frequencies that compose the ABR range from 50 to 1000 Hz (Elberling, 1976, 1979; Kevanishvili & Aphonchenko, 1979; Laukli & Mair, 1981; Suzuki & Horiuchi, 1977; Thornton, 1978). Kevanishvili and Aphonchenko (1979) have suggested that the main spectral components of waves I and II are distributed between 400 and 1000 Hz; wave III between 100 and 900 Hz, and waves IV–VI from 100 to 500 Hz. Hence, it is apparent that the frequency content of the ABR is critical to the selection of appropriate bandpass filtering since the characteristics of the response can be affected by filter bandwidths and roll-off rates.

An additional factor that can confound ABR response identification is that most commercially available evoked potential instruments employ analog filters that are known to cause latency shifts due to phase distortion (Boston & Ainslie, 1980; Lane, Mendel, & Kupperman, 1974). This phase distortion is related both to filter cutoff frequency and slope.

The consequential effects of variations in low-pass (LP) and high-pass (HP) filtering on the ABR have received limited research attention. Jewett and Williston (1971) found no significant differences between responses recorded on-line with filter bandwidths of 0.01–10,000 Hz versus those replayed off-line from an FM tape recorder with LP filter reduction to 2500 Hz; however, they went on to report latency changes following reductions of the bandwidth of from 1.6 to 100 Hz and concluded that the HP setting should be a nominal 1000 Hz. Stockard, Stockard, and Sharbrough (1978) stated that increasing the low-frequency filter settings (3 dB down-point) from 100 to 300 Hz resulted in a progressive decrease in wave latency. Moreover, they noted that the amplitude of the IV/V complex decreased rapidly between low-frequency filter settings of 100 and 300 Hz. Similarly, absolute wave latency was shown to decrease as a result of increasing the high-frequency cutoff from 300 to 10,000 Hz with the most optimal waveform resolution occurring at a high-frequency filter setting of 3000 Hz. Cacace, Shy, and Satya-Murti (1980) have also reported longer latencies with a high-frequency cutoff of 1500 Hz versus 3000 Hz when low-frequency cutoff was held constant at 150 Hz, although wave morphology showed better clarity for the narrower bandpass filter settings.

Figures 5-3 and 5-4 illustrate the effects of changing the filter bandpass on the three ABR response parameters—that is, latency, amplitude, and morphology. These recordings were obtained from normal hearing adults to a 75-dB nHL rarefaction stimulus presented at a rate of 11.1/s. Figure 5-3 shows the effects of changing the low-frequency cutoff when the high-frequency filter setting was maintained at 3000 Hz. Consistent with the findings of Stockard, Stockard, and Sharbrough (1978), increasing the low-frequency setting resulted in a progressive decrease in wave latency, particularly for the more rostral components of the ABR. In addition, waveform amplitude increases in concert with low-frequency cutoff. Finally, the best waveform resolution is shown for the two narrower passbands. Likewise, the responses obtained as a function of manipulating the high-frequency filter (Figure 5-4) again support the findings of Stockard, Stockard, and Sharbrough (1978) and Cacace et al. (1980). Observe that when the high-frequency setting is less than 1500 Hz, wave morphology is totally disrupted with peak V being present only as a remnant. In this example waveform resolution is optimal at a bandwidth of 150–1500 Hz, although the 150 to 3000-Hz setting could be considered clinically acceptable under less ideal electrical environments.

Perhaps the most systematic investigation related to the effects of analog filtering on the ABR in both humans and laboratory cats was reported by Laukli and Mair (1981). They observed

TABLE 5-2.
Differences in filter bandpass used in recording the ABR across 15 published reports

Investigator	Filter Bandpass (Hz)
Jewett and Williston, 1971	10–2500
Lev and Sohmer, 1972	250–5000
Amadeo and Shagass, 1973	10–8000
Martin and Coats, 1973	80–1000
Terkildsen et al., 1973	500–4500
Hecox and Galambos, 1974	80–3000
Picton et al., 1974	10–3000
Starr and Achor, 1975	100–3000[a]
Elberling, 1976	5–5000
Møller and Blegvad, 1976	150–4500
Zollner et al., 1976	350–4000
Rosenhamer et al., 1978	180–4500
Jerger and Mauldin, 1978	300–3000[a]
Gilroy and Lynn, 1978	150–3000[a]
Borg and Lofqvist, 1982	32–3200

[a]Most commonly used filter passbands.

that raising the low-frequency cutoff from 2 to 100 Hz resulted in a loss of the slow component of the response and a decrease in peak latencies. Lowering the high-frequency cutoff from 5000 to 1000 Hz produced uniform latency increases across wave components.

On the basis of these findings, Laukli and Mair (1981) concluded that analog filtering produced significant and complex changes in latency, amplitude, and morphology which could result in diagnostic misinterpretation unless normative data are gathered against which individual clinical patient responses will be compared under the same filter conditions. While they did not specify what those filter characteristics should be, but rather, indicated that a wide filter bandwidth was recommended, it appears that the clearest responses are obtained at filter settings between 150 and 1500 Hz (Figure 5-4), a finding which is in keeping with the findings of Cacace et al. (1980) and Ruth, Hildenbrand, and Cantrell (1982).[1] We hope that future generations of commercially available ABR instrumentation will employ digital filtering to eliminate or minimize phase shifting (Boston & Ainslie, 1980; Dawson & Doddington, 1973; van der Tweel, Estevez, & Strackee, 1980).

[Caveat: Many commercially available ABR systems come equipped with notch filters that are used to reduce the potential electrical interference of 60 Hz line hum. One should be aware that, despite their narrow rejection band, such notch filters may also create phase distortion resulting in latency prolongations even greater than those caused by analog filtering in the amplifiers. Consequently, it is recommended that the practicing clinician avoid using such notch filters if at all possible. Of particular importance here is that if a notch filter is to be used in recording individual patient data, then the same recording conditions must have prevailed during the collection of normative data.]

FIGURE 5-3.
Effect of changing the low-frequency filter cutoff on ABR measurement parameters.

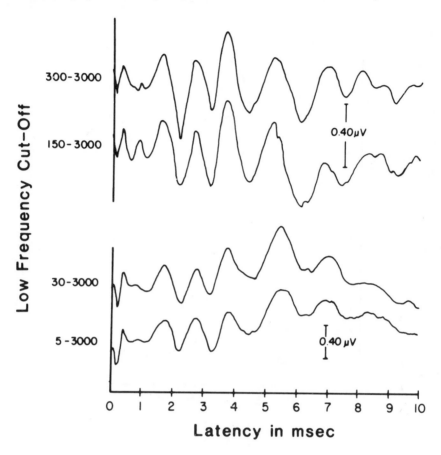

Time Domain Averaging: Number of Samples

Recall from the preceding discussion on bandpass filtering that the absolute voltages of the surface recorded ABR are quite small (less than 1 μV) and are measured from an area with significantly larger neurogenic and myogenic activity. Since the ABR is at most, only 1% of the amplitude of the ongoing EEG activity (Stockard, Stockard, & Sharbrough, 1978), the desired response remains concealed within this background activity.

There are several methods for eliminating unwanted electrical activity and improving the signal-to-noise ratio (SNR) from the desired ABR. Among these are (1) bandpass filtering, (2) artifact rejection, (3) electrode placement, and (4) common-mode rejection; however, the single most powerful tool is time domain averaging (Thornton, 1982).

The absolute number of averages needed for clear response resolution is dependent upon the amplitude of the ABR and amount of unwanted, noncerebral electrical activity. Those subjects with robust ABR amplitudes and low levels of physiologic "noise" may have a clear response after averaging only several hundred trials at high presentation levels. Reduction in stimulus intensity, which results in decreased waveform amplitude, however, necessitates an

FIGURE 5-4.
Effect of changing the high-frequency filter cutoff on ABR measurement parameters.

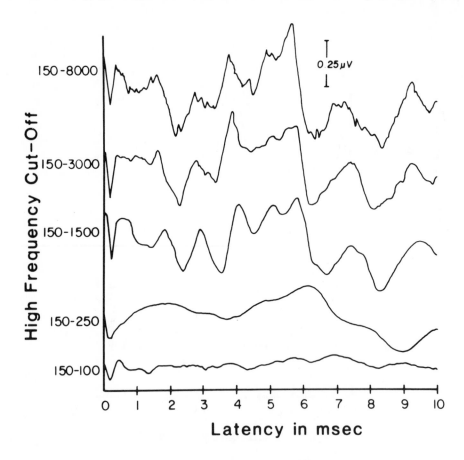

increase in the number of averages to maintain a favorable SNR. Consideration of this concept holds particular importance when the ABR is elicited to low-level stimulation for threshold estimation and when recording the ABR in environments having relatively high electrical ambience, as in the neurological or neonatal intensive care units. (For a detailed review of signal averaging see chapter 3).

To avoid disorganization of waveform morphology and decreased response amplitude it is recommended that (1) at least two averages of 2000 responses be obtained with greater averaging (4000-6000 sweeps) required for threshold measures and myogenically "noisy" subjects, (2) a control (no stimulus input) trial should be performed as a baseline for comparison with the actual response, and (3) artifact rejection of events that exceed the limits of the A-D convertor should be employed.

Stimulus Polarity

The results of empirical investigations concerning the effects of stimulus polarity on the ABR have been ambiguous, at best. The pioneering study of Terkildsen, Osterhammel, and

Huis in't Veld (1973) showed no consistent latency differences between ABRs recorded to both rarefaction and condensation click stimuli. Two years later, Ornitz and Walter (1975) reached the opposite conclusion when they described a consistent shortening in wave V latency on the order of 0.4–0.8 ms to rarefaction versus condensation clicks. In general, research studies have failed to reveal any systematic alteration in the peak latency of wave V with click phase inversion thus confirming the earlier observations of Terkildsen et al. (Borg & Lofqvist, 1982; Kevanishvili & Aphonchenko, 1981; Rosenhamer, Lindstrom, & Lundborg, 1978; Ruth et al., 1982; Stockard, Stockard, Westmoreland, & Corfits, 1979). In light of these data neither rarefaction nor condensation click stimuli seems to have any particular advantage where the identification of wave V is the measuring variable of interest as in the estimation of auditory sensitivity thresholds.

In contrast, several studies have suggested significant effects on the physical characteristics of wave I in the direction of decreased latency, increased amplitude, and improved resolution with the application of rarefaction click stimuli (Kevanishvili & Aphonchenko, 1981; Ruth et al., 1982; Stockard et al., 1979). Obviously, this shortening of wave I latency will influence the subsequent measure of IPLs. Given the importance of wave I in otoneurologic investigation, it would appear more prudent to employ a rarefaction click phase.

In many clinical practices the stimulus is often presented with alternating phase as a means of canceling the confounding effects of electrical artifact and the cochlear microphonic that may be accepted through the recording electrodes. Although alternating polarity does not seem, in our experience, to alter the response characteristics of the ABR (particularly wave I) to the same magnitude as condensation stimuli, it remains that the most optimal responses will be obtained with a rarefaction phase although this remains a matter of clinical preference.

All too often, individuals involved in the measurement of auditory evoked potentials assume that the polarity of a signal generated electrically from their commercial instrument guarantees a similar acoustic polarity when transduced through an earphone. Unfortunately, such is not the case; that is, there does not exist a manufacturing standard for earphone polarity. Thus, selection of a rarefaction phase at the test instrument may result in a positive-going movement of the earphone diaphragm, creating a condensation event. Consequently, it is imperative that the clinician determine the acoustic phase of the stimulus prior to collection of normative data. Cann and Knott (1979) and Staewen, Allison, Harris, Krumholz, and Goldstein (1980) have each described reliable methods for measuring the direction of movement of the earphone diaphragm to define acoustic polarity. More recently, an earphone phase tester (EPT) has become commercially available.[2]

Once acoustic phase is determined, polarization of the earphone can be established by marking that terminal which produces a condensation (+) or rarefaction (−) response with the application of a positive or negative voltage. Both the earphone and its associated cable connectors must be marked accordingly. Failure to correlate the polarity of the signal from the instrument's stimulus generator to that of an earphone diaphragm can result in serious measurement error. Indeed, there is need for a manufacturing standard for labeling the terminals and connectors of transducers used in auditory evoked potential measurements.

Repetition Rate

The effects of changing repetition rate on the latency and amplitude of the ABR among normal subjects have been reported by numerous investigators. Jewett and Williston (1971) were among the first to describe alterations in waveform morphology as repetition rate was increased from 2.5 to 50/s. Pratt and Sohmer (1976) reported decreased amplitudes and increased latencies of N_1–N_5. Similarly, Zollner, Karnahl, and Strange (1976) found a decrease in peak amplitude and an increase in latency for waves N_1–N_5.

In general, increases in rate of stimulation above approximately 20 Hz result in a dimunition in amplitude for the early components of the ABR (waves I–III) with little effect on the more rostral component (wave V) until stimulus rate exceeds approximately 30/s. More importantly, the latency of essentially all ABR components appears to increase by a magnitude of approximately 0.4 ms as repetition rate increases from 10 to 80 Hz (van Olphen, Rodenburg, & Verwey, 1979).

The effect of altering repetition rate progressively from 21.1 to 81.1/s is illustrated in Figure 5-5. Consistent with the findings of most previous investigators (Don, Allen, & Starr, 1977; Fujikawa & Weber, 1977; Gerling & Finitzo-Hieber, 1983; Hyde, Stephens, & Thornton, 1976; Picton, Stapells, & Campbell, 1981; Ruth et al., 1982) the latency of wave V, in particular, increases systematically as repetition rate is changed from 21.1 to 81.1/s.

For clinical practice it appears that the latency of wave V is not seriously affected until stimulus rate exceeds approximately 30/s (Hyde et al., 1976). Consequently, when total test time is critical, as in the development of a latency–intensity function to estimate hearing thresholds in difficult-to-test patients, it is acceptable to use higher rates of stimulus presentation allowing for latency prolongation.[3] Due to the possible compromising effects of repetition rate on response clarity and magnitude of waves I and III, which are important to otoneurologic diagnosis, repetition rates less than 12/s are recommended for evaluating auditory–neural integrity. Of course, it may be desirable to employ fast rates of presentation to detect incipient abnormalities in the brainstem pathway (Gerling & Finitzo-Hieber, 1983; Robinson & Rudge, 1977; Stockard, Stockard, & Sharbrough, 1980).

Stimulus Intensity

The most striking characteristic of the ABR is its sensitivity to the intensity of the acoustic stimulus. A decrease in stimulus intensity results in an increase in response latency of all ABR component waveforms. For a click stimulus, the latency of the most robust wave (V) increases monotonically as stimulus intensity decreases from 90 dB nHL down toward the visual detection threshold of the response. Figure 5-6 presents a latency–intensity function for a normal adult listener. Observe that at the two higher intensity levels (80 and 60 dB nHL) six peaks of the ABR are clearly definable and appear within the expected time domain; however, as intensity is reduced below 60 dB nHL, the earlier waveforms tend to disappear while the most robust wave (V) decreases in amplitude and increases in latency. In general, the magnitude of latency shift for wave V is on the order of 40 μs/dB.

At least two studies (D. E. Rose, personal communication, March 1984; Worthington & Peters, 1980) have calculated the probability of detecting various peak components as function of stimulus sensation level for normal hearers. In both studies, visual detection of wave V was possible in 75% of the cases at intensities between 10 and 20 dB SL and approached 100% at higher stimulus levels. Wave III, on the other hand, was identifiable at levels of approximately 30 dB SL in 50–60% of the subjects. For wave I, Worthington and Peters (1980) reported a response rate of 75% at 50 dB SL, whereas Rose found wave I to be present only 50% of the time for intensities as high as 70 dB SL. This latter finding has important clinical implication for neuroaudiologic diagnosis since wave I represents the electrophysiologic benchmark of the auditory nerve and is used to calculate brainstem conduction time. Consequently, the practicing clinician should take great care to utilize response recording parameters, such as rarefaction polarity, slow repetition rates ($\leq$ 12/s), vertex-earlobe or horizontal electrode placement and intensity levels > 70 dB nHL, that might serve to enhance the detectability of wave I.

In contrast to the earlier waves, the high rate of detectability for wave V at or near the visual detection threshold provides a basis for deriving a latency–intensity series as an aid to estimating hearing threshold in those individuals with whom routine behavioral measurements

FIGURE 5-5.
Changes in ABR characteristics secondary to increasing repetition rate.

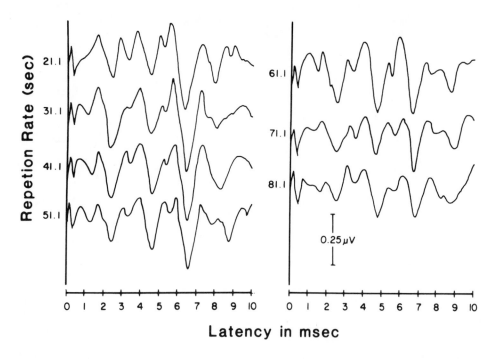

are precluded. Again, it is recommended that each individual facility develop its own normal latency–intensity template for later comparison with patients suspected of hearing loss. As shown in Figure 5-7, group mean and variance data for normal hearers with unremarkable otologic and neurologic history should be calculated for wave V latency. Typically, the latency–intensity function is reserved for wave V alone since it is the ABR component used in the threshold search. As shown in the figure, wave V latency data are plotted within a normal distribution (95% confidence interval) across stimulus intensity.

Of particular importance is that the normalized latency–intensity template developed for clinical use must be representative of the patient population for whom it was intended. For example, since infants show wave V latencies prolonged relative to those of adults, it stands to reason that the normative data should be age stratified. (See chapter 16 for a detailed review of ABR recording in infants.) Unfortunately, it has been our experience that some clinicians compare infant data to adult norms and reach the erroneous conclusion of possible central auditory disorder due to the prolongation of wave V latency at high intensity levels.

Effects of Contralateral Masking

The application of masking in the non-test ear to eliminate crossover of the test stimulus is standard protocol in clinical audiology. Certainly, there is no reason to believe that the possibility of crossover does not exist in ABR testing, particularly since click stimuli are often presented monaurally at moderately high supra-threshold levels. Finitzo-Hieber, Hecox, and Cone (1979) first questioned the need for masking when two adults with unilateral congenital atresia failed to show repeatable ABRs when the impaired ear was stimulated at intensity levels

FIGURE 5–6.
Effect of decreasing stimulus intensity on wave V latency, amplitude, and morphology. Time window is 10 ms.

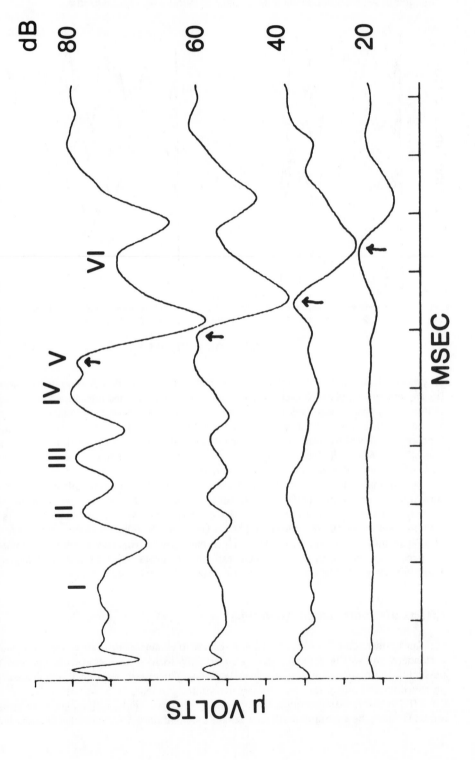

FIGURE 5–7.
Template for wave V latency-intensity function and I-V IPL based on normative data. The shaded area represents ± 2.5 SD. *Note:* This template is based on normative data gathered at the Hospital of the University of Pennsylvania and is not applicable to other test facilities.

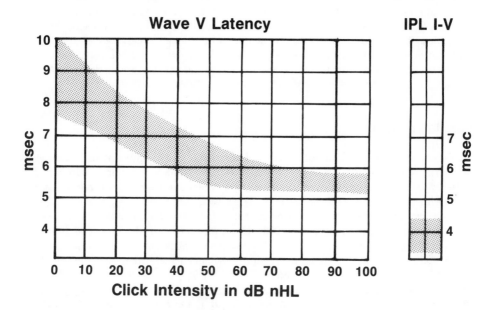

of 100–117 dB peSPL (peak equivalent sound pressure level). Opposite findings were reached by Chiappa et al. (1979) and more recently by Humes and Ochs (1982) who reported recognizable but delayed ABRs which were subsequently ablated with the presentation of masking to the normal ear of patients with unilateral deafness.

Surprisingly, the presentation of a broad-band masker to the non-test ear seems to have only minimal effect on the ABR (Chiappa et al., 1979; Humes & Ochs, 1982; Reid & Thornton, 1983). Rosenhamer and Holmkvist (1983), for example, reported an average latency prolongation on the order of only 0.5 ms for waves III and V when a 90-dB HL broad-band noise was delivered to the contralateral ear of 11 bilaterally normal young female subjects. Reid and Thornton (1983) hypothesized that the short-duration click stimulus and long-duration broad-band masker follow different afferent pathways within the auditory system, thereby explaining the apparent lack of interaction between the two stimuli. Hence, the introduction of a broad-band noise appears to be an effective method for limiting participation of the non-test ear without affecting the desired test ear response.

As has been shown in pure tone audiometry, interaural attenuation values are influenced by such factors as transducer type and activating stimulus. Estimates of interaural attenuation for click stimuli range from 50 dB (Reid & Thornton, 1983) to 75 dB (Humes & Ochs, 1982). As a conservative estimate, therefore, interaural attenuation is considered to be approximately 50 dB for click stimuli. Thus, contralateral masking of the non-test ear should be employed when there is a 50-dB or greater difference between the intensity level of the click stimulus presented to the test ear and the bone-conduction thresholds between 1000 and 4000 Hz in the non-test ear.

An alternative for determining when to mask is to measure the interaural latency differences of corresponding wave components. If this difference exceeds about 1.5 ms, then masking should be introduced in the non-test ear. This criterion is based on the observation that wave V latency is shifted by a magnitude of 0.4 ms/10 dB of intensity change. If crossover occurs at 50 dB nHL, then this should result in a 2.0-ms delay in the contralateral ear.

It is recommended that an effective masking table be constructed using methods and procedures similar to those described by Sanders (1978) for pure tone audiometry, with consideration given to the spectral differences obtained for click stimuli transduced through an electrodynamic earphone. This approach to the masking problem is considerably more systematic and scientifically correct than the simple introduction of a masking level that is chosen somewhat arbitrarily. Remember, there may indeed be no relationship between the numbers denoted on the masking attenuator dial and the actual amount of masking delivered through the transducer (Sanders, 1978; Townsend & Schwartz, 1976).

Transducer Types

Earphone. In routine ABR testing the brief duration (e.g., 100 μs) rectangular wave electric pulse is transduced through some type of standard electrodynamic audiometric earphone (e.g., TDH-39; TDH-49) housed in either circumaural or supraaural cushions. In contrast to those found with pure tone stimuli, the differences between click spectra produced by different earphones may indeed be significant. Most earphones, for example, display two primary resonant peaks somewhere between 3000 and 6000 Hz. Accordingly, if the earphone is damped insufficiently about the resonant frequencies, then the application of a transient signal with an instantaneous rise time will result in "ringing" that can interact with the stimulus of interest. Figure 5-8, taken from Weber, Seitz, and McCutcheon (1981) illustrates the effect of earphone oscillation on the ABR. Observe that for earphone A, which exhibited the least amount of "ringing" and had an acoustic spectrum characterized by a primary resonance at 3004 Hz, the ABR consisted of six clearly discernible waveforms at normal absolute and inter-peak latencies and amplitudes. Conversely, earphone C, which was apparently undamped and processed minimal high-frequency energy beyond 2644 Hz, produced some disorganization in waveform morphology, prolongation in wave latency, and decrease in peak-to-trough amplitude.

On the basis of these findings, it would appear essential for the clinician to define the spectral content of the particular earphone to be used in ABR testing. Moreover, given the observation that earphones are often treated with little regard for the sensitivity of the diaphragm, routine spectral analysis to assess possible alterations in click waveforms should be afforded serious consideration. Failure to follow this recommendation may result in interpretive error since latency prolongation may reflect the physical properties of the transducer and not those of the auditory system. Along these same lines, the clinician should not assume that the two earphones used to transduce the click stimuli are matched relative to their acoustic spectra; that is, spectral analysis should be made on each individual earphone. If the earphones are not matched then only one earphone should be used to record the ABR in both ears.

In addition to the effect of spectral aberrations of the transducer on the ABR, those electrodynamic earphones having low input-load impedance often impart stray electromagnetic fields, which are passed through the recording electrodes only to contaminate the early portion of the ABR in the form of electromagnetic artifact. One common method for reducing stimulus artifact is to enclose the earphone in a conductive material such as mu-metal and to connect the shield to ground. Recently, Hughes and Fino (1979) and Stackenburg and Wit (1983) each described a piezoelectric earphone transducer having electrostatic shielding that not only minimizes stimulus artifact, but also tends to enhance greatly the amplitude of wave I. Figure 5-9 compares ABRs recorded in our electrodiagnostic laboratory with an electrodynamic earphone (TDH-39) to those derived by transducing a rarefaction click through a high-input impedance piezoelectric earphone custom constructed according to the schematics provided

FIGURE 5–8.
Click waveforms, spectra, and ABRs recorded from three electrodynamic earphones (modified with permission from Weber et al. (1981).

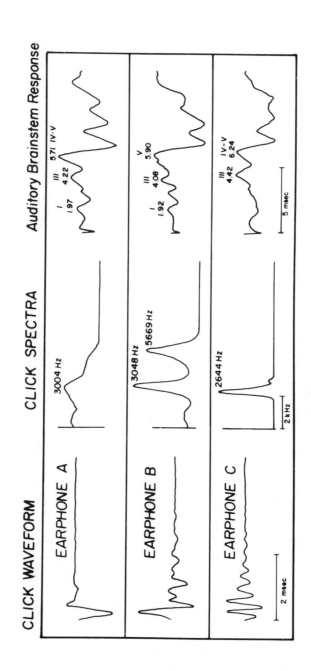

FIGURE 5–9.
Comparison of ABRs recorded to a 75-dB nHL rarefaction click stimulus transduced through a standard audiometric earphone (TDH-39) and a custom-constructed piezoelectric transducer.

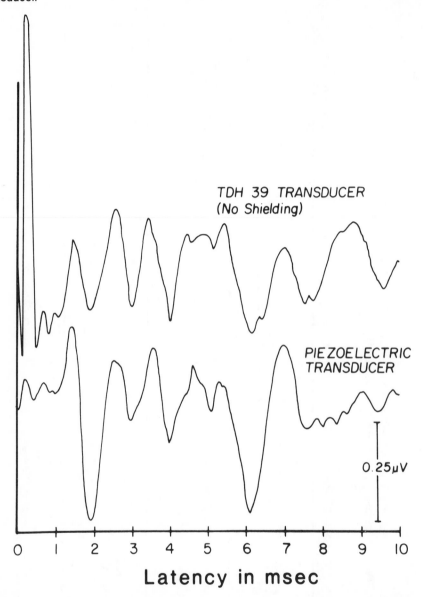

by Stackenburg and Wit. The amplitude of wave I for the piezoelectric earphone is more than twice that obtained with the standard audiometric transducer. Furthermore, this experimental earphone reduced considerably the effects of stray electromagnetic fields as evidenced by the marked reduction in stimulus artifact exhibited for the unshielded earphone recording. Note also that the waveforms are more finely resolved (smoothed) with the piezoelectric transducer.

Sound field. In addition to an earphone, ABRs have also been recorded for signals transduced through a loudspeaker in the sound field. Here, one need be concerned not only with the frequency response of the speaker but also with the time delay that is introduced as a result of the distance between the tympanic membrane and the transducer. For example, a speaker placed at a distance of 0.5 meters from the listener's ear can be expected to introduce a time delay of approximately 0.0015 ms. While this delay may appear singularly negligible, the addition of this increase to that created by other measurement variables can result in a substantial effect on the ABR. Jacobson, Seitz, Mencher, and Parrott (1981) compared binaural earphone-to-sound field generated ABRs and found absolute latencies for all wave components to be prolonged by a significant amount when unfiltered clicks were transduced through a loudspeaker placed one meter from the tragus.

Bone conduction. At times, it is desirable to record the ABR to bone-conducted stimuli in an effort to assess sensorineural reserve. Such is the case when faced with a child exhibiting congenital atresia or microtia of the external ear or one that displays no recordable ABR to air-conducted stimulation. In contrast to air-conducted stimuli, however, research related to ABRs elicited by bone-conducted signals is limited (Cornacchia, Martini, & Morra, 1983; Mauldin & Jerger, 1979; Schwartz & Fadden, 1981; Weber, 1983). In general, bone-conducted ABRs reveal wave V latency delays on the order of 0.5 ms. Mauldin and Jerger (1979) concluded that this latency delay was a result of the effective spectrum of the bone-conducted signal, which showed primary acoustic energy below 2500 Hz. To this end, they recommended subtracting 0.5 ms from the measured bone-conduction wave latency in an effort to provide direct comparison to the derived air-conduction latency values. The average separation in decibels between air-conducted and corrected bone-conducted latency–intensity functions, therefore, yields an estimate of the average air–bone gap from 1000 to 4000 Hz.

Consistent with the effects of earphone spectral differences on waveform latency, amplitude, and morphology, differences among bone-conduction oscillator types, as well as site of placement (i.e., mastoid versus forehead), can also be expected to alter any or all of the ABR parameters. Schwartz and Fadden (1981), for example, presented preliminary data on wave V latency differences obtained for three bone conduction vibrators at two placement sites. Represented in Figure 5-10 are the normalized bone-conducted latency–intensity functions developed for Radioear B-70, B-71, and B-72 bone-conduction oscillators placed on the mastoid. Comparative air-conduction data are also displayed. Results indicate that the earliest wave V latency was obtained for the B-70 followed by that of the B-71. In fact, differences in wave V latency between the B-70 and air-conducted responses were minimal across intensities. While a somewhat similar hierarchy among vibrators was obtained with a forehead placement (Figure 5-11), the latency values for all three bone-conduction transducers were significantly delayed relative both to the air-conduction response and to those derived with a mastoid placement. From these preliminary data, it would appear that the bone-conduction transducer of choice for recording the ABR is the Radioear B-70 placed on the mastoid.

As a final note, the clinician is advised that when a bone-conduction oscillator is connected to the earphone jack of a commercially available evoked potential system, the acoustic output is approximately 40 dB nHL less than the corresponding earphone output at equal attenuator settings. That is, the behavioral threshold for a click transduced through a bone-conduction vibrator will be achieved with an attenuator dial setting of 40 dB for a jury of normal hearers. In addition, the dynamic range of this transducer is only approximately 30 dB; above this level, the oscillator is driven to saturation.

Electrode Location

The recording of auditory evoked potentials requires placement of three or four surface electrodes, two or three of which are connected to the preamplifier inputs with the other electrode

FIGURE 5–10.
Normalized wave V latency-intensity function for a click stimulus transduced through three bone-conduction oscillators with a mastoid placement (Note 4).

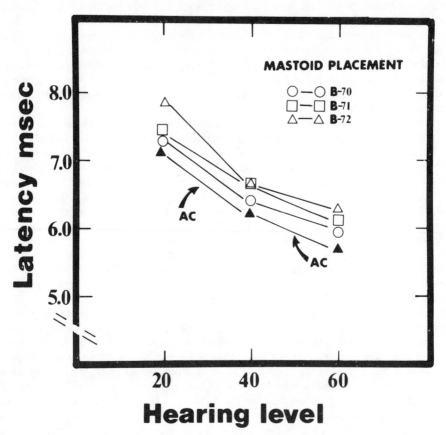

serving as ground. In contrast to electroencephalography (EEG), there does not appear to be general agreement among those involved in the clinical application of ABR as to the most suitable placement for the recording electrodes. Represented in Figure 5-12 is the International 10-20 system proposed by Jasper (1958) in which electrode placements are based on measurements from four standard positions on the head; namely, the nasion, inion, and right and left preauricular sites.

In ABR testing, the electrodes are arranged such that the electrical potential difference is measured between pairs of scalp electrodes (bipolar derivation). In most clinical facilities single-channel ABR recording requires placement of three surface electrodes, two of which are connected to preamplifier inputs with the third serving as ground. The active (positive) electrode is placed on either the vertex (Cz) or high forehead (Fz), while the reference (negative) electrode is adhered to an assumed inactive (neutral) site such as the ipsilateral earlobe (A1, A2) or mastoid (M1, M2) with the contralateral counterpart (earlobe or mastoid) reserved for the ground electrode. Since, in reality, the ABR is a bipolar recording, there does not appear to be a neutral site for the reference (negative) electrode on the scalp that will not pass any stimulus-related electrical activity (Terkildsen, Osterhammel, & Huis in't Veld, 1974). Consequently, it is more

FIGURE 5–11.
Normalized wave V latency-intensity function for a click transduced through three bone-conduction oscillators with a forehead placement (Note 4).

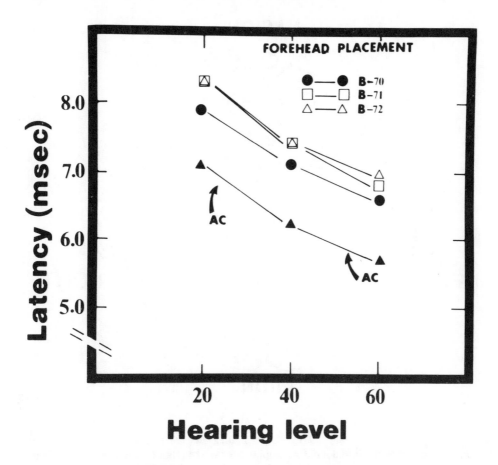

accurate to label these two electrodes as either positive or negative as opposed to "active" and "reference" (Arlinger, 1981).

[Note: In contrast to single-channel recordings, simultaneous bilateral recordings require a four-electrode montage (e.g., Cz-A2; Cz-A1, and Fz as ground].

Although many clinicians continue to use Fz as the site for the positive electrode, research suggests that the single best location is on the vertex (Martin & Moore, 1977; van Olphen et al., 1978; Terkildsen et al., 1974; Terkildsen & Osterhammel, 1981); however, Parker (1981) suggested that the optimal electrode arrangement for measuring all wave components of the ABR was Pz (a parietal site)-to-ipsilateral mastoid with the Cz-to-ipsilateral mastoid representing the second most acceptable pattern. As with all other recording variables, it is important to recognize that changes in electrode position can result in alterations in waveform latency and amplitude.

Of particular importance in neuroaudiologic diagnosis is the ability to record a clearly identifiable wave I whenever possible. Over the years, various special ear canal electrodes have been devised for enhancing the amplitude of wave I via the extratympanic recording of the whole nerve action potential (Durrant, Rosenberg, & Ronis, 1977; Harder & Arlinger, 1981;

FIGURE 5–12.
International 10-20 system for electrode placement. Landmarks most commonly used in ABR recording are A1-A2, Pz, Cz, and Fz.

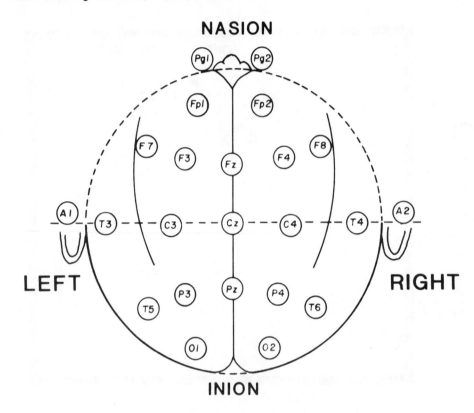

Lang, Happonen, & Salmivalli, 1981; Walter & Blegvad, 1981). Use of these atraumatic intrameatal electrodes tends to double the amplitude of wave I (Harder & Arlinger, 1981; Walter & Blegvad, 1981) without an accompanying change in latency; however, Lang et al. (1981) noted some decrease in the amplitude of waves V and VI. This latter finding could potentially affect the calculation of the relative I–V amplitude ratio. Despite the advantages of ear canal electrode placement for improving the resolution of wave I, such an approach can still be considered somewhat invasive for routine recording of the ABR.

An alternative surface area for placement of the negative electrode to improve the detectability of wave I is the mesial portion of the earlobe. Stockard, Stockard, and Sharbrough (1978) found wave I amplitude to be 1.5 times greater with an earlobe versus a mastoid site for the reference electrode. Our experience has tended to support these findings. Hecox (1980) proposed that wave I amplitude could be enhanced with a horizontal electrode montage with the positive electrode on the contralateral mastoid and the negative electrode on the ipsilateral mastoid. Conflicting evidence has shown no improvement in wave I response amplitude using a horizontal pattern (Ruth et al., 1982).

While there exists no single electrode montage that best records all of the major components of the ABR, many individuals involved in neurodiagnostic work have found that the most acceptable clinical compromise is achieved with a vertex-to-earlobe arrangement. Consistent with the influence of other recording variables on the three measurement parameters of the ABR, it is essential that normative clinical data be established using the same electrode montage as that anticipated for clinical practice so that any aberrations obtained from a patient reflect the true electrophysiologic response of the auditory system rather than variations in recording technique. Of course, as Parker (1981) cautions, the electrode montage that results in the clearest responses among normals may not necessarily correspond to that which is optimal for those with neuropathology.

Bilateral Recording of the ABR

Unlike most other measurement variables that can influence the normal ABR, bilateral recording has received limited research attention (Hashimoto, Ishiyama, & Tozuka, 1979; Rosenhamer & Holmkvist, 1982; Starr & Achor, 1975; Stockard et al., 1979; Stockard, Stockard, & Sharbrough, 1978; Thornton, 1975, 1976). Such simultaneous ipsilateral/contralateral measurements can often facilitate proper identification of component waveforms.

Recordings from the ear opposite that of stimulation show that wave I is often either diminished in amplitude or absent (Rosenhamer & Holmkvist, 1982; Thornton, 1975), whereas wave III can be more attenuated than wave II (Stockard, Stockard, & Sharbrough, 1978). For latency measures, there is a tendency for wave III to have a faster latency, with wave V being slightly prolonged on the order of 0.15 ms relative to its ipsilateral counterpart. Moreover, the I–III IPL is shortened and the I–V IPL increased for recordings obtained on the ear contralateral to click stimulation.

Perhaps the most clinically useful feature of simultaneous ipsilateral/contralateral recordings is the ability to separate the IV–V complex into two distinct waves when morphologic ambiguity exists, as illustrated in Figure 5-13. In the top ipsilateral tracing, wave V appears to be located about one-third of the down portion from the peak of the response. The bottom contralateral response resolves the problem by separating the two wave components, thus verifying that the original site for labeling wave V was correct. Also shown is the reduction in amplitude for waves I and III consistent with the observations of Stockard, Stockard, & Sharbrough (1978).

EFFECT OF SUBJECT CHARACTERISTICS ON THE NORMAL ABR

The preceding section highlighted the relatively large variations in waveform latency, amplitude, and morphology that are produced by only minor manipulations of the controlling measurement variables, thus underscoring the need for individual normative data. In addition to the confounding effects of such procedural variables on the ABR, however, clinically significant alterations in ABR parameters can occur as a result of individual subject differences, pharmacologic factors, and/or physiologic characteristics that are not associated with neurologic disease or auditory disorder.

Age

During the past decade there has emerged a plethora of studies demonstrating the marked alterations in response latency, amplitude, and morphology consequent to physiologic immaturity. It is now well known that infant responses consist of three vertex-positive waves (I, III, and V) having latencies and amplitudes that differ from corresponding adult norms (Cox, Hack, & Metz, 1981; Hecox & Galambos, 1974; Jacobson et al., 1981; Jacobson, Morehouse, & Johnson,

FIGURE 5–13.
Comparison of ipsilateral and contralateral recording of the ABR.

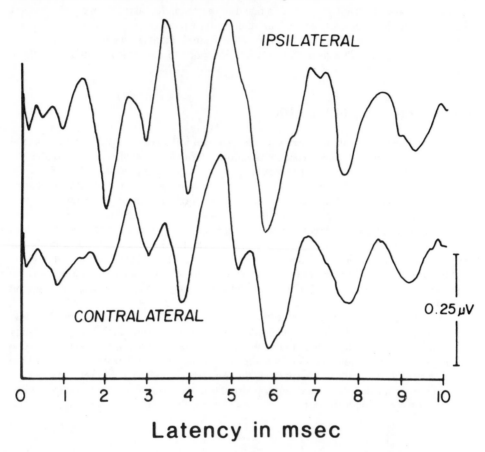

1982; Salamy & McKean, 1976; Salamy, McKean, & Buda, 1975; Schulman-Galambos & Galambos, 1975; Starr, Amlie, Martin, & Sanders, 1977; Weber, 1982). The consensus of these studies is that immaturity in the auditory system is reflected in the ABR by absolute and inter-peak latency delays of the three primary components and a wave I amplitude approximately twice that found in adults, which, accordingly, will have an obviously reducing effect on the I–V amplitude ratio. Such maturational effects become resolved by approximately 12 months of age when the ABR begins to assume characteristics similar to those obtained from adult subjects. (For a detailed review of the ABR in newborns see chapter 16.) In recognition of the differences in wave latency and amplitude on the ABRs recorded from preterm and full-term newborns, adjustments to clinical norms for these measurement parameters are imperative. That is, age-relevant normative data commensurate with the population to be studied is mandatory prior to utilizing this powerful tool to estimate auditory threshold or neurologic integrity either in the well-baby or neonatal intensive care nurseries.

At the opposite end of the age continuum data related to changes in ABR characteristics for individuals beyond the sixth decade of life are both sparse and conflicting. Beagley and Sheldrake (1978) found no increase in latency across subjects grouped according to decades of age from 11 to 79 years who exibited normal hearing. Conversely, Rowe (1978) compared

FIGURE 5–14.
Effect of gender on wave V latency and amplitude (from Jerger & Hall, 1980, with permission).

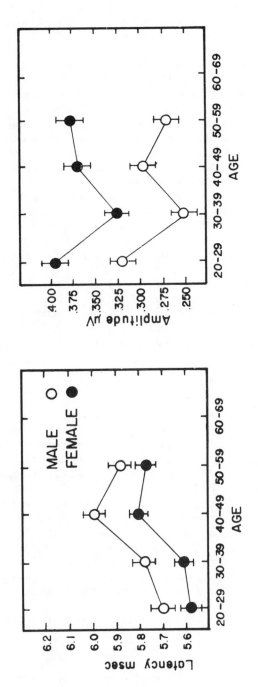

ABR findings for a group of young adults ages 17–33 years to that recorded for subjects ranging in age from 51 to 74 years and found the latter group to exhibit latency delays on the order of 0.30–0.50 ms relative to those obtained from their younger counterparts. According to Thomsen, Terkildsen, and Osterhammel (1978) wave V latency increases at a rate of approximately 0.1 ms per decade of life. More recently, Rosenhamer, Lindstrom, and Lundborg (1980) provided support for the initial findings of Beagley and Sheldrake by reporting no significant differences in wave latency between individuals in the sixth to seventh decades and young adults. Maurizi, Altissimi, Ottaviani, Paludetti, and Bambini (1982) continued the controversy when 14 subjects (mean age of 62 years) with average pure tone thresholds $\leq$ 30 dB HL revealed mean peak latencies for waves I, II, III, and V on the order of 0.20 ms longer than 19 normal hearing adults ranging in age from 28 to 42 years. Moreover, they went on to report that waveform morphology among the total sample of elderly subjects (mean age of 69.5 years) appeared to be more disorganized than that which would be predicted on the basis of pure tone thresholds. A similar latency delay (0.20 ms) in normal hearing subjects between the ages of 20 and 59 years was reported by Jerger and Hall (1980).

While there does not appear to be any overwhelming agreement among investigators as to the relationship between senescence and ABR waveform latency or amplitude, it is reasonable to assume that such alterations could be observed as a result of expected physiological changes that occur within the central auditory nervous system with increasing age. Hansen and Reske-Nielsen (1965) and Kirikae (1965) described reduction of eighth nerve fibers, atrophy of the spiral ganglion, and degeneration of the gangliar cells within the ventral cochlear nucleus, superior olivary complex, and medial geniculate body, all of which are primary generator sites (albeit not necessarily specific) of the ABR. To allow for these changes, the cautious auditory electrodiagnostician will establish a separate normative data base for the geriatric population since the residual effects of high-frequency hearing loss often associated with presbycusis can add further latency delay and thus confuse ABR interpretation (Otto & McCandless, 1983).

Gender

It has been hypothesized that their smaller head circumference, in combination with a foreshortening of the brainstem pathway between the auditory nerve and midbrain, accounts for the phenomenon that females generally present with earlier response latencies than males of the same age (Beagley & Sheldrake, 1978; Goldman, Sohmer, & Godfrey, 1981; Jerger & Hall, 1980; Michalewski, Thompson, Patterson, Bowman, & Litzelman, 1980; Rosenhamer et al., 1980; Stockard, Stockard, & Sharbrough, 1977). Figure 5-14 demonstrates the expected differences in wave V latency between genders as a function of age. When collapsed across age, the average wave V latency for males was 0.14 ms longer than females. Likewise, female subjects displayed waveform amplitudes of a magnitude of 0.080–0.120 μV greater than those of their male counterparts. Regardless of the explanation for this difference in transmission time, the clinical implication of these data is that each facility should generate individual normative latency and amplitude values between genders since application of female norms to male patients could lead to interpretation of delayed waveform latency when none actually exists (Type I error).

Body Temperature

Stockard, Sharbrough, and Tinker (1978) reported on six neurologically and audiologically normal patients subjected to hypothermia during cardiopulmonary bypass surgery who displayed IPLs that exceeded the 99% confidence limit by 0.7–0.9 ms. Since temperatures of about 28–32° C are apparently a common occurrence during such surgical procedures, allowances for possible IPL prolongation should be made if the ABR is recorded intraoperatively (see chapters 13 and 14).

Pharmacologic Agents

The effect of various pharmacologic agents and anesthetics on the ABR has received limited research attention. Stockard et al. (1980) reported a general preservation of all waveform parameters in normal patients undergoing general anesthesia (e.g., halothane, nitrous oxide, meperidine, and diazepam). Similar findings have been reported by Goff, Allison, Lyons, Fisher, and Conte (1977) in humans, and Bobbin, May, and Lemoine (1979) in laboratory animals. More recently, Javel, Mouney, McGee, and Walsh (1982) described changes in waveform morphology following systemic infusion of lidocaine. In our audiologic studies of comatose patients subsequent to closed head injury (Schwartz, Olsen, Berry, & Murray, 1981) we have noted alterations in ABR parameters with increasing barbiturate levels. Finally, as a cautionary note, acute ethanol intoxication has been shown to compromise the ABR in the direction of increased IPLs (Rosenhamer, 1981).

AFTERWORD

This chapter highlights the nonpathologic factors that can influence the measurement parameters of the ABR—namely, absolute and interpeak latencies, peak-to-trough amplitudes, the I-V amplitude ratio, and waveform morphology. While some of these variables may appear to have only minimal effects on the ABR, the synergistic consequences across variables can lead to serious interpretive error. It has been our experience that many clinicians involved in ABR recording are incognizant of such nonpathologic alterations. Indeed, the evidence to support the confounding effects of differences in measurement variables and subject states is compelling and, hence, points to the necessity of establishing individual normative data for each quantitative measure in an effort to avoid clinical misinterpretation. We cannot impress enough upon the beginning auditory electrodiagnostician not to be lulled into a false sense of security at the apparent ease of ABR test administration and interpretation based on either a cursory review of the literature or attendance at a one- or two-day workshop or seminar. On the contrary, the ABR represents a complex interaction of instrumentation and physiological variables that, when understood, will provide the clinician with what has become the most powerful diagnostic tool in audiology today.

Unfortunately, neither a national nor an international standard exists for defining the technical aspects of ABR recording. The recommendation of the task force on evoked potential measurements (Thornton, 1983) represents a first attempt at the development of a standard. Nonetheless, review of those recommendations, summarized in Table 5-3, does not lead us to believe that a technical guideline for ABR measurement similar to that available in other areas of audiology (e.g., audiometric calibration, hearing aid measurement, or ambient noise level) will be available in the near future. In the interim, the selection of filter bandwidths, number of averaged responses, repetition rates, and a host of other variables rests on the shoulders of the individual clinician. Unquestionably, use of this exquisite diagnostic procedure on a clinicopathologic population, in the absence of a firm understanding of the normal response as presented herein, is unjustified.

TABLE 5–3.
Technical and procedural recommendations of Electric Response Study Group task force on ABR measurement

Technical considerations	
Stimulus:	100-ms electric pulse
Transducer:	electrodynamic (e.g., TDH-49) having a relatively flat frequency response
Polarity:	instrumentation should permit monophasic or alternating polarity
Repetition rate:	rates from 1–80/s should be available
Filter pass-band:	30–3000 Hz (3 dB-down points) and a 6 dB/octave roll-off
Computer dwell time:	50 μs (20 KHz sampling rate for a sweep time of 1–20 ms)
Procedural considerations	
Electrode sites:	positive—somewhere between Cz and Fz; negative—ipsilateral earlobe or mastoid (A1-A2); ground—anywhere (No specific recommendation)
Intensity:	90 dB PeSPL
Repetition rate:	one slow rate $<$ 25/s and one rapid rate $\geq$ 50/s
No. of trials:	replicate all averages until corresponding latencies are within ±0.2 ms

Note: From Thornton, 1983.

Completion of this chapter would not have been possible without the assistance of the audiology and clerical staffs of the Speech and Hearing Center at the Hospital of the University of Pennsylvania. We are particularly indebted to our Administrative Secretary, Deborah Y. Wray, who came off maternity leave one month early only to have to wean herself from a typewriter to a computer with word processing capability. Finally, we thank Noreen Daly, a graduate student clinical extern from the Division of Hearing and Speech Sciences, Vanderbilt University, who helped tabulate interlaboratory normative data, compiled references, and, more importantly, served as a reader who represents the target population for whom this chapter is intended.

[1]The recent task force on standardization of evoked potential measurement recommended a wide filter passband from 30 to 3000 Hz (Thornton, 1983).

[2]Grass Instruments, 101 Old Colony Avenue, Quincy, MA 02169.

[3]Fria (1980) calculated that each 20/s increase in repetition rate above 10/s yields a 0.2-ms increase in wave V latency.

REFERENCES

Amadeo, M., & Shagass, Ch. (1973). Brief latency click evoked potentials during waking and sleep in man. *Psychophysiology, 10,* 244–250.

Arlinger, S. (1981). Technical aspects of stimulation, recording and signal processing. *Scandinavian Audiology (Supplement), 13,* 41–53.

Beagley, H. A., & Sheldrake, J. B. (1978). Differences in brainstem response latency with age and sex. *British Journal of Audiology, 12,* 69–77.

Bobbin, R., May, J.G., & Lemoine, R.L. (1979). Effects of pentobarbital and ketamine on brain stem auditory potentials. *Archives of Otolaryngology, 105,* 467–470.

Borg, E., & Lofqvist, L. (1982). Auditory brainstem response to rarefaction and condensation clicks in normal and abnormal ears. *Scandinavian Audiology, 11,* 227–235.

Boston, J.R., & Ainslie, P.J. (1980). Effects of analog and digital filtering on brain stem auditory evoked potentials. *Electroencephalography & Clinical Neurophysiology, 48,* 361–364.

Cacace, A.T., Shy, M., & Satya-Murti, S. (1980). Brainstem auditory evoked potentials: A comparison of two high-frequency filter settings. *Neurology, 30,* 765–767.

Cann, J., & Knott, J. (1979). Polarity of acoustic click stimuli for eliciting brainstem auditory evoked responses: A proposed standard. *American Journal of EEG Technology, 19,*125–132.

Chiappa, K.H., Gladstone, K.J., & Young, R.R. (1979). Brainstem auditory evoked responses; Studies of waveform variations in 50 normal human subjectes. *Archives of Neurology, 36,* 81–87.

Cornacchia, L., Martini, A., & Morra, B. (1983). Air and bone conducted brainstem responses in adults and infants. *Audiology, 22,* 430–437.

Cox, C., Hack, M., & Metz, D. (1981). Brainstem evoked response audiometry: Normative data from the preterm infant. *Audiology, 20,* 53–64.

Davis, H. (1976). Principles of electric response audiometry. *Annals of Otology, Rhinology and Laryngology (Supplement), 28,* 1–96.

Dawson, W.W., & Doddington, H.W. (1973). Phase distortion of biological signals: Extraction of signal from noise without phase error. *Electroencephalography and Clinical Neurophysiology, 34,* 207–211.

Don, M., Allen, A.R., & Starr, A. (1977). Effect of click rate on the latency of the auditory brain stem response in humans. *Annals of Otology, Rhinology, and Laryngology, 86,* 186–195.

Durrant, J.D., Rosenberg, P.E., & Ronis, M.L. (1977). *Efficacy of a non-traumatic ear-canal recording technique (ECochG) in routine audiological evaluations.* Paper presented at the 5th International Symposium of IERASG, Jerusalem, August.

Elberling, C. (1976). Action potentials recorded from the promontory and the surface compared with recordings from the ear canal in man. *Scandinavian Audiology, 5,* 69–78.

Elberling, C. (1979). Auditory electrophysiology: Spectral analysis of cochlear and brainstem evoked potentials. *Scandinavian Audiology, 8,* 57–64.

Fabiani, M., Sohmer, H., Tait, C., Garni, M., & Kinarti, R. (1979). A functional measure of brain activity: Brain stem transmission time. *Electroencephalography and Clinical Neurophysiology, 47,* 483–491.

Finitzo-Hieber, T., Hecox, K., & Cone, B. (1979). Brainstem auditory evoked potentials in patients with congenital atresia. *Laryngoscope, 89,* 1151–1158.

Fria, T.J. (1980). The auditory brain stem reponse: Background and clinical applications. In D.M. Schwartz & F.H. Bess (Eds.), *Monographs in contemporary audiology.* Minneapolis: Maico Hearing Instruments.

Fujikawa, S., & Weber, B.A. (1977). Effects of increased stimulus rate on brainstem response (BER) audiometry as a function of age. *Journal of the American Audiology Society, 3,* 147–150.

Gerling, I.J., & Finitzo-Hieber, T. (1983). Auditory brainstem response with high stimulus rates in normal and patient populations. *Annals of Otology, Rhinology, and Laryngology, 92,* 119–123.

Gilroy, J., & Lynn G.E. (1978). Computerized tomography and auditory evoked potentials: Use in the diagnosis of olivoponto-cerebellar degeneration. *Archives of Neurology, 35,* 143–147.

Goff, W.R., Allison, T., Lyons, W., Fisher, T.C., & Conte, R. (1977). Origins of short latency auditory evoked potentials in man. *Progress in Clinical Neurophysiology, 2,* 30–44.

Goldman, Z., Sohmer, H., & Godfrey, C. (1981). Auditory nerve, brain stem and cortical response correlates of learning capacity. *Physiology and Behavior, 26,* 637–645.

Hansen, C.C., & Reske-Nielsen, E. (1965). Pathological studies in presbycusis. *Archives of Otolaryngology, 82,* 115–132.

Harder, H., & Arlinger, S. (1981). Ear-canal compared to mastoid electrode placement in ABR. *Scandinavian Audiology (Supplement), 13,* 55–57.

Hashimoto, I., Ishiyama, Y., & Tozuka, G. (1979). Bilaterally recorded brainstem auditory evoked responses. *Archives of Neurology, 36,* 161–167.

Hecox, K. (1980). *Brainstem evoked potentials: Neurological applications.* Paper presented at the conference on Auditory Evoked Response in Otology and Audiology, Cambridge, MA, August.

Hecox K., & Galambos, R. (1974). Brain stem auditory evoked response in human infants and adults. *Archives of Otolaryngology, 99,* 30–33.

Hughes, J.R., & Fino, J. (1979). Usefulness of piezoelectric earphones in recording the brainstem auditory evoked potentials: A new early deflection. *Electroencephalography and Clinical Neurophysiology, 48,* 357.

Humes, L.E., & Ochs, M.G. (1982). Use of contralateral masking in the measurement of the auditory brainstem response. *Journal of Speech & Hearing Research, 25,* 528–535.

Hyde, M.L., Stephens, S.D.G., & Thornton, A.R.D. (1976). Stimulus repetition rate and the early brainstem responses. *British Journal of Audiology, 10,* 41–50.

Jacobson, J.T., Morehouse, C.R., & Johnson, M.J. (1982). Strategies for infant auditory brainstem response assessment. *Ear and Hearing, 3,* 263–270.

Jacobson, J.T., Seitz, M.R., Mencher, G., & Parrott, V.F. (1981). Auditory brainstem response: A contribution to infant assessment and management. In G. Mencher & S. Gerber (Eds.), *Early management of hearing loss.* New York: Grune & Stratton

Jasper, H.H. (1958). Report of the committee on methods of clinical examination in electroencephalography. *Electroencephalography and Clinical Neurophysiology, 10,* 370.

Javel, E., Mouney, D.F., McGee, J., & Walsh, E.J. (1982). Auditory brainstem reponses during systemic infusion of lidocaine. *Archives of Otolaryngology, 108,* 71–76.

Jerger, J., & Hall, J. (1980). Effects of age and sex on the auditory brainstem response. *Archives of Otolaryngology, 106,* 382–391.

Jerger, J., & Mauldin, L. (1978). Prediction of sensorineural hearing level from the brain stem evoked response. *Archives of Otolaryngology, 104,* 456–461.

Jewett, D.L., Romano, M.N., & Williston, J.S. (1970). Human auditory evoked potentials: Possible brain stem components detected on scalp. *Science, 167,* 1517–1518.

Jewett, D.L., & Williston, J.S. (1971). Auditory evoked far fields averaged from the scalp of humans. *Brain, 94,* 681–696.

Kavanagh, K.T., & Beardsley, J.V. (1979). Brain stem auditory evoked response III. Clinical uses of bone conduction in the evaluation of otologic disease. *Annals of Otology, Rhinology, and Laryngology (Supplement), 88,* 22–28.

Kevanishvili, Z., & Aphonchenko, V. (1979). Frequency composition of brain stem auditory evoked potentials. *Scandinavian Audiology, 8,* 51–55.

Kevanishvili, Z., & Aphonchenko, V. (1981). Click polarity inversion effects upon the human brainstem auditory evoked potential. *Scandinavian Audiology, 10,* 141–147.

Kirikae, I. (1965). Auditory function in advanced age with reference to histological changes in the central auditory system. *International Audiology, 8,* 221-230.

Lane, R.H., Mendel, M.I., & Kupperman, G.L. (1974). Phase distortion of averaged electroencephalic response. *Archives of Otolaryngology, 99,* 428-432.

Lang, A.H., Happonen, J.H., & Salmivalli, A. (1981). An improved technique for the non-invasive recording of ABR with a specially constructed electrode. *Scandinavian Audiology (Supplement), 13,* 59-62.

Laukli, E., & Mair, I.W.S. (1981). Early auditory-evoked responses: Filter effects. *Audiology, 20,* 300-312.

Lev, A., & Sohmer, H. (1972). Sources of averaged neural responses recorded in animal and human subjects during cochlear audiometry (electrocochleography). *Arch Ohr Nas Kehik Heilk, 201,* 79-90.

Martin, J.E., & Coates, A.C. (1973). Short latency auditory evoked responses recorded from the human nasopharynx. *Brain Research, 60,* 496-502.

Martin, M., & Moore, E. (1977). Scalp distribution of early (0-10 msec) auditory evoked responses. *Archives of Otolaryngology, 103,* 326-328.

Mauldin, L., & Jerger, J.J. (1979). Auditory brain stem evoked responses to bone-conducted signals. *Archives of Otolaryngology, 105,* 656-661.

Maurizi, M., Altissimi, G., Ottaviani, F., Paludetti, G., & Bambini, M. (1982). Auditory brainstem responses (ABR) in the aged. *Scandinavian Audiology, 11,* 213-221.

Michalewski, H.J., Thompson, L.W., Patterson, J. V., Bowman, T., & Litzelman, S. (1980). Sex differences in the amplitudes and latencies of the human auditory brain stem potential. *Electroencephalography and Clinical Neurophysiology, 48,* 351-356.

Møller, K., & Blegvad, B. (1976). Brainstem responses in patients with sensorineural hearing loss. Monaural versus binaural stimulation. The significance of audiogram configuration. *Scandinavian Audiology, 5,* 115-127.

Musiek, F.E., Kibbe, K., Rackliffe, L., & Weider, D.J. (1984). The auditory brain stem response I-V amplitude ratio in normal, cochlear and retrocochlear ears. *Ear and Hearing, 5,* 52-55.

Olphen, A.F. van, Rodenburg, M., & Verwey, C. (1978). Distribution of brainstem responses to acoustic stimulation over the human scalp. *Audiology, 17,* 511-518.

Olphen, A.F. van, Rodenburg, M., & Verwey, C. (1979). Influence of the stimulus repetition rate on brain-stem-evoked responses in man. *Audiology, 18,* 388-394.

Ornitz, E.M., & Walter, D.O. (1975). The effect of sound pressure waveform on human brain stem evoked responses. *Brain Research, 92,* 490-498.

Otto, W.C., & McCandless, G.A. (1982). Aging and the auditory brain stem response. *Audiology, 21,* 466-473.

Parker, D.J. (1981). Dependence of the auditory brain stem response on electrode location. *Archives of Otolaryngology, 107,* 367-371.

Picton, T.W., Hillyard, S.A., Krauz, H.I., & Galambos, R. (1974). Human auditory evoked potentials. I. Evaluation of components. *Electroencephalography and Clinical Neurophysiology, 36,* 179-190.

Picton, T.W., Stapells, D.R., & Campbell, K.R. (1981). Auditory evoked potentials from the human cochlea and brainstem. *Journal of Otolaryngology (Supplement), 9,* 1-41.

Picton, T.W., Woods, D.L., Baribeau-Braun, J., & Healey, T.M.G. (1977). Evoked potential audiometry. *Journal of Otolaryngology, 6,* 90-119.

Pratt, H., & Sohmer, H. (1976). Intensity and rate functions of cochlear and brainstem evoked responses to click stimulation in man. *Archives of Otorhinolaryngology, 212,* 85-92.

Reid, A., & Thornton, A.R.D. (1983). The effects of contralateral masking upon brainstem electric responses. *British Journal of Audiology, 17,* 155-162.

Robinson, K., & Rudge, P. (1977). Abnormalities of the auditory evoked potential in patients with multiple sclerosis. *Brain, 100,* 19-40.

Rosenhamer, H. (1981). Brainstem changes in chronic alcoholism revealed by ABR. *Scandinavian Audiology (Supplement), 13,* 133-134.

Rosenhamer, H., & Holmkvist, C. (1982). Bilaterally recorded auditory brainstem response to monaural stimulation. *Scandinavian Audiology, 11,* 197-202.

Rosenhamer, H. & Holmkvist, C. (1983). Will contralateral white noise interfere with the monaurally click evoked brainstem response? *Scandinavian Audiology, 12,* 11-14.

Rosenhamer, H.J., Lindstrom, B., & Lundborg, J. (1978). On the use of click evoked electric brainstem responses in audiologic diagnosis. I. The variability of the normal response. *Scandinavian Audiology, 7,* 193-206.

Rosenhamer, H.J., Lindstrom, B., & Lundborg, J. (1980). On the use of click evoked electric brainstem responses in audiological diagnosis. II. The influence of sex and age upon the normal response. *Scandinavian Audiology, 9,* 93-100.

Rowe, M.J. (1978). Normal variability of the brainstem auditory evoked responses in young and old adult subjects. *Electroencephalography and Clinical Neurophysiology, 44,* 459-470.

Rowe, M.J. (1981). The brainstem auditory evoked response in neurological disease: A review. *Ear and Hearing, 2,* 41-51.

Ruth, R.A., Hildenbrand, D.L., & Cantrell, R.W. (1982). A study of methods used to enhance wave I in the auditory brain stem response. *Otolaryngology and Head and Neck Surgery, 90,* 635-640.

Salamy, A., & McKean, C.M. (1976). Postnatal development of human brain stem potentials during the first year of life. *Electroencephalography and Clinical Neurophysiology, 40,* 418-426.

Salamy, A., McKean, C.M., & Buda, F.B. (1975). Maturational changes in auditory transmission as reflected in human brain stem potentials. *Brain Research, 96,* 361-366.

Sanders, J.W. (1978). Masking. In J. Katz (Ed.), *Handbook of clinical audiology.* Baltimore: Williams & Wilkins.

Schulman-Galambos, C., & Galambos, R. (1975). Brainstem auditory evoked responses in premature infants. *Journal of Speech & Hearing Research, 18,* 456-465.

Schwartz, D.M., & Fadden, D.M. (1981). *Effect of bone conduction oscillator type and placement on the auditory brainstem response: A pilot study.* Paper presented at the Northeast Regional Meeting of the American Speech-Language-Hearing Association, Philadelphia, June.

Schwartz, D.M., Olsen, K., Berry, G.A., & Murray, B. M. (1981). *Auditory evoked potentials in severe head injury.* Paper presented at the annual convention of the American Speech-Language-Hearing Association, Cincinatti, November.

Staewen, W.S., Allison, D., Harris, K., Krumholz, A., & Goldstein, P. (1980). Determining acoustic condensation and rarefaction of earphones for brain stem auditory evoked responses. *American Journal of EEG Technology, 20,* 133-138.

Starr, A., & Achor, J. (1975). Auditory brain stem responses in neurological disease. *Archives of Neurology, 32,* 761-768.

Starr, A., Amlie, R. N., Martin, W. H., & Sanders, S. (1977). Development of auditory function in newborn infants revealed by auditory brainstem potentials. *Pediatrics, 60,* 831-839.

Stackenburg, M., & Wit, H. P. (1983). Piezoelectric earphone for artifactfree recording of auditory brainstem responses (ABR). *Scandinavian Audiology, 12,* 79-80.

Stockard, J.J., & Rossiter, V.S. (1977). Clinical and pathologic correlates of brain stem auditory response abnormalities. *Neurology, 27,* 316-325.

Stockard, J.J., Stockard, J.E., & Sharbrough, F.W. (1977). Detection and localization of occult lesions with brain stem auditory responses. *Mayo Clinic Proceedings, 52,* 761-769.

Stockard, J.J., Stockard, J.E., & Sharbrough, F.W. (1978). Nonpathologic factors influencing brainstem auditory evoked potentials. *American Journal of EEG Technology, 18,* 177-209.

Stockard, J.J., Stockard, J.E., & Sharbrough, F.W. (1980). Brainstem evoked potentials in neurology: Methodology, interpretation, clinical application. In M.J. Aminoff (Ed.), *Electrodiagnosis in clinical neurology.* New York: Churchill Livingstone.

Stockard, J.J., Sharbrough, F. W., & Tinker, J.A. (1978). Effects of hypothermia on the human brain stem auditory response. *Annals of Neurology, 3,* 368–370.

Stockard, J.E., Stockard, J.J., Westmoreland, B.F., & Corfits, J.L. (1979). Brainstem auditory evoked responses: Normal variation as a function of stimulus and subject characteristics. *Archives of Neurology, 36,* 823–831.

Suzuki, T., & Horiuchi, K. (1977). Effect of high-pass filter on auditory brain stem responses to tone pips. *Scandinavian Audiology, 6,* 123–126.

Terkildsen, K., & Osterhammel, P. (1981). The influence of reference electrode position on recordings of the auditory brainstem response. *Ear and Hearing, 2,* 9–14.

Terkildsen, K., Osterhammel, P., & Huis in't Veld, F. (1973). Far field electrocochleography electrode positions. *Scandinavian Audiology, 2,* 141–148.

Terkildsen, K., Osterhammel, P., & Huis in't Veld, F. (1974). Electrocochleography with a far field technique. *Scandinavian Audiology, 3,* 123–129.

Terkildsen, K., Osterhammel, P., & Huis in't Veld, F. (1975). Far field electrocochleography. Frequency specificity of the response. *Scandinavian Audiology, 4,* 167–172.

Terkildsen, K., Osterhammel, P., & Huis in't Veld, F. (1977). Recording procedures for brainstem potentials. In R.F., Naunton, & C. Fernandez, (Eds.), *Evoked electrical activity in auditory nervous system.* New York: Academic Press.

Thomsen, J., Terkildsen, K., & Osterhammel, P. (1978). Auditory brainstem responses in patients with acoustic neuroma. *Scandinavian Audiology, 7,* 179–183.

Thornton, A.R.D. (1975). Bilaterally recorded early acoustic responses. *Scandinavian Audiology, 4,* 173–181.

Thornton, A.R.D. (1976). Statistical properties of electrocochleographic responses and their use in clinical diagnosis. In R.J. Ruben, C. Elberling, & G. Salomon (Eds.), *Electrocochleography.* Baltimore: University Park Press.

Thornton, A.R.D. (1978). *Methodology and clinical application of brain stem responses.* Proceedings of 3rd International Symposium on Auditory Evoked Responses. Milan: CRS Amplifon Foundation.

Thornton, A.R.D. (1982). AER audiometry: A view from Great Britain. *Hearing Aid Journal, 35,* 14–16.

Thornton, A.R.D. (1983). Standardisation in evoked response measurements. *British Journal of Audiology, 17,* 115–116.

Townsend, T. H., & Schwartz, D.M. (1976). Calculation of effective masking using one octave and one-third octave analysis. *Audiology and Hearing Education, 2,* 27–34.

Tweel, L.H., van der, Estevez, O., & Strackee, J. (1980). Measurement of evoked potentials. In C. Barber, (Ed.), *Evoked potentials.* Lancaster: MTP Press.

Walter, B., & Blegvad, B. (1981). Identification of wave I by means of atraumatic ear canal electrode. *Scandinavian Audiology (Supplement), 13,* 63–67.

Weber, B. (1982). Comparison of auditory brain stem response latency norms for premature infants. *Ear and Hearing, 3,* 257–262.

Weber, B.A. (1983). Masking and bone conduction testing in brainstem response audiometry. *Seminars in Audiology, 4,* 343–352.

Weber, B.A., Seitz, M.R., & McCutcheon, M.J. (1981). Quantifying click stimuli in auditory brainstem response audiometry. *Ear and Hearing, 2,* 15–19.

Worthington, D.W., & Peters, J.F. (1980). Electrophysiologic audiometry. *Annals of Otology, Rhinology, and Laryngology, 74,* 59–62.

Zollner, Chr., Karnahl, Th., & Stange, G. (1976). Input–output function and adaptation behaviour of the five early potentials registered with the earlobe-vertex pick-up. *Archives of Otology, Rhinology, and Laryngology, 212,* 23–33.

Chapter 6

Interpretation: Problems and Pitfalls

Bruce A. Weber

Earlier chapters of this book provide the reader with basic information needed to understand the nature of the auditory brainstem response (ABR) and factors that influence it. The immediately preceding chapter opened the discussion of the clinical applications of ABR audiometry with a consideration of normative data. This chapter considers ABR audiometry as a clinical tool with special emphasis on the problems and pitfalls encountered in the interpretation of the test results. The intent of this chapter is twofold: (1) to provide the reader with practical clinical information and (2) to help dispel the notion that ABR audiometry is a simple procedure that can be readily mastered.

The chapter is divided into two major sections. The first is devoted to ABR as it is used to assess peripheral hearing status and the second considers ABR as a technique for the detection of retrocochlear lesions. Several examples and illustrations are provided for the purpose of preparing the reader for more diagnostic use of ABR described in the remainder of this book.

HEARING ASSESSMENT

Whenever possible the audiologist utilizes behavioral audiometry to determine an individual's hearing status. Behavioral testing with speech and pure tones is preferred over electrophysiological procedures because the responses more fully describe the patient's auditory reception abilities. Unfortunately, there are individuals (e.g., the very young and the multiply handicapped) who cannot be satisfactorily tested with behavioral audiometric procedures. For such patients ABR is often an effective alternative. However, when the ABR is used to evaluate hearing status the examiner and those who read the resulting report should be aware of the technique's limitations and problem areas. Some of these interpretive difficulties are discussed below.

Relationship of the ABR to Behavioral Hearing

There is justification for the view that ABR audiometry is not a test of hearing. Clearly, as its name implies, the ABR is generated at anatomic levels below the auditory cortex, so the response does not reflect the conscious perceptual processing which is normally included in a definition of hearing. The ABR is generated only by a subgroup of auditory fibers called "time keepers," which precisely record time of stimulus arrival (Hecox, Squires, & Galambos, 1976). These fibers probably play a role in such time-related activities as sound localization, but there is a real question about whether their synchronous firings are essential for other aspects of auditory perception. The ABR itself may be only a nonessential by-product (epiphenomenon) of the activity of a small portion of the auditory system. Thus, ABR test results should not be interpreted in the same manner as behavioral audiometric test results.

A patient with a cortical auditory impairment may show abnormal behavioral responses to sound yet demonstrate a normal ABR. Likewise, there is evidence that neurological disorders, such as multiple sclerosis (Robinson & Rudge, 1977), can affect the auditory brainstem and disrupt the function of the timekeeper fibers. This disruption may affect the generation of the ABR while leaving intact those fibers with are essential for other aspects of hearing (Picton, 1978). The difference between behavioral hearing and the ABR is also apparent in the report by Worthington and Peters (1980), which describes four children with no neurologic evidence of brain dysfunction who demonstrated quantifiable hearing and no ABR. Although each of these children possessed some form of auditory disorder, the ABR test results grossly misrepresented the children's peripheral hearing status as measured by behavioral audiometry.

For the vast majority of patients, there is relatively good agreement between ABR test results and behavioral hearing thresholds for frequencies between 2000 and 4000 Hz. One must remember, however, that for all patients the two procedures are tapping the auditory system in markedly different ways. Though most of its major components are generated within the central nervous system, the presence of an ABR cannot be used as an indicator that the patient was consciously aware of the test stimulus. In contrast to behavioral audiometry, which requires a conscious response, the presence of an ABR merely indicates the test stimulus has produced a disturbance in the peripheral hearing mechanism that has been transmitted to the level of the brainstem. It is more appropriate, therefore, to view the results of ABR as estimating the status of the patient's peripheral hearing mechanism. Describing ABR as a test of peripheral hearing, though not totally satisfactory, at least acknowledges that it is not a test of the central aspects of audition, which occur at the level of the cortex. It is easy to forget this fact and conclude that a patient has no hearing problem if ABRs are obtained at a low signal intensity level. The examiner must always remember that significant central auditory problems may exist in a small minority of patients who show normal ABR test results. Even when the examiner is aware of this, he or she may not adequately convey this distinction to parents and other professionals. It is not always easy to discuss these limitations without undermining others' confidence in the value of the test procedure.

Because behavioral audiometry and ABR testing do not tap the auditory system in the same manner, one should not be too surprised when the two procedures produce different test results. When air-conduction and bone-conduction thresholds are not in agreement, it does not imply that one is in error. If ABR audiometry is conceptualized as its own unique *look* at the auditory system, differences between ABR and behavioral testing can be understood as providing useful information. For example, normal ABRs from a nonresponsive child strongly suggest central rather than peripheral reasons for the child's behavior. However, if ABR is thought of solely as a substitute or a double-check for behavioral testing, serious errors in diagnosis can be expected when synchronous evoked potentials from the brainstem fail to accurately estimate a patient's behavioral hearing status.

Time Considerations

Because one of the foremost characteristics of the ABR is its reproducibility, most examiners prefer to replicate each stimulus condition to determine if the pairs of tracings sufficiently superimpose on each other. Good agreement between the two tracings helps ensure that the observed waves demonstrate a response rather than merely reflecting random occurrences. In many instances the two tracings agree well and it is not difficult to decide if a response has occurred. Likewise, very poor agreement between tracings convincingly argues against a detectable response. Unfortunately, there are times when there is some, but not good, agreement between replications of the same stimulus condition. When this occurs during the course of a test, the examiner must make a decision regarding the most appropriate next stimulus condition.

It is at this point that two conflicting goals are encountered. On the one hand, the examiner wants to carefully evaluate the previous tracings in order to decide if stimulus intensity should be raised, lowered, or if an additional run is needed at the same intensity level. On the other hand, ABR is a time-consuming procedure and the examiner must move briskly or testing may not be completed before the patient becomes restless or awakens. Thus, the examiner must attempt to make quick decisions regarding the most appropriate parameters for the next stimulus run even when ambiguous responses are encountered. Because each stimulus run (plus plotting if necessary) adds minutes to the testing time, these decisions cannot be made casually. This is in marked contrast with behavioral audiometry, where just a few seconds are needed to present another test stimulus to help determine if the patient responds at a given intensity level. In ABR, the examiner is continually torn between gathering data as quickly as possible and making certain that the tracings have been carefully examined before moving on to the next stimulus intensity. Decisions regarding appropriate stimulus intensity and when to move to the other ear are not always easy to make. This fact becomes quite apparent to the examiner when trying to interpret marginal quality tracings from a fussy infant who is likely to fully awaken at any moment. Inappropriate use of the test time may result in incomplete and/or misleading test results.

Carefully monitoring the ABR equipment's oscilloscope during each stimulus run can help reduce the difficulty in interpreting the resulting ABRs. A response to the test stimulus should build rather smoothly in computer memory. Thus, by monitoring the memory display in the oscilloscope, the examiner should be able to distinguish between waves which systematically grow in size and those artifacts which appear abruptly during the stimulus run. Waiting until a run is completed before attempting interpretation ignores valuable information. It is also important to monitor the quality of the incoming bioelectric activity from the patient, so the examiner is forced to alternate between observations of patient input and computer memory during each run. Adding a second monitor oscilloscope to the test equipment eliminates this problem.

Subjectivity of ABR Audiometry

Aside from the on-line analysis which must occur during the ABR test itself (as described above), most interpretation consists of an examination of the tracings after the testing is completed. ABR is frequently viewed as an objective procedure because acquisition of the test results is not dependent upon the patient's conscious cooperation. Interpretation of the results, however, is highly subjective. In spite of the use of sophisticated computers and electrophysiologic recordings, the examiner must look at pairs of wavy lines and make a number of very subjective decisions regarding the presence or absence of a response. Whenever possible, the examiner must also attempt to locate component waves of the ABR so that latency measurements can be made. The skill required to make these decisions is frequently underestimated. Though the ABR is highly repeatable and easily recognized in high-quality recording conditions (e.g., with a cooperative normal hearing adult), the response can be very illusive when a hearing-impaired patient is being evaluated. Unfortunately, there is no clear-cut boundary between accurately detecting subtle responses and reading responses into tracings that contain none. Therefore, it is not surprising that some clinicians become frustrated with ABR when their test results do not approach the quality necessary to make easy decisions regarding the presence or absence of a response. With increased experience most examiners can improve their ability to interpret ambiguous ABR tracings, but this skill does not come quickly, especially if the clinician is primarily self-taught. Even the most experienced examiner encounters patients who present test results that are difficult or impossible to interpret. It may be difficult to accept that a long and expensive test session yielded little useful information.

Ideally, the examiner should score ABR tracings without knowledge of stimulus intensity so that this information will not bias interpretive decisions. For example, if the examiner has scored a response at 40 dB HL it is likely that he or she will be biased toward also scoring a response at a higher stimulus intensity (e.g., 60 dB). It is difficult, if not impossible, not to be influenced by this stimulus information. Blind judgments would reduce examiner bias, but are not practical in ABR because one of the most sensitive indicators of a response is the shift in response latency that occurs with changes in stimulus intensity. This latency shift can only be observed when a patient's ABR tracings are examined in relation to stimulus intensity. Without knowledge of stimulus intensity, the examiner would be greatly handicapped in the attempt to judge whether an ABR has occurred. On the other hand, when one does rely on information about stimulus intensity, it is imperative to realize that the test procedure provides no means for evaluating the validity of the judgments made. Control (no-stimulus) runs serve a useful function, but they do not help validate the observer's judgments. This is because there is no real likelihood that a control tracing will be scored as a response. There are objective computerized ABR scoring techniques (Elberling, 1979; Weber & Fletcher, 1980), but these require sophisticated equipment not available in most ABR testing facilities.

Estimating Hearing Threshold from ABR Latencies

In its simplest form, ABR involves the presentation of click stimuli at different intensity levels while detecting the lowest level that produces an observable response. It must always be remembered, however, that the lack of a detectable ABR does not ensure that no response has occurred. For most clinical patients, even sedated ones, it is not reasonable to expect that ABRs will always be detectable at the patient's behavioral hearing threshold. If the patient is restless or if there is excessive contamination from outside sources (e.g., 60 Hz interference), the stimulus may need to be somewhat above behavioral hearing threshold before an ABR can be distinguished from the non-stimulus-related activity. Therefore, absence of a detectable ABR at a given stimulus intensity does not rule out the possibility that the patient responded to the stimulus. A response may have been present, but it could not be observed under the given test conditions.

Because judgments regarding the presence or absence of a response are often not a sufficient analysis of the ABR test results, response latency is also used whenever possible to provide additional information. The latencies of the ABR component waves increase as stimulus intensity is reduced, so it is possible to compare the resulting latency values (usually for wave V) with clinic norms. As shown in Figure 6-1, no ABRs were detected from the patient's right ear below 30 dB HL, but all latency values fall within the normal range. These findings allow the examiner to extrapolate from the test results to conclude that the patient's peripheral hearing in this ear is within grossly normal limits. The left ear also showed responses down to 30 dB HL, but all latencies are extended beyond the clinic norms (area within the box). These findings are consistent with a mild hearing loss. Thus, ABR latencies may provide information not available from the lowest stimulus intensity that produced a detectable response.

Though the use of ABR latency is of clinical value, the technique is not always as straightforward as it may initially appear. Even when it is clear that a response is present, it may not be easy to assign a precise latency value to wave V. There often is a fusing of waves IV and V which results in a mound-shaped wave rather than a distinct peak. There may also be multiple bumps in the region of wave V, so that is is difficult to determine which bump

FIGURE 6–1.
ABR latency/intensity plot for a young child. Wave V latencies for the right ear are shown as circles and x's indicate the latencies for the left ear. The boxed area indicates normal response latencies.

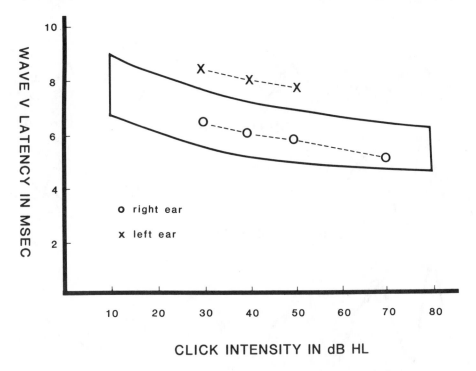

CLICK INTENSITY IN dB HL

is actually wave V. There may also be poor agreement between the two replications at a given intensity level, so that the examiner is forced to make a compromise latency measurement. Further, young infants characteristically show rather cyclic ABRs in which the component waves have similar morphology (Jacobson, Morehouse, & Johnson, 1982); it is not always clear which component waves should be identified as waves III and V. Even when waves can be readily identified and latencies measured with confidence, the precision of the extrapolation technique is markedly reduced when there are only one or two latency values on which to base a threshold estimation.

There is a further complicating factor in the use of ABR latencies to estimate hearing threshold. At intensity levels above about 60 dB HL a population of neural fibers comes into play that is not activated at lower intensity levels. It is likely that these fibers are related in some manner to the inner hair cells, which are less sensitive to noise and toxic agents. Whatever the exact anatomic basis, these fibers demonstrate little latency shift with increased intensity. Thus, a patient with a marked (e.g., 70 dB) hearing loss may show no detectable ABR at low intensity levels, yet demonstrate a clear response with normal latencies at high intensities. It would be a gross error to conclude that normal ABR latencies at the high stimulus levels demonstrate evidence of normal hearing. The extrapolation technique should never be used if there are no ABRs at levels below 60 dB HL. If responses cannot be detected at lower levels, the examiner must confine the analysis to the lowest stimulus intensity that elicited a detectable response.

FIGURE 6–2.
Comparison of three pairs of tracings obtained from a young infant. (A) Tracings obtained during control runs when no stimulus was presented to the patient. (B) Tracings containing a stimulus artifact, but no evidence of a response. (C) Tracings containing an early stimulus artifact and a later response.

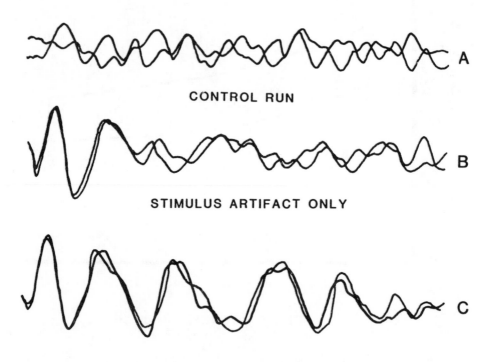

CONTROL RUN

STIMULUS ARTIFACT ONLY

ARTIFACT & RESPONSE

Control Runs

Most examiners obtain at least one pair of control (no-stimulus) tracings at some time during the testing session (see Figure 6-2A). Such tracings are included because they are thought to provide a way of ensuring that the waves seen on stimulus runs are not being produced by nonpatient sources. Any waveform found on a stimulus run which does not also appear on control tracings is routinely viewed as a response originating from the patient. It must be remembered, however, that ABR tracings usually contain some stimulus artifact as well as the response itself. Especially at high intensities, a stimulus run may differ in appearance from a control run, not because of an ABR, but because a stimulus artifact has contaminated part of the stimulus tracing. This is of particular importance when the latter portions of the stimulus artifact appear similar to the wave I component of the ABR (see Figure 6-2B). It is important to remember that the later components of the ABR (usually wave V) have the greatest amplitude. Thus, pairs of tracings containing a response usually show the greatest agreement in the middle and later portions of the tracing (see Figure 6-2C). When the first portion shows the best agreement the examiner should view the "response" with suspicion.

The use of controls creates an additional pitfall: the tendency to apply different quality standards for control and stimulus runs. To conserve memory space within the averaging computer, it is routine clinical practice to discard any tracing that contains unacceptably large contaminating movement artifacts. If large waves develop during a control run, the examiner is likely to terminate averaging because it is known that such waves cannot be a response. The examiner erases computer memory and repeats the run. In contrast, at stimulus intensities where an ABR is anticipated the examiner may be more likely to accept tracings containing large amplitude waves as possible responses because it is difficult to differentiate artifacts from an actual response. As a result, a stimulus run containing significant artifact contamination (but no response) could be erroneously scored as a response primarily because it differs markedly from the less contaminated control runs. If a more stringent criterion for an acceptable tracing is applied to control runs than to stimulus runs, serious interpretation errors can result.

Artifact Rejection

It is often assumed that the quality of an ABR can be determined by examining the number of rejected sweeps that occurred during the stimulus run. The fewer the number of rejected sweeps, the better the quality of the tracing is thought to be. In actuality, just the opposite may be true. The artifact reject function on most clinical ABR test equipment simply throws out any sweep that contains an amplitude that exceeds some acceptable voltage limit. Thus, the amplitude of the incoming electrophysiologic signal from the patient is of critical importance because it determines how great an increase in voltage will be accepted by the test equipment before the artifact reject function comes into play. Imagine a patient from whom the test equipment is recording a low-voltage electrophysiologic signal (see Figure 6-3A). Movement artifacts producing fairly sizeable increases in this signal's amplitude may still not be of sufficient amplitude to exceed the maximum acceptable voltage limits and result in a rejected sweep. Thus, the number of rejected sweeps will be quite small because contaminated samples are included in the averaged response; not necessarily because the input is of high quality. In contrast, an electrophysiologic signal free of stimulus artifacts may have an amplitude that is extremely close to the maximum acceptable limit so that the slightest increase creates a rejected sweep (see Figure 6-3B). In this situation, only the cleanest of the sweeps would be included in the averaged response. Thus, in spite of a large number of rejected sweeps, the tracings in the latter case would be of higher quality than the tracing obtained with a small number of rejected sweeps. Reducing the amplitude of a contaminated signal by lowering the amplifier gain will reduce the number of rejected sweeps. This may give the illusion of improving the quality of the recording, but in actuality, this move will reduce the quality of the resulting ABRs by accepting a more contaminated input. Therefore, it is critical that the amplifier gain (or signal averager sensitivity) be adjusted so that the incoming electrophysiologic signal is very near the artifact rejection threshold.

Even when the amplitude of the input from the patient is properly adjusted, the artifact reject function cannot be expected to eliminate all movement artifacts. Readers can demonstrate this to themselves by testing a cooperative adult under quiet and actively moving conditons. Swallowing, chewing, and eyeblinks can all cause contamination of the ABR tracings in spite of the test equipment's artifact reject function. It is important, therefore, that the examiner realize that the artifact reject capability reduces, but does not eliminate, contaminating artifacts.

FIGURE 6-3.
Effects of the amplitude of the electrophysiologic input from the patient on the rejection of movement artifacts. The artifact reject levels are shown as dashed lines. (A) Small amplitude input containing movement artifacts. (B) Large amplitude input without movement artifacts.

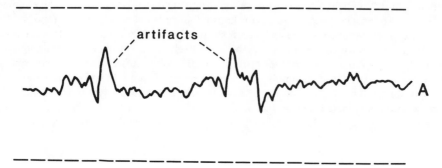

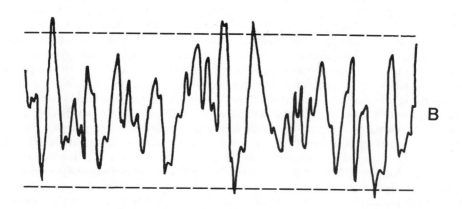

RETROCOCHLEAR TESTING

The ABR is a highly sensitive technique for detecting the presence of a retrocochlear lesion (Bauch, Rose, & Harner, 1982). Rather than attempting to assess peripheral status, as described above, the examiner routinely performs this testing on an individual whose hearing status can be readily assessed with behavioral audiometry. The aim of ABR retrocochlear testing is to stimulate the auditory system with high-intensity (e.g., 80 dB HL) click stimuli in order to clearly define the component waves in the response. Particular attention is given to the latency of the interwave intervals. When wave I cannot be identified, the time intervals from stimulus onset to the appearance of waves III and V are examined for each ear and asymmetry between ears is used to evaluate the status of the eighth nerve and auditory brainstem. Because the patient receiving retrocochlear ABR testing has routinely had a thorough behavioral audiometric evaluation, most of the interpretation problems described earlier in this chapter are of less concern. There are, however, a unique set of pitfalls and some of them are discussed below.

Asymmetrical Hearing

Because the goal of ABR retrocochlear testing is to assess the status of the auditory system central to the cochlea, it is important to minimize the effects of any peripheral hearing asymmetry between the two ears. This is particularly critical when one or both ears are unlikely to produce a detectable wave I which can be used as a temporal benchmark for the initial activation of the neural system.

A technique sometimes used to offset the effects of asymmetrical hearing involves the presentation of click stimuli at equal sensation levels (e.g., 70 dB above the patient's behavioral threshold for the click stimulus at each ear). This approach is used in an attempt to compare latency differences between the two ears independent of any differences in peripheral hearing status. Some problems, however, are engendered by this technique. For patients with a marked (e.g., 60 dB) unilateral hearing loss, the stimulus to the poorer ear cannot be presented at a high sensation level because the maximum equipment output is usually approximately 100 dB. In the above example this would result in only a 40-dB SL click stimulus in the poorer ear. To maintain equal sensation levels for such a patient, a 40-dB SL stimulus would also have to be presented to the better ear. This would result in the use of a much less than optimum intensity level in the better hearing ear in order to maintain equal sensation levels between ears.

Equal sensation levels may be grossly misleading because the ear with the highest threshold may demonstrate a recruitment-like phenomenon. At higher intensity level there may be much less asymmetry between ears than exists at threshold. Thus, equal sensation levels do not ensure equally loud stimuli. To avoid this problem, it is possible to equate the loudness in the two ears using a loudness balancing technique at the desired stimulation level. For example, an 80-dB HL click can be presented to the better ear and the intensity to the poorer ear can be adjusted to match it in loudness. When the hearing in the two ears permits such balancing, this approach avoids the problem of differences in the loudness growth in the two ears. Unfortunately, it also raises another concern: Can behavioral responses be used to balance effective stimulation levels in an electrophysiologic test such as ABR? The answer is clearly "no." One cannot equate the effectiveness of two stimuli in evoking an electrophysiologic response by matching them on some perceptual dimension because different aspects of the click stimulus elicit the two responses.

With unfiltered click stimuli, the frequencies between approximately 2000 and 4000 Hz play the primary role in eliciting the ABR. Frequencies below about 1000 Hz will have a major influence in the patient's behavioral threshold to the click and its loudness, but these frequencies play only a small role in eliciting the ABR. Thus, a patient with a sharply sloping unilateral hearing loss may show a near normal behavioral threshold to the click (and normal loudness levels) in the poorer ear because of good low-frequency hearing. However, equal behavioral thresholds or equal loudness levels for the two ears do not ensure that the level of the click stimuli will be matched in the critical 2000- to 4000-Hz frequency range for eliciting the ABR.

Because there is no satisfactory method for matching the effective level of stimulation to the two ears, it is recommended that equal physical levels be applied. The most convenient method is to use equal attenuator settings (e.g., 80 dB above 0 dB level used for ABR hearing testing). This approach at least provides the examiner with the knowledge that the same physical stimulus was applied to each ear. The problem of hearing asymmetry is thus addressed when the examiner interprets the resulting ABR tracings. This topic is considered later in this chapter.

Peak Picking

The "textbook" ABR tracings usually exhibit clearly defined waves I through V, with each component wave possessing a sharp peak. Precise latency measurements can be readily performed

FIGURE 6–4.
Pairs of tracings obtained from a patient suspected of possessing a retrocochlear lesion. Note how the fusing of waves IV and V obscures the latencies of these waves.

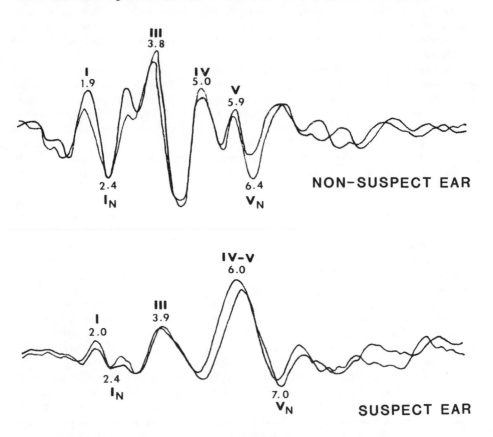

on such ABRs, but clinical patients with significant hearing impairments frequently do not demonstrate such high-quality responses. For patients with a marked high-frequency hearing loss, wave I may be absent and later waves may appear as rounded mounds rather than sharp peaks. In such instances it is impossible to assign any latency to some waves, while only gross approximations (e.g., ± 0.2 ms) can be made on others. Certainly the examiner should not report latency values in hundredths of a millisecond when there is a question about exact peak location.

ABR retrocochlear testing is often conducted on patients with asymmetrical hearing because it is this form of hearing loss which raises questions about a possible retrocochlear lesion in the first place. For such patients it may be easy to assign latencies to waves I, III, and V in the better (nonsuspect) ear, but considerable difficulty may be encountered with the poorer (suspect) ear. There are potential problems when precise latency measurements from one ear are compared with grosser approximations from the other ear. As shown in Figure 6-4 the latency of wave V may be readily distinguished from wave IV in the nonsuspect right ear, but the ABR from the suspect left ear may show a fused IV-V wave which obscured the true location of wave V. If the examiner selects the peak of the IV-V complex as the location of wave V in the suspect ear, an underestimation of its latency will result. Because the examiner cannot merely select the location where wave V is thought likely to be, it is recommended that latencies of other components of the ABR be measured. Often the troughs following waves I and V are quite distinct (see I_N and V_N in Figure 6-4) and provide a sensitive alternative measure of response latency.

When poor or marginal quality tracings are encountered in retrocochlear testing, it is important for the examiner to make every attempt to improve the quality of the recordings during the actual test, possibly including such techniques as reinstructing the patient to remain quiet with the eyes closed, increasing stimulus intensity, increasing the number of sweeps averaged, reducing the stimulus repetition rate, and the inclusion of additional runs. Frequently the analysis of the ABRs can be aided by adding a contralateral recording channel (i.e., forehead or vertex compared with the non-test earlobe or mastoid). Such a recording tends to highlight wave II and often produces a greater separation of waves IV and V than occurs with an ipsilateral recording. Using the forehead or vertex electrode as the patient ground and comparing the electrical activity at the two ears may produce a tracing with a detectable wave I because, in the adult, later components of the ABR are markedly reduced in amplitude. Comparing ipsilateral, contralateral, and horizontal recordings can assist the examiner in the analysis of ambiguous ABR records.

Once the testing has been completed and the patient has departed, the examiner has lost the chance to acquire more test data. Therefore, it is critical that the examiner be satisfied that all essential data have been gathered before testing is discontinued. Many problems in ABR analysis could be eliminated or markedly reduced if a preliminary analysis of the test results were conducted before the recording electrodes were removed from the patient's head.

Interwave Intervals

Although response amplitude, waveform morphology, and the latencies of component waves provide useful clinical information, most examiners rely on extended ABR interwave intervals (IWIs) as the most sensitive indicator of a retrocochlear lesion. A patient's I–III, III–V, and I–V intervals are routinely compared between ears and with clinic norms. Though retrocochlear lesions impacting the eighth nerve or lower brainstem should have their greatest effect on the I–III interval, few clinicians would classify ABR findings as abnormal unless the I–V interval is also abnormally extended. Wave V is included in the analysis because it is usually of larger amplitude and has less interpatient variability than the less stable wave III.

It is convenient to think that the time from stimulus onset to the occurrence of wave I reflects the status of the outer, middle, and inner ears (peripheral conduction time) and the ABR IWIs reflect eighth nerve and brainstem status (central conduction time) free from peripheral contamination. Unfortunately, the situation is not this straightforward. It has been shown that *cochlear* hearing loss causes a greater shift in the latency of wave I than for either wave III or V (Coats, 1978). This greater latency prolongation of wave I results in a reduction in the I–III and I–V IWIs. For some patients this facilitates differential diagnosis because a small IWI is a strong indicator of a cochlear lesion. However, for patients with both a cochlear loss (e.g., a unilateral noise-induced loss) and a possible retrocochlear lesion in the same ear, the clinician must question whether the two disorders may offset one another, resulting in grossly normal IWIs. The matter is further complicated when one remembers that a retrocochlear lesion can disrupt the blood supply to the cochlea, resulting in a combined cochlear and retrocochlear impairment.

Stockard and Stockard (1981) have set some absolute prerequisites for interpreting I–V IWIs between ears. They require that the peripheral hearing in the two ears be equivalent and that the wave I latencies from the ears be within 0.1 ms of each other. Becuase interwave latency differences between ears could be due to peripheral factors, they recommend that IWIs not be compared if the patient's wave I latencies are asymmetric. Though such strict criteria may be reasonable for normal hearing patients with suspected neurologic disorders, they cannot be reasonably applied to patients whose peripheral hearing asymmetry is the primary reason for their referral for ABR audiometry. The examiner who tests hearing-impaired individuals commonly encounters some wave I asymmetry. When such asymmetry is present it must be remembered that some unmeasured peripheral contamination of the I–III and I–V intervals may have occurred.

All ABR labs should have latency norms for waves I, III, and V. However, as mentioned earlier, latency norms for other components of the ABR are also useful when these waves cannot be identified with confidence. In particular, measuring the latencies of the negative trough following wave I (I_N) and the often very large trough following wave V (V_N) can be of real clinical value when wave I is poorly defined or waves IV and V are fused. It is recommended that clinic latency norms be developed for all component waves of the ABR.

Absence of Wave I

When the ABRs obtained from each ear show clearly observable waves I, III, and V, IWIs are usually the first aspect of the response to be examined. Though not without problems, as discussed above, most clinicians believe that these measurements provide the best means for differentiating cochlear and retrocochlear lesions. For some patients, however, all component waves (usually wave I) cannot be observed in spite of recording techniques aimed at enhancing their detectability. When a patient's ABR fails to show a wave I, IWIs obviously cannot be measured. As an alternative measurement, absolute wave V latency (the time from stimulus onset to the appearance of the wave) is used to test for a retrocochlear lesion. If the latency of wave V falls within normal limits, it is reasonably safe to assume that the patient has no clinically significant prolongation of the IWIs. If, however, wave V latencies from one or both ears are extended beyond normal limits, the examiner must attempt to determine whether this prolongation is due to a peripheral hearing impairment or a retrocochlear lesion. Of particular interest is any asymmetry between ears in the absolute wave V latencies. The interaural time difference for wave V is referred to as IT_5 (Selters & Brackmann, 1977).

Because peripheral hearing loss will influence absolute wave latencies, some correction formula must be used with patients with asymmetrical hearing. Selters and Brackmann (1977) and Hyde and Blair (1981) recommend correcting for hearing loss by reducing wave V latency measurement by an amount based on the ear's audiometric threshold at 4000 Hz. Selters and Brackmann suggest subtracting 0.1 ms from wave V latency for every 10 dB increment the behavioral threshold at 4000 Hz exceeds 50 dB HL. Hyde and Blair recommend a 0.1-ms reduction for every 5 dB the 4000-Hz threshold exceeds 55 dB HL. Such correction factors are simple to use and are of definite clinical value, but a nagging question remains: Is a correction factor based on the patient's hearing at only one frequency adequate to offset any hearing asymmetry? It has been shown that audiogram configuration markedly influences wave V latency (Coats & Martin, 1977; Jerger & Mauldin, 1978). Bauch, Rose, and Harner (1981) report that the value of ABR in detecting a retrocochlear lesion is reduced when a hearing loss is present at 2000 Hz. Thus, the clinician using an ABR latency correction factor based on a hearing threshold at a single frequency must be cautious about its applicability to all hearing-impaired patients.

When wave I is absent, causing the absolute latency of wave V to be the sole latency measurement, a conductive hearing loss can greatly complicate the detection of a retrocochlear lesion. A conductive loss may extend wave V latency over 1 ms, a delay which may, in turn, obscure a much smaller wave V latency shift caused by a retrocochlear lesion. It is possible to utilize the size of the air–bone gap on the behavioral audiogram to estimate the extent of the latency prolongation caused by the conductive impairment. However, for patients with ossicular chain disorders, the wave V latency shift is greater than would be predicted from the audiogram (McGee & Clemis, 1982) and significant errors in interpretation could result. With such patients, ABR cannot be used with confidence in retrocochlear testing if no wave I can be identified.

ABR Morphology

It is well known that the effects of a retrocochlear lesion need not be confined to alterations in ABR latencies. Reduction in the stability of the ABR across replication tracings, abnormally small amplitude, or absent component waves and unusual waveform morphology have been observed in patients with retrocochlear lesions (Nodar, Hahn, & Levine, 1980). Because such abnormalities cannot be quantified like the latencies of component waves, the examiner is forced to make some highly subjective decisions. For example, how poor an agreement between successive ABRs is necessary before it is indicative of some retrocochlear lesion? The decision is particularly difficult when the patient's peripheral hearing loss could explain part, if not all, of the poor-quality ABR recording. Therefore, there is often a large gray area between abnormal and atypical normal responses.

The qualitative aspects of the ABR are likely to convey useful clinical information to the experienced examiner. However, there are also a number of non-pathological factors that can also produce highly similar effects on the ABR (Stockard, Stockard, & Sharbrough, 1978). These factors include electrode placement and impedance, movement artifacts, high-frequency interference from other electrical apparatus, the frequency response of the test earphone, filter settings on the test equipment, and stimulus polarity.

It is also worthy of note that tinnitus may also influence the morphology of the ABR. There is evidence to suggest that when tinnitus is present in a single ear, stimulation of that ear may result in poorer quality responses due to the masking effects of the tinnitus (Seitz, Mundy, & Pappas, 1981). This complication further emphasizes that all deterioration of ABR morphology cannot be attributed to a retrocochlear lesion.

CONCLUSIONS

This chapter addresses a number of problems and pitfalls that may be encountered in the analysis of ABR test results. The intent is not to challenge the clinical value of this procedure for either the estimation of peripheral hearing status or the detection of a retrocochlear lesion. On the contrary, ABR appears to have rightfully secured a firm position among clinically useful audiometric procedures. The primary purpose of this chapter is to convey to the reader some of the complexity of ABR analysis and interpretation. It is hoped that it is now clear to the reader that the technique cannot be mastered by reading a single book such as this or by attending a brief workshop. Unfortunately, there is a real shortage of clinical training opportunities, especially for those no longer enrolled in an academic training program. Therefore, it is incumbent upon the individual just beginning his or her acquaintance with ABR to actively seek assistance from those more experienced in the technique. Likewise, experienced users need to give greater attention to how their clinical insights and expertise can be transmitted to those just beginning their work in this area. The clinical value of any technique, especially one as subjective as ABR, depends primarily on the skills of the individual who administers it. Proliferation of ABR without adequate preparation of the examiner may well be its greatest pitfall.

REFERENCES

Bauch, C. D., Rose, D. E., & Harner, S. G. (1981). Auditory brainstem reponses in ears with hearing loss: Case studies. *Scandinavian Audiology, 10,* 247–254.

Bauch, C. D., Rose, D. E., & Harner, S. G. (1982). Auditory brainstem response results from 255 patients with suspected retrocochlear involvement. *Ear and Hearing, 3,* 83–86.

Coats, A. C., (1978). Human auditory nerve action potentials and brainstem responses: Latency-intensity functions in detection of cochlear and retrocochlear abnormality. *Archives of Otolaryngology, 104,* 709–717.

Coats, A. C., & Martin, J. L. (1977). Human auditory nerve action potentials and brainstem evoked responses: Effects of audiogram shape and lesion location. *Archives of Otolaryngology, 103,* 605–622.

Elberling, C. (1979). Auditory electrophysiology: The use of templates and cross correlation functions in the analysis of brainstem potentials. *Scandinavian Audiology, 8,* 187–190.

Hecox, K., Squires, N., & Galambos, R. (1976). Brainstem auditory evoked responses in man. I. Effect of stimulus rise–fall time and duration. *Journal of the Acoustical Society of America, 60,* 1187–1192.

Hyde, M. L., & Blair, R. L. (1981). The auditory brainstem response in neuro-otology: Perspectives and problems. *Journal of Otolaryngology, 10,* 117–125.

Jacobson, J. T., Morehouse, C. R., & Johnson, M. J. (1982). Strategies for infant auditory brainstem response assessment. *Ear and Hearing, 3,* 263–270.

Jerger, J., & Mauldin, L. (1978). Prediction of sensorineural hearing level from the brain stem evoked response. *Archives of Otolaryngology, 104,* 456–461.

McGee, T. J., & Clemis, J. D. (1982). Effects of conductive hearing loss on auditory brainstem response. *Annals of.Otology, Rhinology and Laryngology, 91,* 304–309.

Nodar, R. H., Hahn, J., & Levine, H. L. (1980). Brain stem auditory evoked potentials in determining site of lesion of brain stem gliomas in children. *Laryngoscope, 90,* 258–265.

Picton, T. (1978). The strategy of evoked potential audiometry. In S. E. Gerber & G. T. Mencher (Eds.), *Early diagnosis of hearing loss.* New York: Grune & Stratton.

Robinson, K., & Rudge, P. (1977). Abnormalities of the auditory evoked potentials in patients with multiple sclerosis. *Brain, 100,* 19–40.

Seitz, M. R., Mundy, M. R., & Pappas, D. G. (1981). *The effects of tinnitus on ABR waveforms.* Paper presented at convention of the American Auditory Society, New Orleans.

Selters, W. A., & Brackmann, D. E. (1977). Acoustic tumor detection with brain stem electric response audiometry. *Archives of Otolaryngology, 103,* 181–187.

Stockard, J. E., & Stockard, J. J. (1981). Brainstem auditory evoked potentials in normal and otoneurologically impaired newborns and infants. In C. E. Henry (Ed.), *Current neurophysiology: EEG and evoked potentials.* Miami/Amsterdam: Elsevier-North Holland.

Stockard, J. J., Stockard, J. E., & Sharbrough, F. (1978). Non-pathologic factors influencing brainstem auditory evoked potentials, Part I. *American Journal of EEG Technology, 18,* 177–193.

Weber, B. A., & Fletcher, G. L. (1980). A computerized scoring procedure for auditory brainstem response audiometry. *Ear and Hearing, 1,* 233–236.

Worthington, D. W., & Peters, J. F. (1980). Quantifiable hearing and no ABR: Paradox or error? *Ear and Hearing, 1,* 281–285.

Chapter 7

Conductive Hearing Loss and the ABR

Terese Finitzo-Hieber
Sandy Friel-Patti

The external and middle ears comprise the conductive mechanism. At the lateral end, the auricle, or pinna, is the visible part of the ear which leads inward to the downward sloping, S-shaped, external auditory meatus (EAM). This canal is approximately 25 mm long and 6-7 mm wide in the adult ear. Its primary acoustic function is to channel sound to the middle ear. At its medial end, the EAM is continuous with the tympanic membrane, which serves as a border between the external and middle ears. The primary function of the middle ear is to transform acoustic energy that strikes the tympanic membrane into hydraulic energy of the fluid-filled inner ear. Both developmental variables and pathological conditions of the external and middle ears can alter the efficiency of this transfer mechanism and, as such, affect the auditory brainstem response (ABR).

In the present chapter, traditional problems in the audiometric assessment of conductive versus sensorineural pathology are discussed as they affect the ABR. This section is followed by a review of our ABR experience with common etiologies of conductive hearing loss. Finally, we present data on using ABR to assist in defining the long-term, psychoeducational sequelae of otitis media (OM) in young children.

EFFECT OF CONDUCTIVE PATHOLOGY ON AIR CONDUCTION ABR

Any external or middle ear disorder which interrupts the transmission of sound to the oval window creates an energy loss, resulting in a conductive hearing impairment. Audiometrically, it is characterized by elevated thresholds for air-conducted sound and relatively normal thresholds for bone conduction.

There is a general consensus that conductive pathology prolongs wave component latency for unmasked air conduction stimuli. While there is less agreement on how to predict the degree of the resulting hearing impairment, examining the wave V latency–intensity function (LIF) has been the most common approach (Eggermont, 1982; Finitzo-Hieber, Hecox, & Cone, 1979; Fria & Sabo, 1980; Hecox & Galambos, 1974; McGee & Clemis, 1982). Figure 7-1 illustrates the wave V LIF, with the hatched area reflecting normative values appropriate after 18 months of age. The amount in decibels by which this function is shifted to the right of the normal function in time is considered to be predictive of the conductive loss. Hecox and Galambos (1974) noted that the slope of the LIF in conductive impairment parallels the normal slope. In their estimation, a 1-dB intensity decrease produces a 30- to 60-μs increase in latency, or

© College-Hill Press, Inc. All rights, including that of translation, reserved. No part of this publication may be reproduced without the written permission of the publisher.

FIGURE 7–1.
A wave V LIF. Hatched area represents normal values appropriate after 12 to 18 months of age.

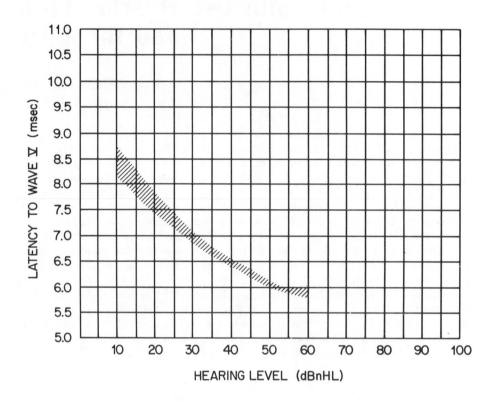

a 0.3- to 0.6-ms latency increase per 10 dB of hearing loss, for the normal subject and the patient with conductive pathology. From the latency prolongation plotted on the LIF in Figure 7-2, a 50-dB conductive impairment would be predicted for the right ear.

Fria and Sabo (1980) compared ABR and audiometric findings using two similar techniques. First, as reported in McGee and Clemis (1982), the patient's wave V latencies were plotted and compared to the normal LIF. Fria and Sabo drew a horizontal line from the normal latency at 20 dB to the patient's LIF. The point where this line intersected the patient's LIF was the estimated conductive hearing impairment. In this way, 7 of 10 subjects had predicted losses that were less than 15 dB different from the 4-KHz pure tone threshold. Using this approach for the example in Figure 7-2 above, the patient's predicted loss would be 41 to 42 dB, compared with his actual loss of 50 dB at 4000 Hz.

In the second approach, when a 0.3-ms delay in wave V latency was established to equal a 10-dB hearing loss, 8 of Fria and Sabo's 10 subjects had a predicted discrepancy less than

FIGURE 7–2.

A wave V LIF for an individual with a right ossicular chain disorder. For this example and in our clinic, 0.4 ms latency prolongation is assumed to equal approximately 10 dB of hearing loss. The patient's latency at 60 dB in the right ear was 8.0 ms; the expected latency at this intensity is 6.0 ms. Therefore, the predicted loss is 50 dB. The obtained pure tone average was 58 dB. The high-frequency average at 1000, 2000, and 4000 Hz was 50 dB.

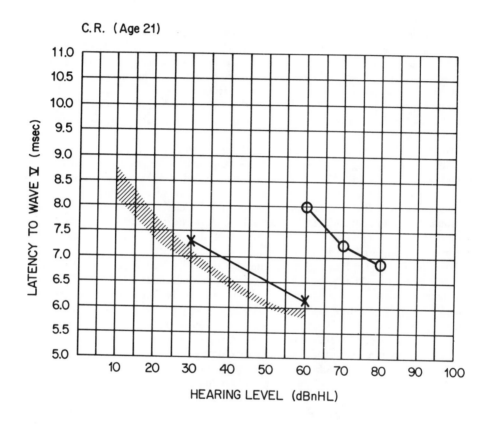

C.R. (Age 21)

LATENCY TO WAVE V (msec) vs HEARING LEVEL (dBnHL)

	500	1K	2K	4K
RE	70	60	40	50
LE	10	5	10	5

15 dB, and for 9 of 10, this was less than 20 dB. While the correlation between latency delay and the 4000-Hz pure tone response was .58, it increased to .81 at 500 Hz. For 70% of the subjects the estimated loss was within 5 dB of the actual loss, except at 4000 Hz where the estimated loss was within 10 dB of actual threshold. Thus for 500, 1000, and 2000 Hz, correlations and predictions were better than at 4000 Hz.

McGee and Clemis (1982), using ABR, also reported good correlation between actual and estimated conductive hearing loss for losses simulated with earplugs and for otitis media. Results for these two groups supported their hypothesis that increased ABR latency was due to simple signal level reduction. However, the LIF overestimated the air–bone gap for ossicular chain disorders. One explanation of the overestimation is that bone-conduction (BC) thresholds in ossicular chain disorders do not represent pure cochlear reserve. Shifts in BC thresholds may be due to mechanical artifact rather than sensory impairment, and this problem is more likely in cases of ossicular chain disorders than for otitis media or external ear impairment (Tonndorf, 1964). When ossicular chain participation is reduced or eliminated in humans, the maximum mechanical bone conduction loss should occur at 1500 to 2000 Hz (Dirks, 1972). Thus, for McGee and Clemis' data, the LIF's relationship to the air-conduction audiogram is perhaps a more accurate estimate of the conductive loss for pure ossicular chain disorders than is the audiometric air–bone gap.

Using a 2000 Hz haversine stimulus, Borg, Lofqvist, and Rosen (1981) correlated the LIF shift with the air–bone gap at various audiometric frequencies. The correlation increased from a low of .45 at 500 Hz and .57 at 1000 Hz to a high of .84 at 3000 Hz and .75 at 4000 Hz. Thus, for their subjects, the least discrepancy was obtained when the conductive loss was measured at 3000 Hz. However, Borg et al. were not able to determine a single correction factor that would totally account for the discrepancy. Because of the nonlinear slope to the LIF, the correction factor depended on the click intensity level, the degree of conductive loss, and the contribution of any sensorineural component.

Eggermont (1982) has criticized approaches that attempt to predict conductive hearing loss from the LIF. He states that because a given latency value will occur for a range of intensities approximately 20 dB wide, the minimum loss detectable will be 20 dB, and the inaccuracy in the amount of loss exceeding this value will be 20 dB. Very mild impairments could remain unidentified and the effects of significant pathology underestimated. In general, the ability to predict the loss within 20 dB does make this figure seem to be a "magic" number. To some extent, clinical evidence supports Eggermont's viewpoint (Fria & Sabo, 1980; McGee & Clemis, 1982; Mendelson, Salamy, Lenoir, & McKean, 1979). For example, Mendelson et al. reported that ABR was more sensitive in identifying acute suppurative otitis media than serous otitis media (SOM). These authors speculated that the difference was related to the milder hearing loss often found in SOM (perhaps with just negative pressure) than acute suppurative otitis media.

Similar findings are seen in infants evaluated in our laboratory. Wave V latency values obtained at 60 and 30 dB for 6- and 18-month-old infants with different tympanogram types are presented in Table 7-1a and b. In the milder cases with negative pressure (type C tympanograms) wave V latency values were similar to latency values obtained with normal type A tympanograms. Mild pathology had little effect on ABR latency. In comparison, although there was considerable overlap, infants with the more acute and less compliant type B tympanograms had longer latencies and statistically higher incidence of absent responses at both 60 and 30 dB when compared to infants with normal type A tympanograms or to infants with negative pressure. Some infants with normal tympanograms also had absent responses at 30 dB. These data include three children with confirmed sensorineural impairment, as well as one case of brainstem dysfunction. While efforts were made to rule out canal collapse in the younger

TABLE 7–1.A
Wave V Latency (ms) for 6-Month-old Premature Infants by Tympanogram Type

	Tympanogram Type			
	A	C	As	B
60 dB	6.74 (.48)	6.74 (.31)	7.06 (.40)	7.22 (.60)
30 dB	7.88 (.48)	8.10 (.53)	8.14 (.33)	8.30 (.44)
Total # (109)	61	10	14	24
% NR 60 dB	0%	0%	7.1%	8.3%
% NR 30 dB	13.1%	0%	15.3%	36.8%

TABLE 7-1.B
Wave V Latency (ms) for 18-Month-Old Premature Infants by Tympanogram Type

	Tympanogram Type			
	A	C	As	B
60 dB	6.32 (.31)	6.34 (.50)	6.13 (.59)	7.10 (.57)
30 dB	7.66 (.38)	7.68 (.56)	7.19 (.37)	8.52 (.54)
Total # (83)	48	10	12	13
% NR 60 dB	4.1%	0%	0%	0%
% NR 30 dB	6.3%	0%	9%	55%

infants, this type of problem would simulate a conductive hearing loss and might have produced a false-positive ABR. Hosford-Dunn, Runge, Hillel, and Johnson (1983) have reported canal collapse in infant populations and speculate that such errors may be elevating the incidence of abnormal ABRs in neonatal screening. Another cause of the normal tympanogram with elevated ABR thresholds could be related to the problems interpreting tympanograms in infants under 7 months of age. Paradise, Smith, and Bluestone (1976) documented the presence of otitis media for infants less than 7 months old with normal tympanograms. These authors speculated that the greater compliance of the infant's external auditory canal was one contributing factor to the false-negative tympanogram findings.

While predictions from the LIF about the degree of simple conductive hearing loss appear reasonably good, as Eggermont (1982) and Borg et al. (1981) caution, these estimations break down as the audiologic picture becomes more complex (i.e., in cases of mixed hearing loss or with primarily low-frequency impairments). Moreover, while a "normal" slope to the LIF with elevated thresholds is consistent with conductive pathology, it is not diagnostic of it. Additional research is needed before this issue is resolved.

ABR AND BONE CONDUCTION

Bone-Conducted Clicks Versus Bone-Conduction Masking

The use of bone conduction to differentiate conductive from sensorineural and mixed losses should be a major research topic in ABR. Yet, until recently, there have been few studies in this area. BC measurement in audiological assessment has been plagued by problems (Dirks, 1972). First, determining the participation of the middle ear to the total bone conduction response is not a trivial issue. Tonndorf (1964), who presents a thorough discussion of this topic, has emphasized the futility of trying to account for all BC phenomena by a single mechanism. Thus, in certain etiologies that may involve the external auditory meatus as well as the middle ear, the degree of sensory reserve may be misrepresented. A well-known, classic example of this problem is seen in otosclerosis with the Carhart notch.

Secondly, for air-conducted ABR click signals, contralateral masking is not necessary below 115–125 dB peak equivalent SPL, as crossover occurs at approximately 70–75 dB (Humes & Ochs, 1982). Such is not the case for bone-conducted stimuli. Masking the participation of the non-test ear is essential with bone-conduction clicks, and is addressed in greater detail in chapter 6.

Other issues important in BC testing include signal calibration, determining consistent vibrator force, and locating the most effective vibrator placement. Furthermore, with a standard bone-conduction vibrator inserted into the earphone jack of most ABR equipment, a 40- to 50-dB reduction in signal intensity results. Thus, the effective dynamic range of the vibrator is limited, and at the higher intensities (50–60 dB), the presence of significant artifact can obscure the brainstem response.

Yet, in infants with aural malformations or severe craniofacial defects, impedance measurements may be precluded. Consequently, an electrophysiological procedure to evaluate sensory reserve may be necessary (Ysunza, Cone-Wesson, & Brattson, submitted for publication). Secondly, for preoperative or intraoperative recordings, bone-conduction stimulation may be preferable to an air-conducted approach (Harder, Kylen, Arlinger, & Ekvall, 1980; Hecox, Malischke, Sauer, Aarenberg, & Kaufman, submitted for publication). Finally, Hooks and Weber (1984) suggest that a combination of air- and bone-conduction screening in the intensive care nursery may be effective in reducing the ABR false-positive rate and in identifying those infants with significant sensorineural impairments.

Bone-Conducted Click-Evoked ABR

Mauldin and Jerger (1979) were among the first investigators to document their experiences with bone-conducted ABR, although investigators had previously reported on bone-conduction stimulation in electrocochleography (Arlinger & Kylen, 1977; Berlin, Gondra, & Casey, 1978; Harder et al. 1980). Mauldin and Jerger identified longer (mean = 0.46 ms) wave V latencies for a one-half cycle of a 3000 Hz sine wave presented through a bone vibrator as compared to an earphone. Like Yoshie (1973), they hypothesized that spectral differences between the acoustic signals were responsible. As shown in Figure 7-3, the spectral content of the two transducers differed in that the bone vibrator had a poorer high-frequency response than the earphone (Weber, 1983). Theoretically, the bone-conduction response would be generated from a more apical region of the cochlea and should result in longer latencies. When the air-conducted signal was low-pass filtered at 2550 Hz and the bone-conduction stimuli remained unfiltered (40 to 20,000 Hz), comparable latencies were obtained. Mean air- and bone-conduction LIFs are displayed in Figure 7-4 for seven normal subjects from our laboratory (using a 100-μs rectangular wave filtered from 300 to 3000 Hz). In general, our results also show about 0.4 ms longer latencies for bone-conducted signals. Boezeman, Kapteyn, Visser, and Snell (1983) found considerably longer latencies (0.9 ms) for bone conduction than did we or Mauldin and Jerger. They speculated that in addition to spectral differences in the transducers, there were differences in travelling time between the air- and bone-conducted signals. In their pilot study, the bone vibrator on the occiput gave shorter latencies than did that on the forehead, suggesting that conduction time and phase differences also need to be considered.

The variability in bone-conduction latency measurement appears to be greater from laboratory to laboratory than that of comparable air-conduction measurement. Indeed, certain investigators (Ysunza et al., submitted for publication) reported that variability within their laboratory was substantial and unacceptable for patient evaluation. Certainly each laboratory needs to establish carefully its own norms in this area and make a decision about clinical measurement. In our experience, while bone-conducted ABR is more difficult and time consuming than air conduction, we have used it successfully in clinical assessment.

Bone-Conduction Masking

Rainville (1955) described a procedure for assessing the status of the sensorineural mechanism that circumvented some of the problems that had plagued bone-conduction audiometry. Instead of measuring bone-conduction thresholds in the presence of air-conducted masking, he reversed the process. Subsequently, Jerger and Tillman (1960) simplified the procedure for audiological assessment. Their technique, known as the SAL (sensorineural acuity level), measures two thresholds: one in quiet, and a second in the presence of bone-conducted noise. The decibel difference between these two thresholds is compared to results obtained for normals. A detailed description may be found in Jerger and Tillman (1960), Tillman (1963), and Jerger and Jerger (1965).

In 1980, Hicks reported an ABR SAL approach to approximate sensory thresholds and bypass the methodologic problems with bone-conduction clicks. Subsequently, Ysunza et al. (submitted for publication) and Webb and Greenberg (1983) reevaluated and extended her findings. In this procedure, the air-conduction ABR threshold is determined for the stimulus selected (click or tone pips), and is referred to as ABR(t). Next, the stimulus is presented 5 dB above ABR(t), and bone-conducted masking is increased until ABR(t) + 5 dB disappears. In normals, subtracting 15

FIGURE 7–3.
Differences in the acoustic spectra of an air-conducted and a bone-conducted click (Weber, 1983).

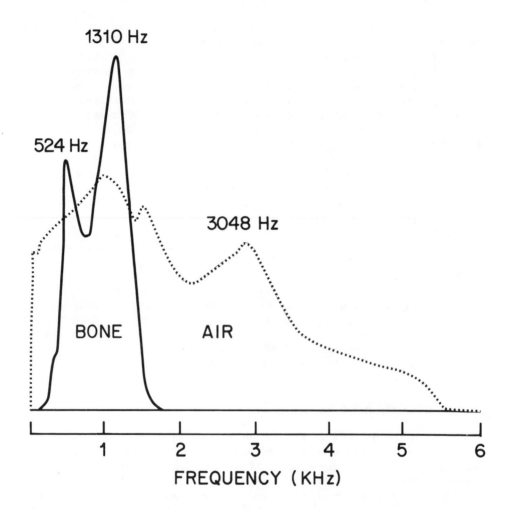

dB from the noise level required to mask $ABR(t) + 5$ gives an estimate of the sensory reserve. Normals and conductives require similar amounts of noise, while the level required for the sensorineural listener is increased.

Such a derived bone-conduction response generally seems to be viewed as a positive development; however, there remain several disadvantages. First, as Webb and Greenberg (1983) point out, test time can be as long as 3 hours. Secondly, $ABR(t) + 5$ dB will be a low-amplitude response, increasing the chance for error. While a theoretical concern could be raised about

FIGURE 7–4.
Mean air- and bone-conduction latencies for seven normal subjects.

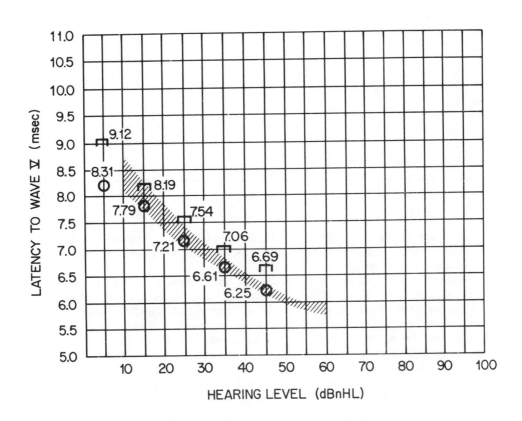

whether a low-pass noise (Figure 7-3) can effectively mask the broader spectrum and higher frequency air-conducted signals, the data do not indicate that this is a problem.

REVIEW OF ETIOLOGIES

External/Middle Ear Malformations

In this section, a review of ABR results in infants and children with confirmed conductive pathologies and/or craniofacial anomalies is presented. An outer or external ear hearing

TABLE 7–2.
Degree of Hearing Impairment for 47 Infants with External Ear Malformations as Predicted by ABR to Air-conducted Clicks

	Opposite (less involved) ear			
	Normal	Mild	Moderate	Severe/Profound
Ear with more severe anomaly				
Normal	19	2		
Mild	1	2		
Moderate	7	4	4	2
Severe/Profound	3		1	2

impairment can be as simple as impacted cerumen in the EAM, as complex as an atresia of the auricle and stenosis of the ear canal, with associated ossicular chain malformations, or as problematic as otitis media.

To identify a subtle ear anomaly, size, position, and landmarks of the auricle should be considered. Jaffe (1977) has simplified the examination of the outer ear by reducing the complexity of the pinna to the presence or absence of three lines (Figure 7-5). Either a missing line or an extra line represents an anomaly. While these subtle malformations do not in themselves obstruct sound, they may be related to more complex ossicular chain anomalies, such as a fixation of one or more of these structures. Both the ossicles and the auricle originate from the first and second brachial arches early in fetal life.

ABR results from our lab are summarized in Table 7-2 for 47 infants with external ear malformations, including atretic pinnas as well as simple preauricular pits or skin tags. Fourteen infants had atretic pinnas of varying degrees. Three were bilateral in nature. The audiological assessment of an infant with this type of problem has been difficult and time consuming, often requiring years of follow-up. Figures 7-6a and b are photographs of a 6-month-old infant with a severe microtia of one pinna. The opposite ear, while dysmorphic, appears less involved. Yet the child had a bilateral conductive impairment when air- and bone-conducted ABR were completed. Indeed, of the 11 infants with unilateral atresias, three had mild impairments and two moderate impairments in their normal appearing or less involved ear.

To be effective, the evaluation for this type of infant must answer two questions: (1) Is there residual hearing on the side of the atresia? and (2) Is hearing in the contralateral ear sufficient for the normal development of speech and language? While polytomography provides information on the anatomical state of the cochlea and middle ear, it does not assess physiological integrity. Air- and bone-conduction ABR can be effective with this population. Masking may be indicated in cases with sensorineural involvement, even for air-conducted clicks.

In 33 infants with sinuses, tags, dysmorphic pinnas, or another associated anomaly (i.e., familial history, craniofacial anomaly), the incidence of hearing loss was 45% with 24% of

FIGURE 7–5.
Pinna inspection simplified to three lines. The longer, outer line represents the helix. The smaller, inner line represents the antihelix, with a superior and inferior portion. The helix terminates inferiorly at the earlobe.

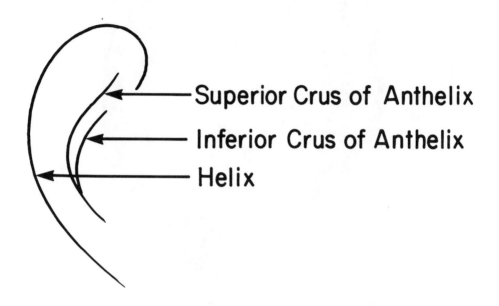

these 33 infants showing evidence of bilateral impairments. In 22 of these infants whose sole craniofacial anomaly was a pit or skin tag, 7, or 32%, had threshold elevations on ABR. Two of the seven children had sensorineural impairments; the remaining five had impairments that were thought to be mixed or conductive in nature. Cremers and Fikkers-Van Noord (1980) report that an individual with preauricular pits only and without affected relatives is likely to have a nongenetic defect. A person with a preauricular pits–branchial clefts–hearing loss triad is likely to be a carrier of an autosomal dominant disorder. For infants with minor anomalies like those seen in our clinic, if immediate habilitation is not indicated, normal language milestones are reviewed with the parents, who are alerted to the need for reevaluation should there be future concern about their infant's development. Genetic counseling is also often suggested.

Otitis Media

The most prevalent middle ear disorder, indeed the most frequent etiology of all hearing impairment in children, is otitis media (OM). Otitis media results from inflammation of the

FIGURE 7–6 a, b.
Unilateral severe microtia (a) of one pinna in a 6-month-old male. The opposite ear (b) is also dysmorphic in appearance.

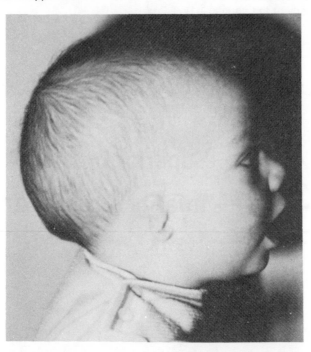

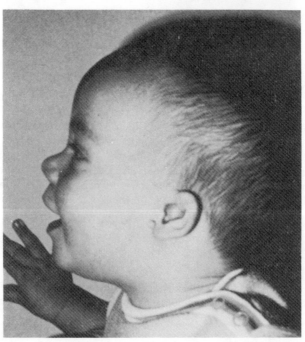

mucoperiosteal lining of the middle ear cleft (Paparella & Shumrick, 1980). In a preliminary analysis of the Greater Boston Collaborative Otitis Media Program, designed to follow prospectively 2600 children from birth, Teele, Klein, and Rosner (1980) report that 71% of the children had one or more episodes of acute otitis media before their third birthday. Thirty-three percent had experienced three or more episodes. Persistence of middle ear effusion (MEE) was frequent.

The hearing loss from OM fluctuates, and is variable depending on both the state and severity of the disorder. In ears with thick effusion from mucoid otitis media, mean air-conduction threshold for 250 through 4000 Hz is 30.8 dB. Hearing is poorer with thick effusion than with thin fluid, where mean air-conduction threshold is 26.8 dB HL (McDermott, Giebink, Lee, Harford, & Paparella, 1983). The audiometric configuration depends on the severity of the disorder with an early stiffness tilt resulting in a rising configuration across frequencies. As fluid accumulates, the mass loading of the ossicles may increase the involvement in the high frequencies. At this point the audiogram is generally flat with perhaps a slight improvement at 2000 Hz (Dobie & Berlin, 1979).

Effects of OM on Language Acquisition

There are three reasons for documenting the effect of otitis media on the auditory brainstem response. First, unrecognized conductive pathology may complicate the detection of retrocochlear pathology, particularly if interaural latency wave V measures are used (McGee & Clemis, 1982). Second, conductive pathology (often OM) exists concurrently with sensory impairments, and could produce an additional 10- to 40-dB threshold elevation in a youngster with significant sensorineural impairment. If unrecognized, it could hinder appropriate habilitation. Ruben and Fishman (1981) report that 6% of 212 hearing-impaired children had either middle ear effusion or a tympanic membrane perforation during their yearly otologic examination. Third, early accurate assessment of the hearing impairment associated with middle ear disease in young infants (0–12 months) has been both frustrating and challenging. The otoscopic examination and impedance measurements have drawbacks in this age group (Paradise et al., 1976).

At issue is whether otitis media, which is a disease with effects that are evaluated on a continuum, has educationally significant sequelae. How severe must the hearing loss be, and for how long, before early language learning is compromised? Conceptually, the hypothesis that there is a link between chronic conductive hearing impairment and normal language development is tenable. The presence of fluctuating changes in hearing means that the young child must deal with conflicting or inconsistent information on which to base his language learning. Indeed, one would expect that a chronic conductive hearing loss during the critical period for language learning would pervade all aspects of rule acquisition in oral language learning: phonology, semantics, and syntax.

Theoretically, an objective measure of hearing, like ABR, should facilitate research in this area. An important initial issue is whether ABR is effective in predicting the presence and/or absence of OM. Two studies have addressed this question (Fria & Sabo, 1980; Mendelson, et al., 1979). Mendelson et al. used otoscopy to validate ABR findings in children with upper respiratory infections. Fria and Sabo's ABR predictions of OM were validated by myringotomy. Consequently, their predictions are likely to be more accurate since myringotomy is superior to otoscopy in confirming the presence of otitis media. Indeed, myringotomy is the test of choice in validity measures relating to otitis media.

The measure of a test's validity to correctly identify a nondiseased ear is referred to as the specificity of the test. A test's accuracy in identifying a diseased ear as abnormal is defined as its sensitivity. Fria and Sabo report that while wave V was 100% sensitive in identifying the presence of OM, its specificity was only 25%. Wave I's sensitivity was 82% and its specificity was 100%. Mendelson et al. report wave I to have a specificity of 94% as compared to 82% for wave V.

Both studies concluded that ABR is able to assist in the identification of OM. Both studies also state that wave I prolongation may be preferable to wave V; however, additional factors need to be considered. First, Fria and Sabo did not compare wave V latencies in the OM group to age-matched normals; they used age ranges. Because wave I is mature by 6 weeks, and wave V maturation takes 12 to 18 months (see chapter 16), wave I is less dependent on age-specific norms than wave V. Thus, as Fria and Sabo themselves suggest, wave V specificity values would likely improve if age-matched controls were used. Second, wave I identification is not without problems. Its advantage in these studies and in other similar research might be reduced or eliminated if subjects with an unidentifiable wave I are included in overall sensitivity and specificity computations. For Fria and Sabo, 5 of 28 subjects (approximately 18%) did not have replicable wave I responses. For McGee and Clemis, 17 of 32 subjects (53%) had no clear wave I responses. Our experience has been similar to that of McGee and Clemis, particularly at hearing levels below 50 dB. Finally, as stated in a previous section, the success of Mendelson et al. predicting OM was somewhat dependent on the severity of the disorder.

With these limitations in mind, we used ABR and tympanometry to evaluate longitudinally the effects of OM and its accompanying fluctuating hearing loss on an infant's early language learning (Friel-Patti & Finitzo-Hieber, 1983; Friel-Patti, Finitzo-Hieber, Conti, & Brown, 1982). Twenty-eight infants were selected for the OM study from a larger study of auditory development in the first 2 years of life (Finitzo-Hieber, McCracken, & Brown, 1984). Although the majority of the 28 subjects were premature infants, all were judged to be developing normally.

At least one ABR was completed prior to discharge from the hospital nursery. Children were reevaluated at 6 weeks and at 6, 12, and 18 months corrected chronological age (age post-term). Language measures were made at 12, 18, and 24 months. Middle ear pathology suspected by either ABR, the pediatric nurse practitioner's examination, and/or tympanometry was confirmed by a pediatric infectious disease specialist using pneumatic otoscopy.

Language development was assessed using the *Receptive–Expressive Emergent Language Scale* (REEL) (Bzoch & League, 1971) and the *Sequenced Inventory of Communication Development* (SICD) (Hedrick, Prather, & Tobin, 1975). During the 12-month visit only the REEL and a detailed parent interview were administered; at the 18- and 24-month visits both REEL and SICD were scored. The speech–language pathologist was unaware of the infant's hearing status at the time of evaluation and later classification.

At the conclusion of the study, the 28 children were placed into one of two groups relative to the number of infections of the middle ear experienced in the first 18 to 24 months of life. The audiologist who completed this classification was unaware of the findings of the speech–language pathologist. Fourteen children who had no more than one episode of otitis media over the course of the study were placed in an otitis-free or control group. Fourteen infants who repeatedly experienced acute middle ear infections with a minimum of three episodes, and fulfilled the definition of Howie et al. for the "otitis-prone" child (Howie, Ploussard, & Sloyer, 1975), were placed in an otitis-prone group. Figure 7-7 is a graph of the mean degree of hearing impairment in the better ear for both groups at each evaluation. The estimation of hearing loss from ABR was made using a 0.4-ms delay in wave V latency to equal 10 dB of hearing loss (40 μs/dB). The otitis-prone group had consistently poorer ABR results at each visit.

FIGURE 7–7.
Mean degree of hearing impairment in the better ear as estimated by ABR for otitis-free and otitis-prone infants.

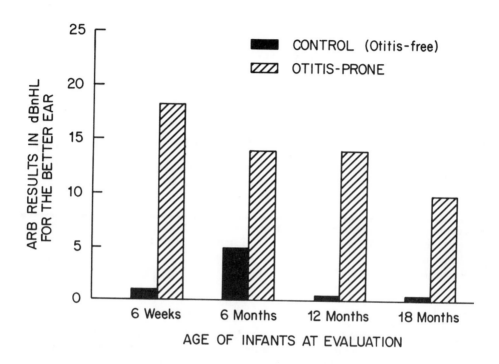

Eleven control subjects (78.6%) had language measures appropriate for their age. Three control children (21.4%) demonstrated some language delay. Two had a mild delay equal to 2 or 3 months; one had a delay greater than 4 months. In contrast, 10 of the otitis-prone children (71.5%) showed language delay. Six (42.9%) had language delays greater than 6 months, and an additional four children (28.6%) were found to show a language delay between 2 and 6 months. Only four children (28.6%) had language skills within normal.

Table 7-3 reveals the rather remarkable correspondence between the degree of hearing loss in the better ear over time, and the severity of the language delay for the 14 otitis-prone children. A significant correlation of .59 was obtained between the mean hearing loss and the language test performance (p is less than .001). Furthermore, receptive language skills correlated more highly ($r = -.65$) with hearing loss than did expressive language skills ($r = -.52$). This finding was also significant at the .001 level of confidence. The long-term degree of conductive hearing loss as predicted by ABR accounted for 42% of the variance in receptive language performance in the 28 children studied.

There are two limitations to our preliminary study. First, the children were drawn exclusively from a lower socioeconomic population. Second, the possible contamination resulting from the neonatal status of prematurity cannot be overlooked. Prematurity alone may place a child

TABLE 7–3.
Conductive Hearing Loss and Language Delay in 14 Otitis-Prone Infants

Subject ^{a}	X dB nHL^b	Language delay
$\underline{1}$	35	+ +
12	30	+ +
$\underline{6}$	26	+ +
11	23	+ +
$\underline{4}$	22	+ +
9	14	
13	14	
14	13	
$\underline{2}$	9	+
7	9	+
$\underline{10}$	4	
8	3	+ +
3	0	+
5	0	+

^{a}Underlined subjects had myringotomy tubes before 18 months.
^{b}Average in better ear at 6 weeks, 6 months, 12 months, and 18 months.
(+)Language delay less than 6 months.
(+ +)Language delay greater than 6 months.

"at risk" for language delay. Our current research controls for these factors. In spite of these limitations, we were encouraged that the degree of hearing loss, predicted by ABR at four regularly scheduled visits in infancy, was strongly correlated with the amount of language delay. Additional longitudinal research in this area could begin in the young infant under 7 months and include ABR to document hearing impairment, or to at least screen the subjects for sensorineural impairment at the onset of the project. With an estimate of the degree of early hearing impairment, additional prospective research should focus on the question of long-term sequelae, including whether there are later auditory perceptual problems and/or reading difficulties associated with an early history of otitis media.

SUMMARY

Simple conductive hearing impairment prolongs the latency of all wave components for air-conduction stimuli. The degree of impairment can be approximated by examining the wave V LIF. However, impedance measurements should be used when age appropriate in conjunction with ABR to improve diagnosis of conductive pathology. If impedance is unfeasible, or if additional clarification is needed, bone-conduction measures (direct or derived) can aid in estimating sensory reserve.

Unrecognized, transient conductive pathology can (1) result in incorrect identification of brain stem pathology, (2) hinder appropriate habilitative intervention for the youngster with sensorineural impairment, and (3) increase the number of intensive care nursery failures and decrease confidence in ABR as a screening tool.

The authors thank Cheryl Cartee who extracted and collated patient information presented here, Ann Syrdal who assisted us in data analysis, and Cindi Jones for her assistance in manuscript preparation. This chapter was supported in part by a grant from the Schering Corporation, Bloomfield, New Jersey, and American Hearing Research Foundation, Chicago, Illinois.

REFERENCES

Arlinger, S., & Kylen, P. (1977). Bone-conducted stimulation in electrocochleography. *Acta Otolaryngologica, 84,* 377–384.

Berlin, C., Gondra, M., & Casey, D. (1978). Bone conduction electrocochleography: Clinical applications. *Laryngoscope, 88,* 756–763.

Boezeman, E., Kapteyn, T., Visser, S., & Snell, A. (1983). Comparison of the latencies between bone and air conduction in the auditory brainstem evoked potential. *EEG and Clinical Neurophysiology, 56,* 244–247.

Borg, E., Lofqvist, L., & Rosen, S. (1981). Brainstem response (ABR) in conductive hearing loss. *Scandinavian Audiology (Supplement), 13,* 95–97.

Bzoch, K., & League, R. (1971). *Receptive–expressive emergent language scale.* Baltimore: University Park Press.

Cremers, C., & Fikkers-Van Noord, M. (1980). The earpits-deafness syndrome: Clinical and genetic aspects. *International Journal of Pediatric Otorhinolaryngology, 2,* 309–322.

Dirks, D.D. (1972). Clinical measurement of bone conduction. In J. Katz (Ed.), *Handbook of clinical audiology,* Baltimore: Williams & Wilkins.

Dobie, R., & Berlin, C. (1979). Influence of otitis media on hearing and development. *Annals of Otology, Rhinology, and Laryngology (Supplement), 88,* 48–53.

Eggermont, J. (1982). The inadequacy of click-evoked auditory brainstem responses in audiological applications. *Annals of the New York Academy of Science, 388,* 707–709.

Finitzo-Hieber, T., Hecox, K., & Cone, B. (1979). Brainstem auditory evoked potentials in patients with congenital atresia. *Laryngoscope, 89,* 1151–1158.

Finitzo-Hieber, T., McCracken, G., & Brown, K. (1984). Prospective controlled evaluation of auditory function in neonates treated with netilmicin or amikacin. *Journal of Pediatrics* (in press).

Fria, T.J., & Sabo, D.L. (1980). Auditory brainstem responses in children with otitis media with effusion. *Annals of Otology, Rhinology, and Laryngology, 68,* 200–206.

Friel-Patti, S., & Finitzo-Hieber, T. (1983). *Recurrent otitis media: Effects on early language.* Invited presentation at the American Speech–Language–Hearing Association Western Regional Conference, Honolulu.

Friel-Patti, S., Finitzo-Hieber, T., Conti, G., & Brown, C.K. (1982). Language delay in infants associated with middle ear disease and mild, fluctuating hearing impairment. *Pediatric Infectious Disease, 1,* 104–109.

Harder, H., Kylen, P., Arlinger, S., & Ekvall, L. (1980). Pre-operative bone-conducted electrocochleography in otosclerosis. *Archives of Otolaryngology, 106,* 757–762.

Hecox, K., & Galambos, R. (1974). Brainstem auditory evoked responses in human infants and adults. *Archives of Otolaryngology, 99,* 30–33.

Hecox, K., Malischke, M., Sauer, R., Aarenberg, R., & Kaufman, I. *Intraoperative electrophysiologic monitoring of the auditory system: Technical factors.* Submitted for publication.

Hedrick, D.L., Prather, E.M., & Tobin, A.R. (1975). *Sequenced inventory of communication development.* Seattle: University of Washington Press.

Hicks, G.E. (1980). Auditory brainstem response: Sensory assessment by bone conduction masking. *Archives of Otolaryngology, 106,* 392–395.

Hooks, R., & Weber, B. (1984). Auditory brain stem responses to bone conduction stimuli in premature neonates: A feasibility study. *Ear and Hearing, 5,* 42–46.

Hosford-Dunn, H., Runge, C., Hillel, A., & Johnson, S. (1983). Auditory brain stem response testing in infants with collapsed ear canals. *Ear and Hearing, 4,* 258–260.

Howie, V.M., Ploussard, J.H., & Sloyer, J. (1975). The "otitis-prone" condition. *American Journal of Diseases in Children, 129,* 676–678.

Humes, L., & Ochs, M. (1982). Use of contralateral masking in the measurement of the auditory brainstem response. *Journal of Speech and Hearing Research, 25,* 528–535.

Jaffe, B. (1977). *Hearing loss in children.* Baltimore: University Park Press.

Jerger, J., & Jerger, S. (1965). Critical evaluation of SAL audiometry. *Journal of Speech and Hearing Research, 8,* 103–128.

Jerger, J., & Tillman, T. (1960). A new method for the clinical determination of sensorineural acuity level (SAL). *Archives of Otolaryngology, 71,* 948–953.

Mauldin, L., & Jerger, J. (1979). Auditory brain stem evoked responses to bone-conducted signals. *Archives of Otolaryngology, 105,* 656–661.

McDermott, J. C., Giebink, S., Lee, C. T., Harford, E. R., & Paparella, M. (1983). Children with persistent otitis media. *Archives of Otolaryngology, 109,* 360–363.

McGee, T.J., & Clemis, J.D. (1982). Effects of conductive hearing loss on auditory brainstem response. *Annals of Otology, Rhinology, and Laryngology, 91,* 304–309.

Mendelson, T., Salamy, A., Lenoir, M., & McKean, C. (1979). Brainstem evoked potential findings in children with otitis media. *Archives of Otolaryngology, 105,* 17–20.

Paparella, M., & Shumrick, D. (1980). *Otolaryngology: Vol. II: The ear.* Philadelphia: Saunders.

Paradise, J., Smith, C., & Bluestone, C. (1976). Tympanometric detection of middle ear effusion in infants and young children. *Pediatrics, 58,* 198–210.

Rainville, M. (1955). Nouvelle methode d'assourdissement pour le releve des courves de conduction osseuse. *Journal Français Otorhinolaryngologique, 4,* 851–858.

Ruben, R., & Fishman, G. (1981). Otological care of the hearing impaired child. In G. Mencher, & S. Gerber (Eds.), *Early management of hearing loss,* 105–120. New York: Grune & Stratton.

Teele, D., Klein, J., & Rosner, B. (1980). Epidemiology of otitis media in children. *Annals of Otology, Rhinology, and Laryngology,* Supplement 68, *89,* 5–6.

Tillman, T. (1963). Clinical applicability of the SAL test. *Archives of Otolaryngology, 78,* 20–32.

Tonndorf, J. (1964). Animal experiments in bone conduction: Clinical conclusions. *Annals of Otology, Rhinology, and Laryngology, 73,* 659–678.

Webb, K.C., & Greenberg, H.J. (1983). Electrophysiologic techniques in audiology and otology: Bone-conduction masking for threshold assessment in auditory brain stem response testing. *Ear and Hearing, 4,* 261-266.

Weber, B. (1983). Masking and bone conduction testing in brainstem response audiometry. *Seminars in Hearing, 4,* 343-352.

Yoshie, N. (1973). Diagnostic significance of the electrocochleogram in clinical audiometry. *Audiology, 12,* 504-539.

Ysunza, A., Cone-Wesson, B., & Brattson, A. Bone-conducted clicks vs. bone-conducted masking for BAEP pediatric audiological evaluations. *International Journal of Pediatric Otorhinolaryngology.* Submitted for publication.

Chapter 8

The Effect of Cochlear Lesions on the ABR

Martyn L. Hyde

INTRODUCTION

The auditory brainstem response (ABR) waveform depends upon the underlying spatiotemporal distribution of neuroelectric events in the cochlear nerve and brainstem pathways. This pattern originates within the cochlea, so any factor which affects cochlear output can affect the ABR. In this chapter, changes in the ABR which are associated with cochlear pathology are outlined.

Pure tone hearing loss of cochlear origin does not affect cochlear output in a causative sense, but is itself a result a change in cochlear signal processing. Two possible outcomes of a cochlear disorder are abnormal pure tone audiometric thresholds and ABR changes. These may show a correlation; because pure tone thresholds are relatively easy to measure, it is convenient to pretend that hearing loss "causes" ABR changes, and to discuss the "dependency" of the ABR on the pure tone audiogram. It is important to remember that we are relating two complex and poorly understood phenomena, each affected in some way by the underlying pathology.

The ABR and the pure tone audiogram each have many features, and to quantify relationships between them, important parameters of each must be selected. If the hearing loss is purely sensory and if we restrict our attention to, for example, thresholds at 500, 1000, 2000, and 4000 Hz, a set of four numbers contains all the audiometric information. The problem is how to express it; the usual method is to reduce the set by taking simple linear combinations, such as the mean of some or all of the numbers to represent an average hearing loss, or differences to represent contour features such as slope. The results may then be further degraded into categories such as "flat," "high-slope," and so forth. The point is that the audiogram is actually a multidimensional quantity, but when it is used to explain changes in the ABR, it is forced into some simple form with an inevitable loss of information. Another point is that the audiogram elements are interrelated; the 2000 Hz threshold will correlate with the 4000 Hz threshold, for example, and the slope will correlate with its components. These factors can cause problems in isolating specific audiogram features that affect the ABR.

The ABR itself has many parameters, and it is natural to focus on those used clinically, such as the latencies of prominent vertex-positive peaks. These are neither the only measures nor necessarily the ones which relate most strongly to the audiogram, but they are the most common.

FACTORS UNDERLYING AUDIOGRAM–ABR RELATIONSHIPS

Many factors can influence the association, or lack thereof, between the audiogram and the ABR. These factors are poorly understood, and the literature is frequently contradictory.

Stimulus Characteristics

The ABR depends upon both cochlear input and the state of the cochlea. Thus, the stimulus is extremely important because it determines the potential pattern of cochlear excitation. Some of these issues are covered by Gorga et al. in chapter 4 of this volume, and will be summarized here.

Envelope. The stimuli used for pure tone audiometry and ABR measurements differ. For the former, long-duration tones with shaped and gradual onset and offset envelopes are used to minimize the spectral spread of stimulus energy. The standard ABR wave series is not elicited by such stimuli; rather, more rapid stimulus onset is required to promote increased synchrony of neuroelectric events. The most commonly used stimuli are clicks, obtained by exciting the headphone with a rectangular voltage pulse. These stimuli have the fastest possible onset, leading to well-synchronized neural activity and clear ABR waveforms.

Spectrum. Unfortunately, clicks are relatively difficult stimuli to control and quantify. They have a broad acoustical energy density spectrum at the tympanic membrane, and will excite a much larger region of the cochlear partition than a pure tone of comparable intensity. Thus, there is a distinction between pure tone audiometry and ABR measurement on purely acoustical grounds. The effective spectrum is determined by the combined system of the headphone coupled to the external ear canal. Different headphones may give different spectra, affecting the cochlear excitation pattern and the ABR (Laukli, 1983). Even if the spectra are similar, the time history of the pressure profile may vary over transducers. This can also change the ABR, which is intimately related to the detailed stimulus time history, rather than simply to its spectrum.

Cochlear excitation pattern. The stimulus evokes a traveling wavefront which progressively excites a considerable length of the cochlear partition and the associated hair cells. The velocity of the traveling wave decreases apically, and the innervation density also varies, so the number of primary neurons activated per unit time depends on cochlear position. If the ABR is a weighted linear summation of activity at the electrode evoked by each elementary neuroelectric event, the major contributions to the overall response come from those cochlear regions where excitations are most highly synchronized, especially basal regions. Another factor is the tuning characteristic of primary auditory neurons, which typically has a steep high-frequency segment, and a more gradually sloping tail toward low frequencies (Evans, 1983). This suggests that low-frequency stimuli may excite neurons tuned to higher frequencies, whereas the converse is less likely. Both of the above effects may lead to discrepancies between the acoustical spectrum of the stimulus and its effective cochlear excitation pattern.

Polarity. The initial polarity of the click stimulus may affect the pattern of cochlear excitation. The use of alternating-polarity clicks has been criticized on the grounds that differences in the ABR evoked by compression and rarefaction clicks may summate to give unpredictable results (Stockard & Stockard, 1983). The situation is complicated by possible interactions between hearing loss profile and the cochlear excitation pattern associated with each type of click.

Intensity. While the acoustical stimulus spectrum is independent of intensity, the cochlear excitation pattern is undoubtedly intensity dependent, shifting to higher frequencies as the intensity is raised (Don & Eggermont, 1978). Intensity is of particular interest because the pattern of change in ABR latency with stimulus intensity, that is, the intensity–latency function, has been proposed as a tool for the differentiation of site of lesion.

ABR Source Patterns in the Normal and Disordered Cochlea

Much of the evidence for distributed cochlear sites of ABR initiation comes from the important *derived response* technique using filtered masking noise and waveform subtraction (Don & Eggermont, 1978). From such studies, it is widely belived that the ABR is a simple summation of contributions from specific regions of the cochlea. The patterns of derived response latency change are fairly consistent with cochlear traveling wave properties. It is possible to allocate a weighting of the contribution from various cochlear regions to the overall response; for a click stimulus at moderate intensity, it appears that wave V has contributions from regions extending to low frequencies, whereas wave I has a more basal weighting. Both weightings are likely to be intensity dependent in the normal cochlea. For example, a 70 dB click appears to excite a very broad range of the cochlear partition, from 8000 through 500 Hz (Don & Eggermont, 1978). This range is still apparent at 40 dB, but the excitation converges to the 1 to 2 kHz region at 10 dB.

The validity of the derived-ABR concept is widely accepted, but is not proved conclusively. There are various possible sources of nonlinearity both of cochlear masking mechanisms and in auditory brainstem pathways. The fact that derived ABRs summate to precisely the unmasked ABR is merely a necessary consequence of the underlying arithmetic. Validation studies are suggestive, but not conclusive. It is possible that the patterns of cochlear excitation which actually occur for unmasked stimuli may differ from those revealed by the derived response method. Nevertheless, its findings are plausible and represent a reasonable model on which to base interpretation of some of the effects of hearing loss.

Given this summation model of the normal ABR, it follows that pathologic depletion of contributions to the ABR from specific cochlear regions may have quite complex effects on the click response waveform. Insofar as pure tone hearing loss reflects these cochlear changes, a fact which is itself not understood, the associations between the audiogram and the ABR can be expected to be complex. Cochlear dysfunction might affect the various waves of the ABR differently. For example, high-frequency hearing loss may exert a greater effect on wave I than on wave V, because of the more basal cochlear generation pattern of wave I. A reduction in interpeak latency (IPL) for waves I and V would be expected, and has been reported (Coats, 1978). Other configurations of loss may exert unpredictable effects on individual ABR components. Also, it must be remembered that wave V latency is affected by summation mechanisms at several synapses, and this may alter the final result of change in the source pattern. The possibilities are almost endless, and these issues are certainly not well understood.

Another source of complication in relating pure tone thresholds and ABR properties is the change in tuning characteristics of primary neurons, a change which is often associated with some types of cochlear hearing loss (Evans, 1983). Loss of tuning will change the cochlear source pattern, especially by increased basal spread. Loss of tuning is often correlated with pure tone threshold shift, but there are cases in which the correlation breaks down.

A further possibility is that cochlear output might be inadequately synchronized as a result of cochlear pathology, yet the pure tone thresholds may be normal. It must be remembered that this issue of neural synchrony may underlie many apparent discrepancies between the audiogram and the ABR; while normal ABR development apparently requires an abrupt and substantial change in the firing rate of many neurons simultaneously, normal pure tone sensitivity may not have that requirement. This effect is apparent in retrocochlear lesions, such as acoustic tumor, and in demyelinating disease. It is certainly feasible that unrecognized disorders of cochlear output timing may underlie some of the reported cases of idiopathic ABR absence.

A more radical possibility is that the afferent neuronal populations that mediate the ABR to transients such as clicks may be different, either wholly or in part, from those that mediate psychoacoustic response to pure tone stimuli. This differentiation may occur at any level in the afferent pathway, and there is certainly ample evidence of obvious functional differentiation at the cellular level, as the system ascends.

Clearly, attempts to relate the ABR and pure tone thresholds will require close attention to underlying physiologic mechanisms of *both* phenomena. For example, if we try to relate ABR generation to specific cochlear regions, then we must consider the evidence that the pure tone audiogram itself relates to cochlear place (Don & Eggermont, 1978). In cases of steep low-frequency hearing loss the pure tone threshold may be mediated by cochlear events that are more basal than the region normally associated with the nominal stimulus frequency. If a so-called *frequency-specific* stimulus such as a tone pip were used to elicit the ABR, it might also reflect the cochlear place change, whereas if a masking approach were used to force a *place-specific* ABR, quite different results could occur.

In spite of the above litany of reasons why simple and consistent relationships between the audiogram and the ABR should not be expected, a few limited empirical relationships having clinical utility can be described: It is not necessary to understand phenomena in order to use them empirically.

The two major areas of current ABR clinical application in which the effects of cochlear hearing loss are important are in the investigation of retrocochlear lesions, where the loss may confound ABR interpretation, and in auditory threshold estimation, where the extent of correspondence between perceptual and ABR thresholds is the main question. Useful reviews have been given by Rosenhamer (1981), Eggermont (1983), and Hall (1984).

COCHLEAR HEARING LOSS AND OTONEUROLOGIC INVESTIGATION

The ABR parameters most often used otoneurologically are the absolute latencies of vertex-positive peaks, inter-peak latencies, and interaural latency differences. Diagnostic criteria for retrocochlear lesion detection are based primarily upon an increase in absolute or interpeak latencies, or on a significant departure of interaural differences from zero.

The issue is the extent to which cochlear hearing loss is associated with changes in any of the above measures, and whether the changes alter the diagnostic criteria and the accuracy of decisions.

It is obvious that a profound cochlear hearing loss affecting all frequencies implies such extensive cochlear dysfunction that there may be no effective cochlear output at all, even at the highest available stimulus intensities. There will be no ABR waves, and this finding has no diagnostic value at all. On the other hand, when the audiogram is normal, the finding of no ABR strongly implies that there is a lesion affecting the cochlear nerve. Most cases of interest fall between these two extremes, wherein the hearing loss will be associated with intermediate effects on the ABR that must be differentiated from the effects of a retrocochlear lesion.

The click stimuli at the moderate or high intensities that are used in most otoneurologic investigations have their *effective* excitation maxima in the 1000 to 4000 Hz region. Careful inspection of derived narrow-band ABRs (Don & Eggermont, 1978) suggests that while contributions from higher and lower frequency regions affect the ABR waveform as a whole, the latency of wave V is dominated by contributions from the 2000 to 4000 Hz region, and that suppression of 500 and 1000 Hz contributions would have its major effect on the vertex-negative wave following wave V, as well as on wave VI. There is no convincing evidence in the literature that low-frequency hearing loss affects common ABR parameters.

When cochlear hearing loss occurs in the 2000 to 4000 Hz region, effects on the high-intensity click ABR are to be expected, and have been widely reported (Rosenhamer, 1981; Selters & Brackmann, 1977). Most published data refer to the wave V latency, which is generally reported to increase as hearing loss increases. The most common audiogram parameter selected as a correlate of wave V latency is the pure tone threshold at 3000 or 4000 Hz.

There is a lack of consensus about the exact form of the latency increase. The data of Selters and Brackmann suggest that latency is constant for hearing losses less than about 50 dB, but increases for greater losses. Regression line fitting to their data yields a rate of latency increase of about 0.015 ms/dB, although they proposed a smaller slope as the basis for a purely empirical latency correction factor in differential diagnosis of retrocochlear lesions. Rosenhamer (1980) found a rate of latency increase of about 0.01 ms/dB, starting at about 30–40 dB.

Some of the discrepancies in reports of cochlear hearing loss effects on wave V latency may be attributable to uncontrolled variables, one of which is the age of the subject. In a group of 180 patients with cochlear hearing loss studied in our laboratory, it was found that in patients with 4000 Hz thresholds better than 50 dB, the major variable accounting for intersubject latency variation was the age of the subject. For losses over 50 dB, the major contributing variable was hearing loss. Grouping the subjects by age and hearing loss revealed the dependency of latency on both variables; the bivariate surface is as shown in Figure 8-1. Age and hearing loss effects interact, so that the effect of hearing loss depends on age. For young subjects, latency increases in an accelerating fashion for losses greater than about 40 dB. For elderly subjects, the latency starts off at higher values and does not begin to increase further until much larger hearing losses are encountered. If the age variable is not controlled, then the observed effects of hearing loss can vary in an unpredictable manner; various age distributions may produce the variable results reported by others.

With regard to diagnostic criteria for retrocochlear lesion detection, the above model suggests that not only is the latency correction process nonlinear, but it must take account of age. For interaural latency criteria, the correction required in a young adult is greater than that required in an elderly patient with the same pure tone audiogram.

The observed nonadditive latency behavior is consistent with the notion that both aging and cochlear hearing loss deplete or otherwise modify a partially common and presumably cochlear population of responding units. The model also implies that the depletion can occur without necessarily changing the pure tone threshold.

The question of whether the slope of high-frequency hearing losses influences the ABR elicited by high-intensity clicks is complex, and the literature is inconsistent. Jerger and Mauldin (1978) reported that the slope of the audiometric contour correlates better with wave V latency than with the average loss severity, whereas Rosenhamer (1981) found no clear slope effect when hearing loss at 4000 Hz was controlled. The data underlying the age/hearing loss model described above also failed to reveal a slope effect when severity was tightly controlled; the 4000 Hz threshold was the major determinant of latency increase, regardless of slope. The resolution of this question requires very careful analysis, partly because slope and severity are intimately related, and their correlation will depend in particular upon the degrees of hearing loss included in the study sample. The use of average hearing loss as a controllable severity measure is questionable; if average loss were controlled to, say, 50 dB, a wide range of slopes would be possible, and the slope effect could be examined. Increase in latency with increasing slope might indicate that slope is important, but another possibility is that the 4000 Hz threshold really determines the latency, and controlling average loss does not adequately control 4000 Hz. The slope effect may be an illusion based upon inappropriate choice of the severity measure.

Figure 8–1.

A bivariate surface showing the dependency of wave V latency upon both age and pure tone hearing loss at 4 kHz. Stimuli were 85 dB nHL alternating-polarity clicks at 20/s. The surface was fitted to data from 180 males with cochlear impairment. The data suggest that the latency increase is nonlinear with both hearing loss and age, and the two effects are not additive.

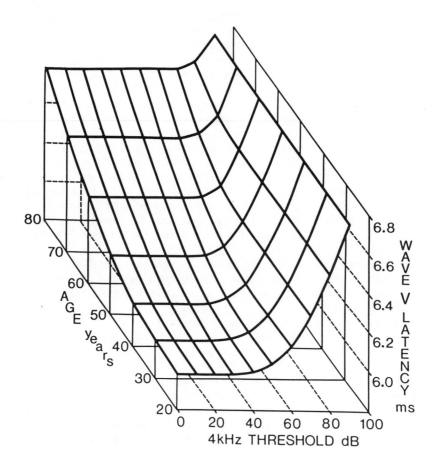

THE CLICK ABR INTENSITY-LATENCY FUNCTION

Flat Hearing Loss

The effect of cochlear hearing loss at a fixed high intensity is of special interest, but is a small part of the broader picture relating wave V latency to both hearing loss and stimulus intensity. For the case of flat cochlear hearing loss in young adult subjects, the effects are shown schematically in Figure 8-2. This figure is an attempt to assemble some of the reported data in an illustrative manner; because of the limited sample sizes and variations of case material and methodology across studies, some aspects of the figure are speculative. The curves are generally consistent with reported effects (Galambos & Hecox, 1978; Yamada, Kodera, & Yagi, 1979).

The leftmost dotted curve represents the wave V intensity–latency function for clicks in normal-hearing subjects, derived by Picton, Stapells, and Campbell (1981) from the results of many laboratories. The other dotted curves represent, for comparison purposes, the latency functions in the presence of 20, 40, and 60 dB of flat conductive hearing loss, assuming that such losses are equivalent to a corresponding reduction in the effective stimulus intensity. Note that the curves are *not* exactly parallel to the normal curve, as is often stated, because the normal curve is nonlinear. The solid curves, moving left to right, show the effects of 20, 40, 60, and 80 dB of flat cochlear hearing loss. ABR thresholds are starred. The main features of the solid curves are that the slope is increased immediately above ABR threshold; for mild and moderate losses, the latency is normal at high stimulus levels, the ABR threshold moves closer to the hearing loss value as the latter increases, and the latency at threshold is reduced with increasing loss. The last point is difficult to prove because of the rapid latency changes with small intensity increments near threshold, but is plausible on the basis of increasingly basal excitation as the physical intensity of the threshold stimulus increases.

The latency shift functions discussed earlier for fixed click intensities in otoneurologic investigations can be derived from Figure 8-2 by taking vertical cuts at the desired stimulus intensity. It is apparent that the effects of increasing cochlear hearing loss will decrease as the intensity is raised, and that latency correction procedures for retrocochlear lesion detection will be intensity-dependent.

It is also apparent that any inference of the type of hearing loss on the basis of the curvilinear shape of the intensity–latency function is quite problematic. For conductive losses, and for a fixed click intensity range in dB nHL, the slope increases as the hearing loss increases; to distinguish between the conductive and cochlear curves, for a given hearing loss severity, it is essential to define the ABR threshold very accurately and to derive the slope over a specific decibel range based on the threshold. For cochlear loss, a quite misleading slope measurement may be obtained if the stimulus range chosen for latency measurements is even 10 dB above the true ABR threshold. In the author's experience, differentiation of the hearing loss type on the basis of latency functions can be unreliable in the *individual* patient, in spite of the fact that clear *average* differences between groups of patients with conductive and cochlear hearing losses can be demonstrated.

The effects of hearing loss on other ABR measures such as IPL I–V are even less well understood than the effects on wave V latency. With the usual periauricular recording electrode sites, wave I is frequently absent, even for high click levels if hearing loss exceeds 50 dB at 4000 Hz. There is evidence that IPL I–V decreases as click intensity decreases in normal hearing subjects (Stockard & Stockard, 1983), apparently consistent with the well-documented latency behavior of wave I from electrocochleographic studies. There is no universal agreement on this issue. The detailed effects of cochlear hearing loss on IPL I–V as a function of intensity

Figure 8–2.
A model of the effects of flat hearing loss on the click intensity-latency function for wave V. Dotted curves (left to right): normal ears and ears with 20, 40, and 60 dB of flat conductive hearing loss. Solid curves (left to right): ears with 20, 40, 60, and 80 dB of flat cochlear hearing loss. ABR thresholds are starred.

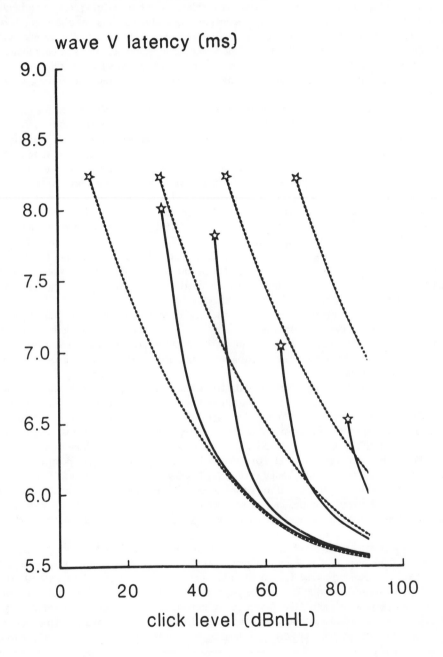

are largely unknown, though Coats (1978) has reported IPL reductions in the presence of high-frequency cochlear hearing loss, using an endomeatal electrode to enhance wave I.

Steep Hearing Loss

What are the effects of steep high-frequency cochlear hearing loss on the latency of wave V? We shall assume that hearing loss effects can be conceived in terms of a filtering action on the pattern of response contributions arising from the various regions of the cochlea. A high-frequency loss will depress basal contributions, tending to cause latency increase. Precipitous high-frequency loss might be expected to produce latency delays compatible with the time taken by the cochlear traveling wavefront to traverse the inactive basal region. Supporting evidence for this comes from high-pass noise-masking studies (Don & Eggermont, 1978), and from patient data (Galambos & Hecox, 1978).

A precipitous loss above 4000 Hz will not have a marked effect, because contributions from such regions are overwhelmed by that of the 1000- to 4000-Hz region. Such a loss starting at 2000 Hz will have a strong effect, modeled schematically in Figure 8-3. Again, the lower dotted curve is the normal intensity–latency function, and the upper dotted curve is what would be obtained if the effect of the loss were a *fixed* latency increase. The size of the increase has been exaggerated, for illustrative purposes, and the apparent increase in distance between this curve and the normal one as intensity increases is an optical illusion. Another possible result is shown as the heavy solid curve, which develops the full delay at high click levels but tends toward more normal values as the click level is decreased. The rationale for this difference is that at high intensities the normal cochlear excitation maximum lies at 2000 to 4000 Hz, which will be inactivated by the precipitous loss, whereas at low click levels the excitation shifts to the 1000 to 2000 Hz region, which is little affected by the loss. There is at present insufficient information to resolve these alternative forms, and the difference between them would only be apparent at click intensities near the ABR threshold.

Many patients with steep high-frequency losses do not have profound loss at frequencies above 4000 Hz, but may plateau or even reverse. Very different behavior of wave V latency would be expected if the loss is, say, 60 dB at 4000 Hz and above, compared to that if the loss were profound at those frequencies. The reason is that the high-intensity click will now be adequate to excite the basal region of the loss. The latency function that might result in such a case is shown as the heavy broken curve in Figure 8-3. At low click intensities, it follows the solid curve mentioned above, but as the intensity exceeds the high-frequency loss, the basal regions become strongly active and the latency begins to return rapidly to normal values.

In the case of a more gradually sloping loss, the pattern may be very difficult to interpret because of interaction between the intensity-related change in stimulus excitation pattern and the hearing loss. The overall picture is one of extreme complexity, if the variety of possible audiometric contours, loss etiologies, and measurement methods is taken into account.

Effects for Stimuli Other than Clicks

Recently, there has been a trend toward the use of more place-specific stimuli for otoneurologic investigations in an attempt to avoid some of the physical and physiologic problems of clicks and their interaction with hearing loss (Laukli, 1983). At present, there is relatively little agreement about which alternatives to the click are most appropriate; whatever the choice, a body of data concerning hearing loss effects remains to be developed. The effective cochlear excitation patterns of transient stimuli other than clicks, and the effects of intensity, hearing loss, and changes in cochlear tuning have yet to be elucidated (see Stapells et al., chapter 9).

Figure 8–3.
A model of the effects of high-frequency hearing loss on the click intensity-latency function for wave V. Lower dotted curve: normal hearing. Upper dotted curve: a constant latency increase associated with precipitous high-frequency loss. Solid curve: an alternative form which incorporates a basal shift in cochlear excitation weighting with increasing click intensity. Heavy broken curve: a possible effect of moderate high-frequency loss.

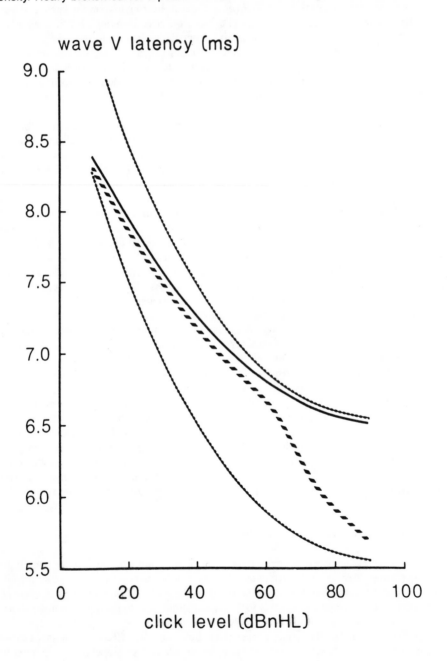

The Effect of Etiology of Cochlear Hearing Loss

There are few definitive data concerning quantitative differences between etiologies of cochlear dysfunction in relation to effects on the ABR. One problem with such studies is the need to carefully exclude effects of a particular disorder that are acting at sites other than the cochlea. For example, in presbycusis it would be extremely difficult to unravel the effects on the ABR attributable to cochlear and more central degeneration. A similar difficulty would occur in otosclerosis with associated sensory hearing loss, and in retrocochlear lesions that may influence the cochlea, such as by impairing the vascular supply.

To the extent that etiology of cochlear damage is related to the profile of the pure tone audiogram, studies which segregate the case material on the basis of the audiometric contour may give insight into effects of etiology. However, if quantitative relations between the audiogram and ABR changes are shown to be consistent across etiologies, then the value of an etiologic analysis is limited; the audiogram is a much more concrete entity to relate to the ABR than are etiologic inferences, which are often highly circumstantial. At present, the writer is unaware of studies with sufficient case volume and controls to indicate that exclusively cochlear etiologies may have different ABR effects above and beyond those attributable to audiogram differences. Such effects are certainly possible, however, and may underlie some of the intersubject variation in ABR effects associated with given patterns of loss severity and contour.

ESTIMATION OF COCHLEAR HEARING LOSS WITH THE ABR

The second area of concern is the use of the ABR to approximate the audiogram. This is dealt with in depth by Stapells et al. in chapter 9 of this volume, so only major points will be outlined.

Here, we are concerned primarily with using the ABR "threshold" to estimate the true sensory threshold. This is an empirical matter, in that there is no a priori reason for perception of sound to correspond exactly with detection of gross electrical activity at a remote electrode. Rather, the "true" threshold is estimated statistically on the basis of observed correlations. The accuracy of the estimate will depend on many factors, such as the level of electrical noise in the recordings, the stimulation and recording parameters, interpretive skill, the type of patient, and the nature of the pathology.

The use of click stimuli in the ABR is inherently limited by the wide-band nature of the click excitation. In cochlear hearing loss which is flat in the 1000 to 4000 Hz range, the use of the click is relatively meaningful, because the audiogram can be accurately expressed by a single number. The accuracy of the ABR threshold estimate probably increases slightly for increasing amounts of hearing loss; in the presence of substantial flat cochlear loss, the slope of the ABR intensity–amplitude function tends to increase, with the result that ABRs are usually detectable at only 5 dB above the click threshold. When hearing is normal, on the other hand, the stimulus may need to be 10 or 20 dB SL before the ABR is detectable.

Because most click generation systems cannot produce click levels greater than about 95 dB nHL without distortion or nonlinearity, flat losses greater than about 85 dB cannot be measured reliably by ABR methods.

When the hearing loss is not flat, the audiogram is not adequately represented by a single number. In such cases, the click is a highly questionable tool for threshold estimation. Because the audiometric contour is usually unknown in any patient having ABR testing for audiometric purposes, it follows that the click is of questionable utility in almost every case.

The correlation between click ABR threshold and such approximations as the *average hearing loss* will depend upon the distribution of severity and contour in the study sample. Hearing losses below 1000 and above 4000 Hz will have little effect on the click ABR threshold, but the intervening frequency range will definitely influence it. Because the click is wide-band, the ABR threshold will probably correlate best with not an average loss but with the best of the pure tone thresholds in the 1000 to 4000 Hz range, but there have been no statistically adequate reports on this point.

There is an increasing trend towards the use of *frequency-specific* ABR methods. The current debate concerns the accuracy with which various ABR procedures can estimate the audiometric threshold at specific frequencies. There are many approaches to the problem, including the following: control of the acoustical spectrum of a transient stimulus, the use of frequency-modulated stimuli, control of the cochlear response region by masking, including high-pass and bandstop (band-reject, notch-filtered) masking, and other methods based on more advanced mathematical concepts, such as deconvolution and algebraic decomposition.

A fundamental distinction must be recognized between frequency specificity and place specificity. Frequency specificity is a property of a stimulus, having its roots in Fourier analysis and relating to the degree of concentration of the stimulus energy–density spectrum. Place specificity, on the other hand, is a property of the cochlear excitation pattern produced by the stimulus. In the normal cochlea, a frequency-specific stimulus may be place-specific, at least at low intensities; this is almost a matter of definition, since our concepts of cochlear place arise primarily from studies using tonal stimuli. However, we now know that in the disordered cochlea, frequency specificity of the stimulus does not necessarily imply that the excitation is located at the usual place. The effective "place" may be different, and not necessarily predictable. As Don and Eggermont (1978) have noted, conventional pure tone audiometry makes no special attempt to control these place changes; nor, of course, is place controlled in the everyday reception and analysis of speech or other signals. The apparent ability to control the place of excitation, for instance, in masking paradigms, implies not only that thresholds obtained using frequency-specific and place-specific paradigms may differ, but also that greater insight into cochlear disorders may be gained. This may arise from the place-specific procedures per se, or from their relationships to frequency-based procedures.

There is considerable doubt that it is possible to obtain threshold measurements that are adequately frequency specific over a wide range of severities and contours of cochlear hearing loss using simple transient acoustical stimuli such as tone pips. Some of these issues are reviewed in this volume, and have been described elsewhere (Gorga & Worthington, 1983; Jacobson, 1983). A great deal of research is required in order to establish appropriate and generally valid procedures.

In connection with the ABR, the question arises as to what is, or is not, properly considered to be part of the ABR. For example, Davis and Hirsh (1979) introduced the concept of the SN_{10} response, a prominent vertex-negative wave which could serve as an audiometric tool. SN_{10} is easily seen in response to brief tone pip stimuli, especially if steep high-pass filtering of the EEG is used in the recording. As indicated by Hyde, elsewhere in this volume, in most cases SN_{10} arises from phase distortion of the energy in wave V itself. Accordingly, SN_{10} is indeed part of the ABR, and whatever reservations are applied to the frequency or place specificity of wave V also apply to SN_{10}.

There is a variation across subjects in the prominence of the SN_{10} component in wide-band records, and if such records are strongly high-pass filtered, oscillatory activity extending through 20 ms latency or more can be induced. Accordingly, part of the middle latency response and 40-Hz event-related potential may, in fact, be ABR.

STUDIES OF COCHLEAR SIGNAL PROCESSING

The pure tone audiogram is extremely limited as a predictor of the difficulty a patient will experience in real-life situations such as the reception of speech in a background of competing speech or noise. Pure tone sensitivity loss is apparently a rather gross and insensitive indicator of cochlear damage. Indeed, there may be normal thresholds in the presence of serious communication problems, and it is probable that some disorders labeled as "central" may have at least partial origins in subtle cochlear dysfunction which is not tapped by conventional audiometry. There is increasing emphasis upon disorders of frequency selectivity or of temporal processing as potentially more sensitive and predictive indices of cochlear dysfunction. A problem with more complex psychoacoustical techniques is that they are either unreasonably difficult, lengthy, or are strongly confounded by extraneous variables when applied to patients. Here, electrophysiological methods may prove to be very valuable, because of their relative objectivity and efficiency. It has been demonstrated, for example, that cochleographic study of cochlear frequency selectivity is feasible in humans, and an important question is whether useful measures of this feature of cochlear function can be obtained noninvasively by ABR methods. A few studies have given promising results and it is to be expected that activity in this area will become intensive. It is interesting to note that lack of place specificity, which is a serious problem in the ABR, may turn out to be a powerful concept in more detailed analysis of cochlear dysfunction.

At present, it is too early to say what the ultimate contribution of the ABR will be to a better understanding of cochlear dysfunction, to quantifying its perceptual sequelae, and to more refined diagnosis and rehabilitation. The history of ABR research and development suggests two things: that there will be a useful contribution, and that current methods and interpretations will rapidly become outdated.

REFERENCES

Coats, A.C. (1978). Human auditory nerve action potentials and brain stem evoked responses. Latency–intensity functions in detection of cochlear and retrocochlear abnormality. *Archives of Otolaryngology, 104,* 709.

Davis, H. & Hirsh, S.K. (1979). A slow brain-stem response for low-frequency audiometry. *Audiology, 18,* 445-461.

Don, M., & Eggermont, J.J. (1978). Analysis of click-evoked brainstem potentials in man using high-pass noise masking. *Journal of the Acoustical Society of America, 63,* 1084-1092

Evans, E.F. (1983). Pathophysiology of the peripheral hearing mechanism. In M.E. Lutman & M.P. Haggard (Eds.), *Hearing science and hearing disorders.* New York: Academic Press.

Galambos, R., & Hecox, K.E. (1978). Clinical applications of the auditory brainstem response. *Otolaryngologic Clinics of North America, 11,* 709-722.

Gorga, M.P., & Worthington, D.W. (1983). Some issues relevant to the measurement of frequency-specific auditory brainstem responses. *Seminars in Hearing, 4,* 353-362.

Hall, J.W. (1984). Auditory brainstem response audiometry. In J. Jerger (Ed.), *Hearing disorders in adults.* San Diego: College-Hill Press.

Jacobson, J.T. (1983). Effects of rise time and noise masking on tone pip auditory brainstem responses. *Seminars in Hearing, 4,* 363-373.

Jerger, J., & Mauldin, L. (1978). Prediction of sensorineural hearing level from the brain stem evoked response. *Archives of Otolaryngology, 104,* 456.

Laukli, E. (1983). Stimulus waveforms used in brainstem response audiometry. *Scandinavian Audiology, 12,* 83–89.

Picton, T.W., Stapells, D.R., & Campbell, K.B. (1981). Auditory evoked potentials from the human cochlea and brainstem. *Journal of Otolaryngology, 10,* Supplement 9.

Rosenhamer, H. (1981). Auditory evoked brainstem electric response (ABR) in cochlear hearing loss. In T. Lundborg (Ed.), *Scandinavian symposium on brain stem response (ABR). Scandinavian Audiology,* Supplement 13.

Selters, W.A., & Brackmann, D.E. (1977). Acoustic tumor detection with brain stem electric response audiometry. *Archives of Otolaryngology, 103,* 187.

Stockard, J.E., & Stockard, J.J. (1983). Recording and analyzing. In E.J. Moore (Ed.), *Bases of auditory brain-stem evoked responses.* New York: Grune & Stratton.

Yamada, O., Kodera, K., & Yagi, T. (1979). Cochlear processes affecting Wave V latency of the auditory evoked brainstem response: A study of patients with sensory hearing loss. *Scandinavian Audiology, 8,* 67–70.

Chapter 9

Frequency Specificity in Evoked Potential Audiometry

David R. Stapells
Terence W. Picton
Marilyn Pérez-Abalo
Daniel Read
Andrée Smith

INTRODUCTION

The *frequency specificity* of an audiometric measurement indicates how frequency independent a measure at one frequency is of the measures at other frequencies. The term is usually applied to the evaluation of auditory thresholds. When frequency specificity is poor, the threshold at one frequency may be inaccurately measured because of responses mediated by other frequencies. This chapter discusses many aspects of frequency specificity in brainstem response audiometry. We shall try to link them all together by bedtime.

Electrophysiological Audiometry

The auditory evoked potentials are the electrical responses of the nervous system to auditory stimuli. These responses are recorded at some distance from the cells being activated by the auditory stimuli, and represent the overlapping field potentials of these cells. Because of this overlapping, the evoked potentials (EPs) are largest when cells are activated synchronously, and when the activated cells are sufficiently organized geometrically to create large fields at a distance. Because most neuronal responses contain both negative and positive components, they are more easily evoked by the onset than by the continuation of the stimulus (Elberling, 1976). Because different neurons may be activated at different thresholds, the EPs are best evoked when the onset of a stimulus is sufficiently rapid to activate both high- and low-threshold fibers simultaneously. Furthermore, the shorter the latency of the EP, the briefer the stimulus that evokes it. Even when the stimulus is prolonged the response is evoked only by the onset of that stimulus. The most commonly used stimuli in evoked potential audiometry are therefore clicks and brief tones.

Acoustics of Brief Stimuli

Brief auditory stimuli are quite different from the long-lasting pure tones used in conventional audiometry. Clicks produced by passing a brief square wave through an earphone have a broad frequency spectrum with a null value at the frequency equal to the reciprocal of the square wave duration (Pfeiffer, 1974). The flatness and the upper frequency cutoff of the spectrum are determined by the transfer function of the earphone. Brief tones have a concentration of energy at the nominal frequency of the tone and sidebands of energy at higher and lower frequencies (Burkard, 1984; Laukli, 1983b). The periodicity of these sidebands is determined by the duration of the tone, whereas the relative energy in the sidebands is determined by the rise and fall times of the tonal envelope. The spread of energy to frequencies other than the nominal frequency of the tone is termed "spectral splatter" (Durrant, 1983). Several approaches to a reasonable compromise between the brief duration of the tone and its frequency specificity are available (Davis, Hirsh, Popelka, & Formby, 1984; Gabor, 1947; Harris, 1978), but none can completely prevent spectral splatter. Distortion of the stimuli during passage through the middle ear may further broaden their effective frequency spectrum. Because both clicks and brief tones contain energy over a range of frequencies, responses to these stimuli may be evoked by any of the frequencies present in their spectrum.

Frequency Analysis in the Cochlea

The frequency content of an auditory stimulus is analyzed in the cochlea by several mechanisms. Because of the physical properties of the basilar membrane and the cochlear fluids, a wave travels from the base of the cochlea toward the apex (von Békésy, 1960). The higher frequencies in the sound will vibrate only the basal regions of the basilar membranes; the lower frequencies will vibrate all the regions of the basilar membrane but mostly the apical regions. This traveling wave results in a *place* coding for frequency on the basilar membrane. There are three important corollaries to this analysis: First, the traveling wave has a finite velocity that decreases as it moves along the basilar membrane. The wave takes approximately 5 ms to travel from the base to the apex of the human cochlea. Responses to low-frequency sounds are initiated later than those to high-frequency sounds. Second, the traveling wave is asymmetrical. High frequencies activate only the high-frequency region of the basilar membrane but low frequencies activate both basal and apical regions. Thus the traveling wave acts as a sequential low-pass filter. Third, because of the decreasing velocity of the traveling wave, the extent of basilar membrane specifically activated by a particular frequency increases as the wave moves from base to apex. The mapping of frequency to distance along the basilar membrane is approximately logarithmic.

As well as the traveling wave, there may exist a "second filter" that makes the normal neuronal response more specific to one "characteristic" frequency than would be expected from an initial evaluation of the traveling wave. Gorga and Worthington (1983) have recently discussed this second filter theory. The second filter may derive from some extra tuning of the basilar membrane, some complex interaction between inner and outer hair cells, or both of these phenomena. The effect of this second filter is to add a low-intensity tip onto the broad high-intensity tuning curve of the auditory nerve fiber response. In cochlear pathology this tip is reduced. The thresholds for activating the nerve fibers are elevated, but once reached the activation is similar to when the tips were present.

The phase locking of neuronal discharges to the periodicity of an auditory stimulus is an additional means for providing frequency information. This type of analysis is probably basic to most of pitch perception. The auditory brainstem responses (ABR) have not been extensively evaluated in the context of this type of frequency analysis. The *frequency following potential* (Huis in't Veld, Osterhammel, & Terkildsen, 1977; Moushegian, Rupert, & Stillman, 1978) may reflect the locking of brainstem neurons to low-frequency stimuli. Since it is only evoked by low-frequency stimuli with intensities greater than 40 dB above threshold, it is not very helpful in evaluating frequency-specific thresholds and will not be further discussed.

Masking

Masking has been used in several evoked potential techniques for obtaining frequency-specific thresholds. It is therefore important to review briefly some of the present concepts of masking. The "line-busy" hypothesis proposes that the response of neurons to the masking stimulus makes them unable to respond further when the masked stimulus is presented. This theory, particularly when one considers the effects of adaptation to an ongoing masking stimulus (Smith, 1979), can explain most masking phenomena. There remain, however, some phenomena that are difficult to explain in this way and require the further postulation of "suppression" (Geisler & Sinex, 1980; Pickles, 1982). Suppression occurs when the presence of one stimulus does not activate a fiber but decreases its sensitivity to another stimulus. Suppression may involve similar processes to those mediating "two-tone inhibition" (Sachs & Kiang, 1968). Most studies of the mechanisms of masking have been performed in normal cochleas. Exactly how masking is changed in pathological cochleas is unknown. It is possible that pathology may invalidate some of the assumptions underlying the use of masking to increase frequency specificity (Gorga & Worthington, 1983), although there is, as yet, no evidence of this. A final aspect of masking that should be considered is the "spread of masking." Because of the asymmetry of the traveling wave, low-frequency stimuli are able to mask higher frequency stimuli (by busy-line mechanisms) but not vice versa (Egan & Hake, 1950).

Adding and Averaging

We now switch from the acoustic noise that may mask our perception of sound to the background electroencephalographic (EEG) and electromyographic (EMG) noise that obscures our recognition of the EPs. The ABR is too small to recognize in the background EEG and EMG, and must be recorded by averaging. Averaging assumes that a signal (the EP) remains constant each time a stimulus is presented, whereas the noise (background EEG and EMG) is different. The basic principle of averaging is that, as the sweeps are added together, the amplitude of the noise obscuring the signal increases less rapidly than that of the signal (see Hyde, chapter 3).

It is important to realize that averaging can never totally eliminate the background EEG and EMG noise. There will also be some residual unaveraged noise remaining in any averaged evoked potential (Picton, Linden, Hamel, & Maru, 1983). This residual noise must be considered when one adds two waveforms together or subtracts one waveform from another. In these manipulations, one does not divide by 2 as one does in averaging (but beware the simplicity of push-button computers). If the residual noise components in the two waveforms being combined are independent, the residual noise of their sum or difference will have a root mean square value which is $\sqrt{2}$ times that of the two original waveforms.

BRAINSTEM RESPONSES TO CLICKS

The most common stimulus in auditory brainstem response audiometry is a broad-band click. While some frequency-specific auditory threshold data can be gained from the click response, more information is available if the clicks are presented with various masking stimuli. This section discusses responses to unmasked clicks, the controversial literature concerning the brainstem responses to clicks in notched noise, and finally, two *derived response* techniques: the first based on masking with high-pass noise, and the second based on masking with pure tones or bandpass noise.

Unmasked Clicks

Although the ABR to broad-band clicks cannot provide accurate information about hearing threshold levels at different frequencies, it nevertheless provides important audiometric information. The threshold for the click-evoked potential can give a rough idea of the overall threshold for hearing, while the latency–intensity function for wave V can provide some insight into the etiology and audiometric configuration of a hearing loss.

Several reports have indicated that the click-ABR threshold correlates best with hearing threshold at 2000–4000 Hz (Coats & Martin, 1977; Jerger & Mauldin, 1978; Yamada, Kodera, & Yagi, 1979; Yamada, Yagi, Yamane, & Suzuki, 1975). These results should be viewed with caution since these responses (with the exception of those of Coats and Martin) were obtained using a short sweep of 10 ms and/or a high, low-frequency cutoff setting ($>$100 Hz). The components of the brainstem response that derive from the low-frequency regions of the cochlea may have latencies of 15 ms or more, and have their major electrical energy at frequencies below 100 Hz. These cautions notwithstanding, the most recognizable components of the click-ABR response derive from the 2000- to 4000-Hz region of the cochlea. This is because high-frequency regions of the cochlea are located close together in an area of the basilar membrane where the traveling wave has relatively high velocity, resulting in a more synchronized discharge and a higher amplitude response.

The *latency-intensity* function for wave V can also provide information that is helpful in determining the nature of a hearing loss. The normal latency of wave V in response to broad-band clicks changes from about 5.6 ms at 80 dB nHL to about 8.2 ms at 10 dB nHL (Picton, Stapells, & Campbell, 1981). The standard deviation of this latency increases from about 0.2 ms at high intensity to about 0.3 ms at low intensity. The normal click latency–intensity function has an average slope of about 40 μs/dB. However, the function is somewhat curved and the slope at high intensities may be as low as 10 μs/dB while, at low intensities, as high as 60 μs/dB.

There are two basic types of abnormal latency–intensity functions (Galambos & Hecox, 1978; Picton, Woods, Baribeau-Bräun, & Healey, 1977; Yamada et al., 1975; Yamada et al., 1979). These are illustrated in Figure 9-1. The first type of abnormal function is one in which wave V occurs within normal limits at high intensities. When the intensity is decreased there is either a rapid increase in the latency of wave V outside normal limits or an abrupt disappearance of the response (Figure 9-1A). This abnormality indicates a cochlear hearing loss and is usually associated with recruitment. The second type of abnormal latency–intensity function is one in which the entire function is skewed to the right of the normal limits. There are three different causes of this finding. First, a conductive hearing loss will displace the latency–intensity function by an amount approximately equivalent to the hearing loss (Figure 9-1B). A similar shift of the latency–intensity function may result from a steep high-frequency cochlear hearing loss (Figure 9-1C). In this case, the displacement is not due to the decreased intensity of sound reaching the cochlea but is due to the traveling wave delay to reach a responsive low-frequency region of the cochlea. In a sense, the function is skewed upward rather than to the right. The slope of this latency–intensity function may be slightly less than normal (Galambos & Hecox, 1978). About 1 ms of the total 3.5-ms change in latency from 80 dB to threshold is caused by an apical shift of the region of the basilar membrane responsible for wave V (Picton et al., 1981), and this would not occur in patients with a high-frequency hearing loss. In these patients there is little if any apical shift since the basal regions of the cochlea are not functioning. A third cause of a delayed wave V latency–intensity function is the presence of retrocochlear dysfunction that slows neural conduction between the ear and the generator of wave V (Figure 9-1D). Distinguishing between these three causes of a skewed latency–intensity function requires additional information. Impedance audiometry and/or the recording of brainstem responses to bone-conducted stimuli (Mauldin & Jerger, 1979) are helpful in demonstrating a conductive hearing loss. An abnormally delayed wave I–V interpeak latency is helpful in indicating a

FIGURE 9–1.
Latency–intensity functions for wave V of the auditory brainstem response. Two basic types of latency–intensity function are shown. See text for the descriptions. Part A shows the audiogram and latency–intensity functions for a patient with Meniere's disease. The open circles represent the results for the left ear and the closed circles the results for the right ear. On the latency–intensity graphs the dashed lines represent the normal values obtained in our laboratory plotted at ± 2 SD. Part B shows the results obtained in a patient with a conductive hearing loss. The filled circles represent the results obtained using air-conducted stimuli, and the open triangles represent the results obtained by bone conduction. Part C illustrates the results obtained in a patient with a steep high-frequency hearing loss. Part D indicates the results obtained in a patient with an acoustic neuroma.

Illustration continued on following page.

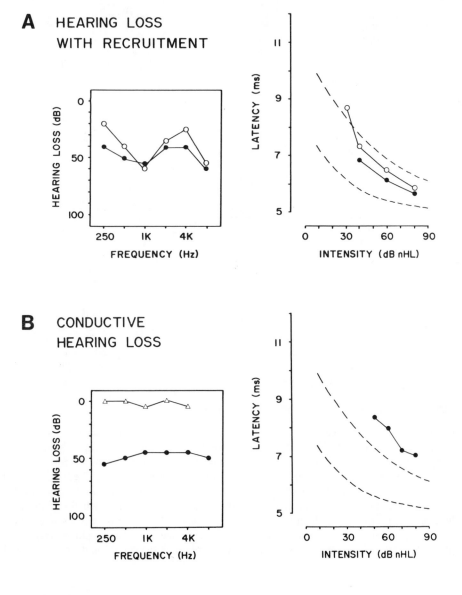

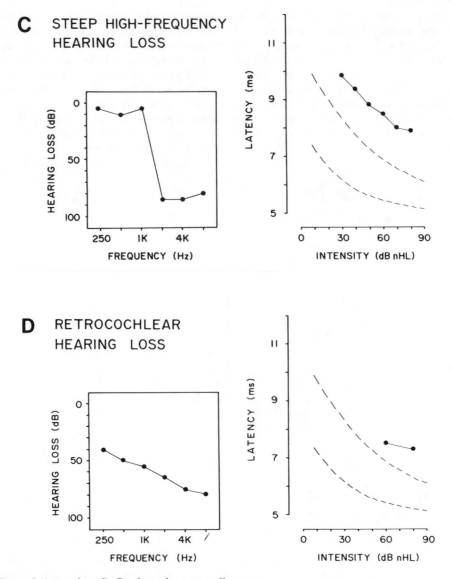

Figure 9–1 (continued). See legend on preceding page.

retrocochlear hearing impairment. These results may be difficult to obtain since bone-conduction EPs are technically demanding and since, particularly in high-frequency hearing losses, the first component of the brainstem response may be too small for accurate measurement.

Click ABRs are therefore an important part of objective audiometry. These responses can provide (i) an evaluation of the retrocochlear pathways; (ii) a general idea of auditory sensitivity, particularly at the higher frequencies; and (iii) some suggestion about whether a peripheral hearing loss is conductive, high frequency, or recruiting. There are several disadvantages to limiting the evaluation to unmasked clicks only. Individuals with hearing losses restricted to particular frequencies may show normal ABRs. Normal thresholds and latency–intensity functions for click-evoked ABRs can be recorded from ears having significant losses between 500 and 6000 Hz (Picton, Ouellette, Hamel, & Smith, 1979; Yamada et al., 1979). Furthermore, the residual low-frequency sensitivity in a patient with a severe high-frequency loss cannot be assessed with these responses. Finally, the click-evoked ABR cannot provide the information about hearing at different frequencies that is necessary for the proper fitting of hearing aids. Several techniques have therefore been devised to improve the frequency specificity of the click-evoked brainstem potential. These techniques involve various types of masking: notched noise, high-pass noise, and pure tones or bandpass noise.

Clicks in Notched Noise

Notched noise is broad-band noise in which one band of frequencies has been stopped or rejected. It allows responses to frequencies within the notch while masking responses to frequencies outside the notch. The effective depth of the notch is limited by the spread of masking from low-frequency edge of the notch; because of the traveling wave hydrodynamics, low frequencies mask regions of the cochlea that respond to higher frequencies. This type of masking was initially used in human neurophysiology by Eggermont and Odenthal (1974) to assess the frequency specificity of the auditory nerve response. Figure 9-2 illustrates the use of notched noise with both clicks and brief tones.

It is theoretically possible to distinguish different frequency components in the click ABR by using notched noise to restrict the responses to particular frequency regions. Unfortunately, the results are quite confusing. Pratt and Bleich (1982) found that waves III and V of the ABR remain clearly defined with notched noise masking, that the latency of wave V increased by about 0.6 ms from its latency in the unmasked condition, and that there was no significant effect of the frequency of the notch on the latency of the wave V. This latter effect was unexpected. One would have anticipated an increased latency of the response with decreasing frequency of the notch. Furthermore, Pratt, Ben-Yitzhak, and Attias (1984) reported that the thresholds for the responses obtained in this manner did not correlate very well with the results of pure tone audiometry in a group of patients with hearing loss. In contrast, van Zanten and Brocaar (1984) found that the latency of the response to clicks in notched noise increased with decreasing frequency of the notch. At 70 dB, for example, they found that the latency of wave V increased from 6.6 to 10.2 ms as the center frequency of the notch decreased from 4000 to 500 Hz. Stapells (1984) also demonstrated this expected latency change from 6.2 to 10.6 ms. Three technical aspects could have caused these contradictory results. First, the notch-width in each study differed; Pratt and his colleagues used a one-half-octave notch, van Zanten and Brocaar a 5/3-octave notch, and Stapells a full-octave notch. Second, EEG filter settings were different; Pratt and his colleagues used a 100-Hz low-frequency cutoff compared to 10 Hz for van Zanten and Brocaar and 25 Hz for Stapells. This cutoff could have made the broader, later components of the response less recognizable. Third, the levels of masking noise were adjusted differently in each of the experiments. In Stapells, the level of masking was adjusted to 5 dB above the maximum level required for perceptual masking in 10 normal subjects. In the other two experiments, the level of masking was adjusted by determining what level was required to make the ABR unrecognizable. However, van Zanten and Brocaar used binaural stimulation, which produces larger responses than monaural stimulation and may have provided a more accurate assessment of the levels of noise required for masking. The results of Pratt and Bleich may therefore have been caused by some degree of undermasking. Burkard and Hecox (1983a) and Moore (1983) have demonstrated that the ABR remains with only a slightly greater latency when the intensity of white noise is raised to a level close to but not quite sufficient for perceptual masking.

To evaluate the effects of the width of the notch and the level of the masking noise on the click ABR in notched noise, a second set of experiments was performed. The stimuli were 100-μs rarefaction clicks presented through TDH-49 headphones at 50/s and at 60 dB nHL

FIGURE 9–2.
Auditory brainstem responses recorded using notched noise. On the left are shown the responses to clicks in notched noise and on the right the responses to brief tones in notched noise. The upper part of the figure represents diagrammatically the frequency spectra of the stimuli (dotted area) and the masking noise (black area). The frequencies in this spectra are plotted from high to low frequency. This is done to make the diagrams compatible with the diagrams of the traveling wave which goes from the base (high frequency) to apex (low frequency) of the cochlea. The area shaded by horizontal lines represents the spread of masking into the notch from its low-frequency edge. In the lower portion of the figure are plotted the evoked potentials recorded from a single subject to 60-dB nHL clicks on the left and 60-dB nHL 500-Hz tones (2–1–2) on the right. Each tracing represents the average of 2000 responses recorded from vertex to mastoid with negativity at the vertex plotted as an upward deflection. Wave V of the brainstem response is indicated by the triangle. The response is much larger to tones than to clicks. Since the stimuli were presented at a rate of 39/s, wave V is superimposed upon a 40-Hz response that is most apparent in the tone-evoked potential, where there is a roughly sinusoidal wave with a positive peak at approximately 5 ms and a negative peak between 15 and 20 ms.

Illustration continued on following page.

Clicks in Notched Noise

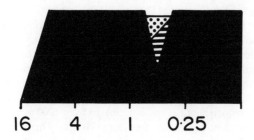

16   4   1   0·25   kHz

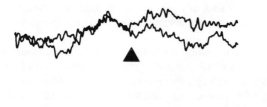

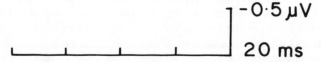

−0·5 µV

20 ms

Figure 9–2 (continued).

Tones in Notched Noise

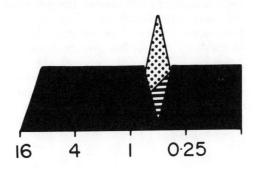

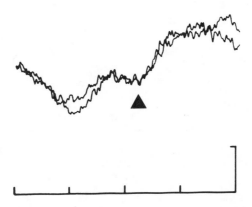

(96 dB peak SPL). Psychophysical studies had indicated that the intensity of white noise required to mask the perception of these clicks ranged in 10 normal subjects from 77 to 83 dB SPL (Stapells, 1984). ABRs were recorded using noise levels (measured prior to notching) of 88, 83, 78, and 73 dB SPL. There were two other variables: the center frequency of the notch (500 or 2000 Hz), and the width of the notch (0.5, 1, or 2 octaves). Three of the eight subjects examined showed expected results. At intensities below the level necessary for masking there were two components in the response to clicks in noise notched at 500 Hz, one at the latency appropriate to the 500-Hz region and one at an earlier latency. At higher levels of masking, the earlier component of the response disappeared. The waveforms from one subject are presented on the left of Figure 9-3. In the other five subjects, the earlier component of the response persisted even at levels of masking above those required (before notching) to mask either the perception of the click or the brainstem response. The responses of one subject of this type are illustrated in the right part of Figure 9-3. The width of the notch had no definite effect on the responses. Since the TDH-49 earphone has a steep drop-off above 5000 Hz, the possibility existed that there was some energy in the click at high frequencies that was not masked by the white noise.

FIGURE 9–3.

Brainstem responses to clicks in notched noise. Responses from two subjects are shown. Each tracing represents the average of 8000 responses recorded between vertex and mastoid, with negativity at the vertex being represented by an upward deflection. The responses were evoked by 60-dB nHL clicks presented at a rate of 50/s in notched noise (NN) that had intensities of between 73 and 88 dB SPL (measured prior to notching). The intensity level of the unnotched noise required to mask the perception of the click stimuli was 80 dB SPL for the first subject and 82 dB SPL for the second subject. In the first subject the brainstem response to clicks presented in noise notched at 2000 Hz shows a prominent vertex positive wave at 7.5 ms (filled triangle) that persists as the intensity of the noise is increased. A small component with a latency of approximately 11 ms (open triangle) is visible only at the lower intensities of masking. In response to the clicks presented in noise notched at 500 Hz the opposite effect occurs. The early component is only visible at the lower intensities and the later component persists at all intensities. The second subject shows somewhat different results to clicks presented in noise notched at 500 Hz. Both components of the response persist at all intensities.

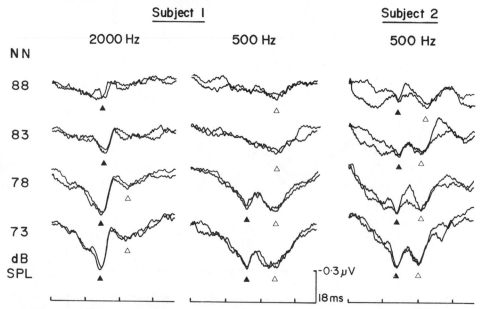

To test this hypothesis, we filtered both the noise and the click with a low-pass filter set at 5000 Hz and a 96-dB/octave slope. The responses to the clicks in the 500-Hz notched (NN) were unchanged.

Despite the complexity of these data, some conclusions can be drawn from our results. First, a late component in the ABR persists with high-intensity, 500-Hz notched masking and is not clearly evident in the response obtained with 2000-Hz notched masking. This component has a broad morphology and probably would have been attenuated severely by the 100-Hz, high-pass cutoff filters used by Pratt and his colleagues. Second, there is a peak in the response to clicks presented in 500-Hz notched noise that has a latency similar to that of the 2000-Hz response. This peak occurs in all subjects when the levels of the masking noise are low, and in some subjects even at high levels of masking. The persistence of this wave at high levels of masking is extremely difficult to interpret if masking is assumed to be based only on "busy-line" mechanisms. However, if one considers that masking may also be partly caused by suppression, then the removal of some of the masking noise at one frequency might decrease the suppression of responses at other frequencies. This removal of suppression might be most evident at the higher frequency region of the cochlea, either because of the particular organization of the suppression mechanism or because that area produces more synchronized responses.

As well as being extremely complex, the ABR to clicks in notched noise is very small, probably related to the spread of masking from the low-frequency edge into the notch (Picton et al., 1979). Using the notched noise with slopes of 48 dB/octave, we examined the effective depth of the notch by recording the improvement in click psychophysical thresholds in the notched and unfiltered noise conditions. The average improvement was only 4, 5, and 7 dB for the noise with notch widths of 0.5, 1, and 2 octaves, respectively. In a study of 10 normal subjects using masking SPL levels of 28 dB greater than nHL of the click and one-octave notches (Stapells, 1984), the average amplitude of the response at 70 dB nHL was 0.18 μV across the frequencies 500, 1000, 2000, and 4000 Hz. This small size of the response makes it very difficult to recognize. In these 10 subjects and in 10 hearing-impaired patients response thresholds significantly overestimated those obtained from pure tone audiometry and were much more variable than those obtained with other EP tests. The ABRs to clicks in notched noise, therefore, do not hold much promise as a technique for objective audiometry.

Derived Responses Obtained Using Clicks in High-Pass Noise

High-pass noise has been widely used to evaluate the frequency specificity of auditory responses since its initial introduction by Teas, Eldridge, and Davis (1962). The traveling wave in the cochlea and the response pattern of single auditory nerve fibers show a very steep high-frequency edge. Noise in the high-frequency regions can therefore mask the responses of high-frequency fibers without affecting fibers with lower characteristic frequencies. This specificity of masking differs from that of low-pass masking where there is a spread of masking into the higher frequencies.

Very regular changes can be noted in the ABR to clicks when high-pass masking noise is used. The response remains relatively unchanged in the presence of masking noise that has been high-pass filtered as low as 4000 Hz. Lowering the cutoff frequency causes the earlier waves I to IV to disappear, leaving only wave V clearly recognizable (Don & Eggermont, 1978; Thümmler, Tietze, & Matkei, 1981). The latency of wave V increases as the response is limited to regions further and further along the basilar membrane by decreasing the cutoff frequency of the high-pass noise. High-pass cutoffs as low as 500 Hz still result in a clear wave V with a latency about 4 ms later than the latency in the unmasked response (Don & Eggermont, 1978; Thümmler et al., 1981).

The relative contributions of each region along the basilar membrane to click ABRs can be obtained by sequential subtraction of the recorded responses using high-pass noise with decreasing high-pass cutoff frequencies. Subtraction of the response in high-pass noise at one cutoff frequency from the response at a higher cutoff frequency leaves a "derived response" to the frequencies between the two cutoff settings. This process is illustrated in Figures 9-4 and 9-5. Derived responses representing a full-intensity series for each audiometric frequency were obtained using high-pass noise masking cutoffs from 8000 to 500 Hz. This technique was first applied to human electrocochleography by Elberling (1974) and has subsequently been used in analyzing the human ABR (Don & Eggermont, 1978; Don, Eggermont, & Brackmann, 1979; Eggermont & Don, 1980; Parker & Thornton, 1978a,b,c). The basic assumption of this technique is that the response evoked through the region of the cochlea that has lower frequencies than the cutoff of the high-pass noise is unaffected by the masking noise. Although there is little spread of masking from high- to low-frequency regions in the cochlea related to the traveling wave, there are definite interactions in the cochlea and in the brainstem between sounds of

FIGURE 9–4.
Derived brainstem responses obtained using high-pass masking. On the left of the figure are shown the brainstem responses to 70-dB nHL clicks presented at a rate of 39/s either alone or in the presence of high-pass masking with the cutoff settings at 4000, 2000, 1000, and 500 Hz. Each tracing represents the average of 2000 responses recorded from vertex to mastoid, with negativity at the vertex being represented by an upward deflection. The diagrams to the left of the tracings represent the spectra of the click (dotted area) and the masking noise (black area). On the right are shown the derived responses obtained by sequential subtraction of the responses obtained using decreasing filter settings for the high-pass noise. On the far right of the figure are shown diagrammatically the narrow-band frequency areas that theoretically activate the derived responses.

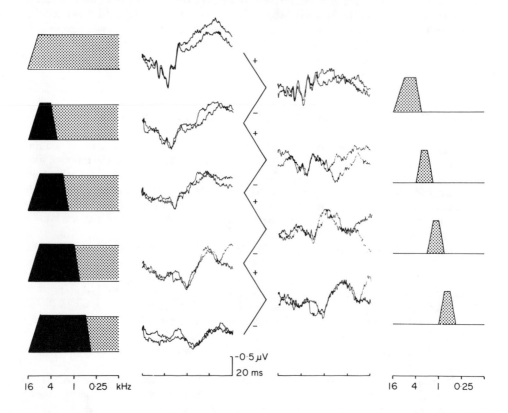

different frequencies. Nevertheless, the derived responses obtained using this technique have definite frequency specificity as demonstrated by masking within the frequency band of the derived response (Parker & Thornton, 1978b) and by evaluating patients with hearing losses at specific frequencies (Don et al., 1979).

As the center frequency of the narrow-band derived response decreases, there are changes in the latency and morphology of the response. Wave V latency increases by approximately 4 ms as the center frequency decreases from 4000 to 500 Hz (Figures 9-4 and 9-5). The higher frequency (2000 and 4000 Hz) waveforms show small early responses (waves I and III) at high intensities, but below 2000 Hz the waveforms show only a broad wave V component. At 70 dB nHL, the derived responses from the 2000- and 4000-Hz regions of the cochlea are most

FIGURE 9–5.
Derived response waveforms. These derived responses were obtained from the same subject illustrated in the previous figure. They represent the derived responses at each of the frequency bands obtained using clicks that decreased in intensity from 70 to 0 dB nHL. There is a recognizable wave V (arrows) at 500 Hz down to 40 dB and at the other frequencies down to 20 dB nHL.

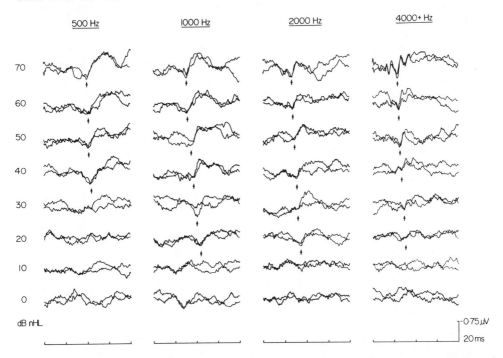

similar to the unmasked response, suggesting that the basal region of the cochlea provides the greater contribution to the high-intensity unmasked response. Little change in the amplitude of wave V occurs with changes in center frequency, although the response is smuch sharper at the higher frequencies. The early studies of these derived brainstem responses reported that thresholds were predicted with 10–20 dB of normal threshold (for the unmasked click) at 1000, 2000, and 4000 Hz and at about 30 dB for 500 and 8000 Hz (Don et al., 1979). The elevated threshold and the high levels of noise required for masking permitted only a 40-dB range to be evaluated at the extreme frequencies.

Normal thresholds for the derived response technique are generally within 15–25 dB of those obtained using pure tone audiometry (Stapells, 1984). However, one major problem with the technique is that the derived responses are difficult to recognize in the background EEG noise. This lack of clarity is due primarily to the increased noise levels introduced when one waveform is subtracted from another. As discussed in the Introduction, this subtraction process increases the noise level by a factor of approximately 1.4. A further problem with the derived response technique is that the high levels of noise required to mask high-intensity clicks can cause temporary threshold shifts. Although high levels of noise can be presented for very brief periods to normal subjects without affecting cochlear function, it is difficult to predict what might happen in patients with pathological cochleas. Our experience has indicated that noise levels of greater than 108 dB SPL should not be used in patients with hearing loss (Stapells, 1984). Since we have found that the intensity of the white noise in decibels SPL required to mask a click stimulus is 27 dB greater than the nHL of the click, this requirement limits the intensity of the click to 80 dB nHL. Another difficulty with the technique is that it requires more on-line recording time than other techniques and extra time after the recording for the subtraction procedures. When responses are derived off-line, one cannot be sure whether a threshold has been reached, thus requiring a full-intensity series at each frequency. Even if one were able to calculate the derived responses on-line, it would still be necessary to record extra waveforms to allow for the subtraction process. As well, derived responses require storage and subtraction capabilities which many clinical averaging systems do not presently possess.

These disadvantages notwithstanding, the derived responses obtained using high-pass masking are probably the most frequency-specific responses available. There is no spread of energy related to the brevity of the stimulus because the frequency-determining high-pass noise is continuous during the recording. Since the steep edge of the auditory nerve fiber response curve remains even in pathological cochleas, the basic technique is valid for patients with hearing loss.

Derived Responses Obtained Using Tonal or Narrow-Band Masking

Another technique for obtaining derived responses uses tonal masking. Berlin and Shearer (1981) recorded the responses to 10/s 60-dB nHL clicks alone and in the presence of continuous pure tones with intensities of 10 to 40 dB SL. They reasoned that the continuous pure tone would activate those neurons responding specifically to that frequency and prevent them from responding to the broad-band click. If the masking effect were mediated in the cochlea, then subtracting the response to the combined click and tone from the response to the click alone could yield a derived response equivalent to the tone response. If the masking effect were partially central, the results would be more complex, but there would still be a different waveform to indicate the masking effect of the pure tone. Their results did not, however, show any derived responses significantly larger than the differences between replications of the click-evoked potentials. Two aspects of this experiment are worth considering when interpreting these negative results. First, the waveforms were recorded after averaging as few as 1,024 responses. Although this yields appropriate noise levels for the elementary brainstem responses, the different waveforms would have noise levels of 1.4 times greater, easily obscuring a small derived response. Second, the tone may have been insufficiently intense to alter the response of the auditory units to the clicks. Burkard and Hecox (1983a) found that levels of broad-band masking below 40 dB SPL had little effect on the click-evoked ABR. It is therefore possible that the 10- to 30-dB SL tones used in this experiment would have had no definite masking effect.

Pantev and Pantev (1982) performed a similar experiment but used pure tones with SL intensities equal to or greater than the intensity of the click. Their initial experiments indicated a derived response with a wave V latency appropriate to the frequency of the tone when the SL intensity of the tones were 0–20 dB greater than the intensity of the click. At these masking levels for a 50-dB click, the 500- and 1000-Hz derived responses had peak latencies of 9–10 and 7–8 ms, respectively. These derived responses changed in latency by approximately 2 ms when the clicks were decreased in intensity from 70 to 20 dB. When the intensity of the masking tone was increased to more than 20 dB greater than that of the click, there was evidence of spread of masking. The 500-Hz derived response had early peaks apparently related to higher frequency regions of the cochlea that were affected by the spread of masking from the 500-Hz tone.

We decided to examine this technique using narrow-band noise rather than pure tones. Rarefaction clicks were presented at an intensity of 70 dB nHL (106 dB peak SPL) and a rate of 21/s. The intensity of broad-band noise required to mask these clicks varied between 88 and 90 dB SPL. Broad-band noise of 98 dB SPL was band-pass filtered with a two-thirds-

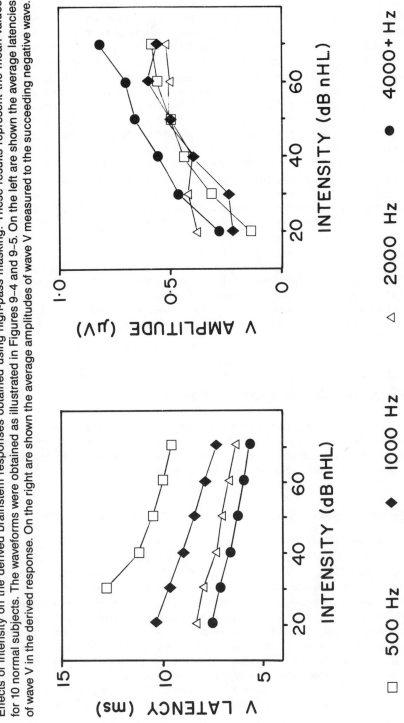

FIGURE 9-6.
Effects of intensity on the derived brainstem responses obtained using high-pass masking. These results represent the mean values for 10 normal subjects. The waveforms were obtained as illustrated in Figures 9-4 and 9-5. On the left are shown the average latencies of wave V in the derived response. On the right are shown the average amplitudes of wave V measured to the succeeding negative wave.

□ 500 Hz ◆ 1000 Hz △ 2000 Hz ● 4000+ Hz

octave width centered at either 500 or 2000 Hz. The EEG was recorded using a bandpass of 25–3000 Hz and 4000 trials were averaged for each response. Sample results are shown in Figures 9-7 and 9-8. The 500-Hz derived response shows a prominent wave V at about 9 ms, but it also produced earlier components similar to those in the response to the unmasked click. These components are probably caused by the spread of masking from the 500-Hz narrow-band noise into the 1000- to 4000-Hz frequency region of the cochlea. They were larger, that is, the masking was greater, when the relative intensity of the masker was increased (Figure 9-8). When the narrow-band masker had a much lower intensity than the click (third tracing on the right of Figure 9-8), there were no clearly recognizable frequency-specific components of the response (cf., Berlin & Shearer, 1981) although there were possibly some earlier components. We evaluated the effects of intensity in five female subjects using noise at 28 dB SPL (measured before filtering) greater than the nHL of the click and found the following average wave V values at 500 Hz: 70 dB—8.4 ms; 0.4 μV and 40 dB—9.9 ms, 0.2 μV; and at 2000 Hz: 70 dB—5.5 ms, 0.6 μV and 40 dB—6.4 ms, 0.4 μV. These results are somewhat different from those obtained using high-pass masking; the latencies are approximately equivalent. The amplitude of the 500-Hz response is, however, smaller than that obtained using high-pass noise masking. This is probably caused by components in the 500-Hz response deriving from higher frequency regions of the cochlea because of the spread of masking. The negative-going wave that follows the wave V from these higher frequency regions would overlap and attenuate the positive wave V from the 500-Hz regions. This spread of masking is not a problem when using high-pass masking techniques. Both techniques involve subtraction, and therefore increase the noise levels of the recording. Masking the tones or narrow-band noise can be done at higher intensities than those possible using high-pass noise masking. Although this latter capability is a distinct advantage, the complexities of the spread of masking suggests that high-pass masking is at present the better approach.

BRAINSTEM RESPONSES TO TONES

The most direct approach to obtaining frequency-specific thresholds is to use frequency-specific stimuli. Many researchers have therefore recorded brainstem responses to brief tones. This section considers these responses and discusses the problem of tonal spectral splatter. Several techniques are reviewed that may provide frequency-specific thresholds.

Unmasked Tones

There are three main brainstem responses to brief tones: wave V, SN_{10}, and the 40-Hz potential. Brief high-frequency tones elicit brainstem responses which are similar to those evoked by clicks (Terkildsen, Osterhammel, & Huis in't Veld, 1973, 1975). Early researchers found that responses to low-frequency tones were difficult to identify and were probably mediated by the basal regions of the cochlea (Davis & Hirsh, 1976). Subsequent research, however, showed that the brainstem response to a low-frequency stimulus was identifiable. This broad vertex-positive wave could be recorded to within 10–20 dB of threshold provided that the high-pass filter setting of the amplifier was lowered to 0.5 Hz from the usual 100–150 Hz (Suzuki, Hirai, & Horiuchi, 1977; Suzuki & Horiuchi, 1977). Davis and Hirsh (1979), using a high-pass filter set at 40 Hz, found the vertex-negativity following wave V to be the most prominent component of the ABR to low frequency tones. They called this wave the "slow negative wave at 10 ms" or SN_{10}. Stapells and Picton (1981) investigated the effects on the brainstem response to 500-Hz tones of varying the cutoffs of the high-pass filters from 10 to 100 Hz. They recorded the largest

FIGURE 9–7.

Derived responses obtained using narrow-band masking. In the top section of the figure are shown the responses to 70-dB nHL clicks presented at a rate of 21/s. Each tracing represents the average of 4000 responses recorded between vertex and mastoid with negativity at the vertex represented by an upward deflection. In the middle section of the figure are shown the responses to the click presented together with narrow-band noise centered at either 500 or 2000 Hz. The narrow-band noise is represented on the left by the dark area. The area shaded with horizontal lines represents the spread of masking from the narrow-band noise into the higher frequencies. In the lower section of the figure are shown the difference waveforms obtained by subtracting the masked response from the response to the click without masking. In the response obtained using the 500-Hz masking noise there is a broad late vertex positive wave with a peak latency of around 9 ms (indicated by the triangle). The frequency scale for the diagrammatic spectra on the left is arbitrary but goes from high frequency (H) on the left to low frequency (L) on the right, as in the other figures of this chapter.

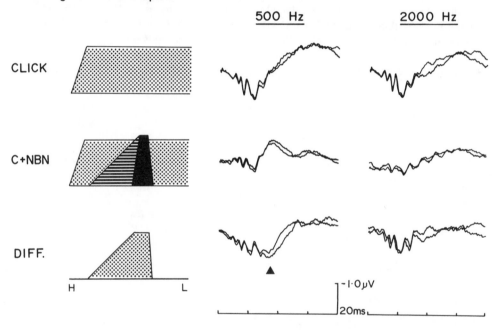

brainstem responses using a high-pass filter setting of 10 Hz. The major component of this response was a broad vertex-positive wave. The use of increased high-pass filter settings, particularly when combined with high roll-off slopes, resulted in responses of lower amplitude and a distortion of the response so as to accentuate the vertex negative wave following wave V. Results of the study recommend using a wide bandpass on the amplifier and recording wave V for tones of all frequencies. Galambos, Makeig, and Talmachoff (1981) recently reported a sinusoidal response to brief tones presented at a rate of 40 Hz. They interpreted this response as the superimposition of wave V and the middle-latency components of the auditory evoked potential. The origin of the response is unknown, but it may, in part, reflect activity of the brainstem reticular formation because of its sensitivity to changes in arousal (Klein, 1983a).

Brief tones differ from clicks in two important characteristics: rise time and frequency content. Two kinds of brief tones are commonly used in brainstem response audiometry—

FIGURE 9-8.
Derived responses obtained using narrow-band noise (NBN) at different intensities. On the left is shown the brainstem response to 70-dB nHL clicks recorded from vertex to mastoid with negativity at the vertex represented by an upward deflection. Waves I, III, V are indicated with the filled triangles. On the right are shown the derived responses obtained using narrow-band noise centered at 500 Hz. The derived responses were calculated according to the procedures illustrated in Figure 9-7. The click intensities are indicated in decibels nHL, and the intensity of the narrow-band noise is indicated in decibels SPL measured prior to band-pass filtering. In the top tracing, when the narrow-band noise is relatively loud, there is no clear component generated at a latency appropriate for the 500-Hz region. There are two earlier components indicated by the diamonds, the first of which has a latency equivalent to the wave V of the unmasked click response and the second of which may represent a component deriving from the 1000-Hz region of the cochlea. In the second tracing there is a recognizable wave (indicated by the open triangle) that occurs at a latency appropriate for the 500-Hz response. In the third tracing when the intensity of the masking is less than the intensity of the click there is no definite response in the 500-Hz latency region. In the bottom tracing, obtained using low-intensity clicks, there is a broad vertex positive wave that occurs at a latency appropriate for a low-intensity, 500-Hz response.

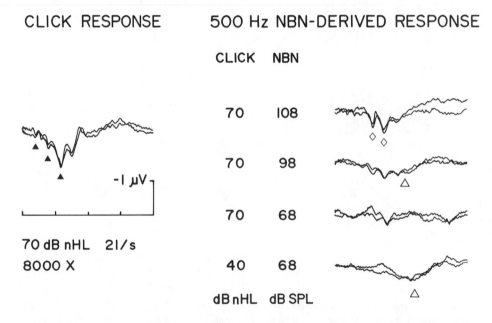

those with rise times comprising a constant number of cycles, and those with rise times lasting a constant time regardless of the frequency of the stimulus. The advantage of the former is that the spectra of tones with different frequencies are equivalent when plotted on a logarithmic frequency axis; that is, the bandwith of the energy in the tone, expressed in octaves, is constant across frequency. Davis and his colleagues (1984) have recommended tones having rise and fall times of 2 cycles each and plateau durations of 1 cycle—the "2-1-2" tone. The advantage of the constant rise time tone is that once the traveling wave delays have been accounted for, the initiation of the auditory impulse occurs at an approximately equivalent time for each frequency. We have recommended using tones with 5 ms rise times regardless of their frequency (Stapells & Picton, 1981).

The rise time of a stimulus affects both the latency and the amplitude of the brainstem response. The longer the rise time of the stimulus, the longer the latency of wave V. Brinkman and Scherg (1979) have introduced the concept of a "virtual trigger time," which represents the point in the rise time of a stimulus at which the majority of nerve fibers innervating the generators of the brainstem response are activated. This virtual trigger time is a function of the rise time, the intensity, and the frequency of the stimulus. Increasing the rise time of a tone while keeping the slope of the rise constant causes no significant alteration in the latency or amplitude of the brainstem response after a critical duration is reached (Kodera, Marsh, Suzuki, & Suzuki, 1983; Suzuki & Horiuchi, 1981). This critical duration is approximately 2 ms for 2000-Hz tones and 4 ms for 500-Hz tones. For tonal stimuli, the amplitude of brainstem responses decreases with increasing rise times, the major changes occurring when rise times exceed 5 ms (Stapells & Picton, 1981). The latency of wave V in response to a brief tone shows complex variations with the rise time, frequency, and intensity of the tone (Jacobson, 1983; Stapells, & Picton, 1981). A high-intensity, low-frequency tone with a rapid rise time has extensive spectral splatter and evokes a dominant early response through the high-frequency regions of the cochlea. The effects of rise time on the responses to broad-band noise stimuli are much simpler. No change occurs in the amplitude of the unmasked response to broad-band stimuli when rise time is increased (Brinkman & Scherg, 1979; Hecox, Squires, & Galambos, 1976). A recent study by Hecox and Deegan (1983) used high-pass noise techniques to demonstrate that rise time has a specific effect on the latency of wave V that is independent of the place in the cochlea mediating the response. They found that a change in rise time from 2 to 5 ms caused an increase in latency of approximately 0.5 ms. Stapells and Picton (1981) found a similar change for high-frequency tones but a 1.5-ms change for 500-Hz tones. The change in latency of wave V caused by varying the rise time of a tone is composed of both a specific rise-time effect and an effect of decreasing spectral splatter with longer rise times. The latter effect is most evident for high-intensity, low-frequency tones.

Changing the frequency of the tone causes very significant changes in the brainstem response. These effects can be seen in Figure 9-9, which shows the responses of one subject to tones of 500 and 2000 Hz. The peak-latency of wave V is longer in response to low-frequency tones than to high-frequency tones. The increased latency reflects, in part, the time taken by the traveling wave to reach the low-frequency regions of the basilar membrane near the apex of the cochlea. The magnitude of this latency difference depends upon the intensity of the tone. At 120 dB peak SPL (about 90 dB nHL) a tone of 2000 Hz evokes a wave V latency of approximately 1 ms earlier than does a 500-Hz tone, whereas at 70 dB SPL the latency is about 3 ms earlier (Stapells & Picton, 1981). This relationship to intensity is most easily interpreted on the basis of the spread of energy in the tone and traveling wave. The relatively early responses to high-intensity, low-frequency tones are probably mediated by the high-frequency region of the cochlea. This spread of energy away from the nominal frequency of the tones becomes subthreshold when stimulus intensity is decreased and the tone then evokes a response through the region of the cochlea specific to its frequency. When the spread of energy in the tone to other regions of the cochlea is prevented by notched noise masking, the latency–intensity functions for low-frequency tones are roughly parallel to those for tones of higher frequency. The effects of notched noise on the latency and amplitude of the brainstem response to 1000-Hz tones are illustrated in Figure 9-10. The amplitude of the brainstem wave V remains relatively constant across frequencies provided that the recording amplifiers have a sufficiently low high-pass cutoff. Indeed, there is a tendency for the response to be larger for lower frequency stimuli, regardless of whether the rise time is specified in terms of a constant number of cycles (Coats, Martin, & Kidder, 1979; Stapells, 1984) or a constant rise time (Klein, 1983a; Kodera et al., 1977; Stapells & Picton, 1981).

There are several means of evaluating the frequency specificity of the brainstem response to brief tones. One method is to compare unmasked tonal responses to those obtained by notched

FIGURE 9-9.
Evoked potentials to brief tones. This figure plots the brainstem responses to brief tones presented at a rate of 39/s with rise and fall times equal to two cycles of the frequency and plateau durations of one cycle. Each tracing represents the average of 2000 responses recorded between the vertex and the mastoid with negativity at the vertex represented by an upward deflection. In the top half of the figure are shown the evoked potentials to 500-Hz tones and in the bottom half of the figure are the responses to 2000-Hz tones. Three responses are given at each intensity: responses to tones presented ALONE, tones presented in notched noise (NN), and tones presented in white noise (WN). The filled triangles indicate wave V in the brainstem response. The masking noise decreases the amplitude of the responses at both frequencies and increases the latency of wave V to 500-Hz tones at high intensity. There is little change in the latency of the response at 2000 Hz. A 40-Hz response can be seen in the responses to 500-Hz tones. This goes from positive in the first part of the tracing to negative at the end of the tracing.

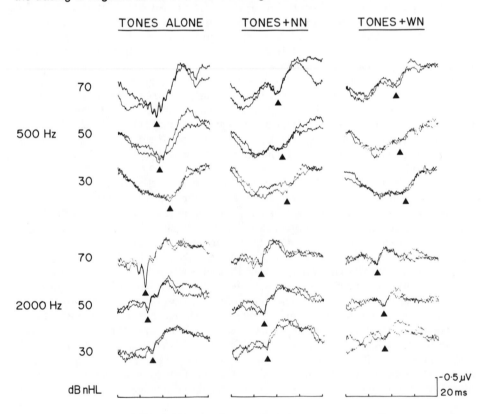

noise. Notched noise serves to limit the responsiveness of the cochlea to regions of the basilar membrane specific to the nominal frequency of the tone (Picton et al., 1979). Notched noise significantly alters the response when tones have intensities of greater than 80 dB peak SPL (Picton et al., 1979; Stapells & Picton, 1981). At these intensities there are components in the response that are mediated through frequencies in the spectrum of the brief tone that are outside of the nominal frequency of the tone. Notched noise can also demonstrate the decreased frequency specificity of tones with short rise times (Jacobson, 1983; Stapells & Picton, 1981). Other approaches use high-pass noise to mask out the contribution of the high-frequency regions

FIGURE 9–10.
Brainstem responses to tones alone and in masking noise. On the left of the figure are graphed the latencies of wave V of the brainstem response to 1000-Hz tones with rise and fall times of 2 ms and plateau durations of 1 ms. Tones were presented either ALONE, in NOTCHED NOISE, or in WHITE NOISE. At low intensities the latencies are similar but at high intensities the latency of the unmasked response is shorter than the latency of the response to tones presented in masking noise. On the right of the figure are plotted the amplitudes of wave V measured to the succeeding negative wave. Each of the measurements graphed represents the average of 10 normal subjects.

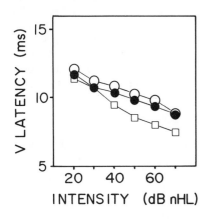
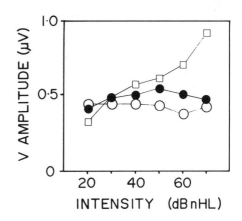

□ ALONE   ● NOTCHED NOISE   ○ WHITE NOISE

of the cochlea (Burkard & Hecox, 1983b; Jacobson, 1983; Kileny, 1981; McDonald & Shimizu, 1981). These studies demonstrate that the responses to high-intensity, low-frequency tones are largely mediated by the basal turn of the cochlea. Klein (1983b) and Folsom (1984) have used pure tone masking to assess the frequency specificity of the brainstem responses to brief tones. Klein measured the level of pure tone masking necessary to reduce the slow wave component of the brainstem response by half. These measurements provide an inverse assessment of how much energy in the brief tone at the frequency of the masking tone is evoking the response. Klein found that frequency specificity was reasonably achieved for tones with rise and fall times of 3 ms up to intensities of 80 dB SPL, except at 250 Hz, where the frequency specificity was very widespread. Folsom measured the change in latency of wave V caused by the pure tone masking. He found that 40-dB SL filtered clicks at 1000 and 4000 Hz (three cycle rise and fall times and one cycle plateau) showed good frequency specificity, but at 60 dB SL (approximately 95 dB SPL) there was a high-frequency spread of cochlear activation. A final means of evaluating the frequency specificity of the response to brief tones is to record these responses in patients with hearing losses that are signficantly different across frequencies. There are several reports of patients whose high-frequency thresholds were significantly underestimated because responses were mediated through the spread of energy in high-frequency tones to the low-frequency regions of the cochlea where their hearing was much better (Picton, 1978; Picton et al., 1979; Suzuki et al., 1981). Such a patient is illustrated in Figure 9-11. This difference between the ABR threshold and the threshold obtained during conventional pure tone audiometry does not happen in patients with low-frequency hearing losses because the pure tone audiogram in these patients may also underestimate the actual loss. As their intensity is raised, low-frequency pure tones can be heard

FIGURE 9–11.
Brainstem responses in a patient with a steep high-frequency hearing loss. In this patient the thresholds obtained during pure tone audiometry (PTA) were 20 dB at 1000 Hz and 80 dB at 2000 Hz. This figure represents the brainstem responses to tones presented either ALONE or in notched noise (NN). There is little difference in the responses obtained for the 1000-Hz tones. However, the responses obtained using 2000-Hz tones show a marked difference in threshold when the tones are presented alone or in notched noise. When the 2000-Hz tones are presented alone responses are recognizable down to 50 dB nHL. These responses are probably mediated by frequency spread to the 1000-Hz region of the cochlea. The 2000-Hz response at 70 dB is very similar to the 500-Hz response at 40 dB. Notched noise prevents this frequency spread and gives a threshold at 90 dB that is just above the threshold obtained using pure tone audiometry. In each of the tracings recognized as a response wave V is indicated by a filled triangle. The unusually large responses (open triangles) noted at 30 and 20 dB for the 1000-Hz tones in notched noise may represent 40-Hz potentials. A 40-Hz potential is also apparent in the response to 90-dB, 2000-Hz tones in notched noise, where it goes from negative in the early portion of the tracing to positive at the end.

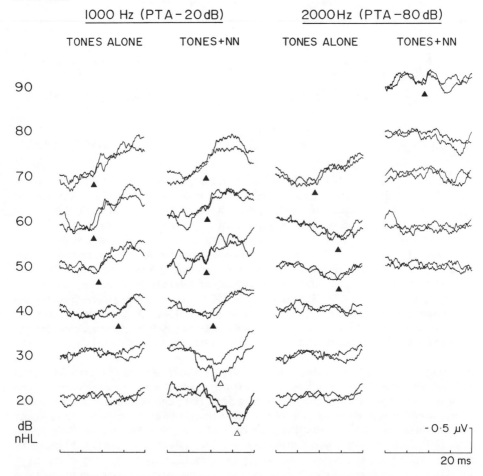

through the basal regions of the cochlea. The steepness of a low-frequency hearing loss never exceeds 40 dB/octave on a pure tone audiogram (Gravendeel & Plomp, 1960; Schuknecht, 1960; Vanderbilt University Hereditary Deafness Study Group, 1968).

In summary, brief tones in isolation may not evoke frequency-specific brainstem responses. At high intensities, they may evoke responses that are mediated by regions of the cochlea that are most sensitive to frequencies other than the nominal frequency of the tone. Some of the techniques that have been used to demonstrate the lack of frequency specificity to brief tones may also be used to ensure that these responses are frequency specific. These are considered in the following sections.

Tones in Notched Noise

As we have discussed earlier, notched noise can be used to restrict the responsiveness of the cochlea to frequencies within the notch. Picton et al. (1979) recorded ABRs to tones in notched noise using rise and fall times of 1 ms and a two-octave notch width. Although the slope of the filters creating the notch was 48 dB/octave, the effective notch was reduced to about 27 by the spread of masking from the low-frequency edge of the notch (Figure 9-2). The advantage of using tones rather than clicks is the lower intensity of the noise necessary to mask responses outside of the notch. In this study, SPL noise levels (before filtering) of 15 dB below the peak SPL of the tone were found to provide effective masking even in patients with steep high-frequency hearing losses. Recently, we used 2-1-2 tones and a one-octave notch and found that noise levels can be reduced by a further 8 dB to 23 dB SPL below the peak SPL of the brief tone. To mask clicks, the SPL intensity of the noise must be greater than 13 dB below the peak SPL of the click; compare the 14 dB found by Burkard and Hecox (1983a) and the 15 dB found in notched noise reported earlier in this chapter. The difference is even more striking if one considers that since the tones concentrate their energy in one frequency region, they have much lower thresholds than the broad-band clicks. Normal threshold for a click is 36 dB peak SPL (Stapells, Picton, & Smith, 1982), and for a 2-1-2 500-Hz tone is approximately 25 dB peak SPL (Davis et al., 1984—21 dB; Stapells, 1984—28 dB). Thus, for a 60-dB nHL click, masking levels of at least 83 (96-13) dB SPL are required but for 60-dB nHL 2-1-2 500-Hz tones, masking levels of 62 (85-23) dB SPL can be used (see Figure 9-2). Tones in notched noise provide a greater concentration of stimulus energy at the frequency under examination than do clicks in notched noise. This leads to a larger but no less frequency-specific response. Furthermore, because much of the frequency spread in the tone is overmasked, there is probably little effect of the suppression mechanisms that may confuse the response to clicks in notched noise.

Notched noise has different effects on the responses to tones of high and low frequencies. These are illustrated in Figures 9-9 and 9-10. Notched noise does not significantly alter the latency of wave V to tones of 2000 and 4000 Hz but it does reduce the amplitude of the response at high intensities. These effects are most easily explained by the removal of an underlying broad response to the low-frequency spread of energy in the tone. The removal of this broad component does not alter the peak latency, which is measured at the sharp deflection initiated by the well-synchronized, high-frequency region of the cochlea. However, the amplitude measured from the peak positivity to the succeeding negativity is reduced. Some degree of masking at the frequency of the notch could also contribute to the decrease in amplitude. Notched noise significantly increases the latency and decreases the amplitude of the response to high-intensity tones of 1000 and 500 Hz. This is because of the removal of the early sharp wave that is evoked by the spread of energy into the high-frequency regions of the cochlea and is superimposed upon the broad wave V evoked from the low-frequency regions.

The ABR to tones in notched noise can provide an accurate assessment of the pure tone audiogram even in patients with steep hearing losses (Picton et al., 1979), as is presented in

Figure 9-11. In this patient, the 2000-Hz thresholds for the tones without masking underestimate the severe hearing loss, but tones in notched noise provide a reasonable estimate of the elevated threshold. The tuning curves of auditory nerve fibers in pathological cochleas may differ from normal by the absence of a specific tip and by a decreased fall-off of threshold toward the low frequencies. As pointed out by Gorga and Worthington (1983), this difference may interfere with the mechanisms of notched noise masking, although our experience has so far shown no evidence of this. Tones in notched noise have been used to assess hearing impairment in infants (Alberti, Hyde, Riko, Corbin, & Abramovich, 1983; Stockard, Stockard, & Coen, 1983). The technique appears to be practical in infants but its accuracy in patients of this age is not yet known.

A simpler approach to masking the energy spread in brief tones is to use unfiltered white noise (Picton et al., 1979). White noise causes effects similar to those of notched noise, except that the amplitudes of the response are reduced, as illustrated in Figures 9-9 and 9-10. Although white noise has the advantage of simplicity, notched noise is more appropriate when measuring responses near threshold.

Tones in High-Pass Noise

The responses to low-frequency tones are more frequency specific when presented in high-pass masking noise. High-pass masking prevents the contribution of basal cochlear regions which could be activated either by traveling wave hydrodynamics or by the spread of energy in the spectrum of the brief tone. This approach has been used by Jacobson (1983), Kileny (1981), and Laukli (1983a). Its advantage over notched noise is based on the lack of any spread of masking from high to low frequencies; therefore, very little masking occurs at the frequency of the tone. Furthermore, the overall intensity of high-pass noise is less than that of notched noise and therefore, produces less stapedius reflex effect which could result in an attenuation of hearing at low frequencies. The disadvantage of this approach is that it is inappropriate for high-frequency tones where the lack of specificity is in the opposite direction to that controlled by high-pass noise. High-frequency brief tones may evoke responses through the spread of energy into the low frequencies. It is possible that a compromise would be to use notched noise at the middle and high frequencies and high-pass noise for the lowest frequency to be examined.

We investigated the effects of high-pass noise on the combined brainstem wave V and 40-Hz response to 500-Hz tones. Tones with rise and fall times of 5 ms and a 5-ms plateau were presented at a rate of 40/s either alone or in the presence of high-pass noise. Tone intensities were 100, 80, and 60 dB peak equivalent SPL (nHL is approximately 24 dB). The high-pass noise had a cutoff at 1300 Hz and a slope of 60 dB/octave. The noise was presented at SPL intensities (before filtering) of 0, 10, and 20 dB below the peak equivalent SPL of the tone. Complete masking of the tone by unfiltered broad-band noise required SPL intensities of 8 dB greater than the peak equivalent SPL of the tone. For the high-intensity tones, the high-pass masking noise caused a decrease in the amplitude of the overall response and an increase in the latency of wave V. These results are shown in Figure 9-12. This effect was not due to a stapedius reflex since it occurred at all levels of the high-pass noise. The wave V latency change is caused by the traveling wave delay. The amplitude change indicates that at high intensities, the 40-Hz response to 500-Hz tones derives from basal and apical regions of the cochlea. This indicates that the spread of energy to the high-frequency regions of the cochlea, by spectral splatter or by traveling wave, had become subthreshold. These results are therefore compatible with those reported by Döring (1983), who found that high-pass noise had no effect on the 40-Hz response to a 50-dB HL 500-Hz tone. However, results suggest that there is a decreasing frequency specificity for the response with increasing intensity of the tone.

FIGURE 9–12.
Evoked potentials to tones in high-pass noise. At the top of the figure are shown, on the left, a diagrammatic representation of the frequency spectrum of a brief 500-Hz tone and, on the right, its brainstem and middle-latency evoked potentials. In the middle and lower parts of the figure are shown the results obtained using high-pass masking noise to eliminate the high-frequency spread of the energy in the brief tone. The high-pass masking noise decreases the overall amplitude of both the wave V component and the 40-Hz response. Furthermore, it increases the latency of wave V. The brief tones had rise and fall times of 5 ms each and a plateau duration of 5 ms and were presented at a rate of 40/s. The overlapped responses to two different tones are recorded in one 45-ms sweep. Each tracing represents the average of 2000 evoked potentials recorded from vertex to mastiod, with negativity at the vertex represented as an upward deflection. Wave V of the brainstem response is indicated by the triangles. The dotted lines show the latency of wave V evoked by the unmasked tones. With masking the latency increases.

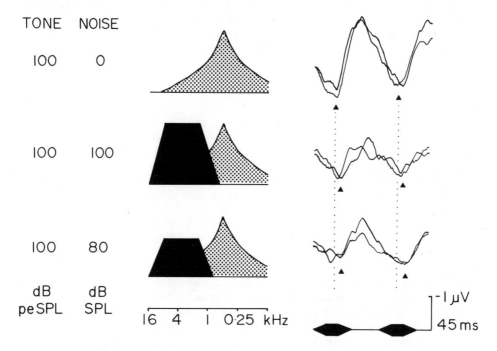

Decomposition of the Brainstem Response to Brief Tones

Helfer and Gerken (1983) have recently proposed a technique that decomposes tonal ABRs into the responses to the high-, middle-, and low-frequency regions of the energy in the tones. They recorded brainstem responses to three haversine stimuli of 500, 1250, and 5000 Hz and pointed out that the response to any of the stimuli could be considered as having regional components from various areas of the cochlea. The actual waveform for each component could be estimated by the relative intensities of the different frequencies in the acoustic spectrum of the stimuli. Once the responses to each tone are known for different intensities, a series of algebraic equations can be constructed along the lines of, "the recorded waveform to a 5000 Hz tone of intensity x dB is equal to the 5000 Hz regional component at intensity x dB plus the middle-frequency regional component at an intensity x–y dB and a low-frequency regional component at an intensity x–z where y is the difference in intensity in the stimulus spectrum from 5000 Hz to 1250 Hz and z is the difference from 5000 to 500 Hz". This series of algebraic equations can be solved to give expressions for each of the regional components. These can then be calculated by appropriately adding and subtracting the waveforms recorded to tones at different frequencies and intensities. The latencies obtained using this technique are similar to those obtained by measuring derived responses by high-pass masking. The advantage of the technique is that it does not require any masking noise. It therefore does not entail the assumption that the response to a stimulus outside of the frequencies being masked is unaffected by the masking. Despite the relative success of the different masking techniques, it is always possible that in certain patients or under certain conditions there may be unexpected interactions between the masking noise and the stimulus that invalidate the procedures. One disadvantage of the decomposition technique, however, is that there may be differences between the spectra of the tone at the earphone and at the eardrum. Another disadvantage is that the noise levels of the responses are increased by the square root of the number of waveforms added or subtracted to obtain them. Finally, the technique depends upon there being no interaction between the responses to the different frequency components of a stimulus, an assumption that, although less demanding, is basically similar to that required of the masking techniques.

CONCLUSIONS

This final section considers the experiments on frequency specificity with reference to the introductory principles of the chapter. The masking procedures used with brief stimuli are related to frequency analysis in the cochlea by the concept of *place specificity*. Some recommendations are proposed on the basis of recording efficiency—a parameter that derives from the principles of averaging. Finally, some comments are made about these recommendations in the context of clinical audiometry.

Frequency and Place

The frequency specificity in the ABR is intimately related to the place specificity in the cochlea where the response is initiated (Starr & Don, in press). Frequency specificity and place specificity can, however, lead to quite different results. The pure tone audiograms of patients without any functioning cells beyond the first turn of the cochlea do not show an absence of hearing but only a mild to moderate hearing loss at the low frequencies. The traveling wave allows the low frequencies to be received by regions of the cochlea normally specialized for high-frequency hearing. Evoked potential techniques that obtain their frequency specificity by masking are in fact place specific. In these particular patients, place-specific measurements show a severe hearing loss at low frequencies that is not present in the pure tone audiogram. In trying to prevent the spread of energy in the spectrum of the click or brief tone from evoking a response, the masking has also removed the spread of energy in the traveling wave which allows low-frequency sounds (without any spectral splatter) to be received by high-frequency regions in the cochlea. Responses obtained using brief tones without masking do not have this problem. They will give quite similar results to the pure tone audiogram provided that the spread of energy in the brief tone is less than the spread of activation that results from the traveling wave. The main difficulty with this approach is that there is a spread of energy in the tones from high to low frequencies as well as from low to high. High-frequency thresholds on the pure tone audiogram may therefore be significantly underestimated when the high-frequency hearing loss has a steepness of greater than the approximately 30-dB/octave spread of energy in a brief tone. It is interesting to note that the spread of energy in brief tones is within the recommended standards for clinical audiometers that was set on the basis of the traveling wave effects (American National Standards Institute, 1973). Clinical audiometers, however, far exceed these standards and allow us to detect very steep high-frequency hearing losses. The information available through place-specific threshold techniques is much more helpful than that available through frequency-specific techniques. The pure tone audiogram can be reasonably accurately derived from the place-specific thresholds, but not vice versa.

Recommendations

When considering the best approach to obtaining frequency-specific thresholds by means of the ABR, one must assess both frequency specificity and recording efficiency. Efficiency reflects how quickly a reasonable signal-to-noise ratio can be obtained so that a response (or its absence) may be recognized. Efficiency is increased by increasing the size of the response and by decreasing the amplitude of the background noise (Picton et al., 1983). Although the technique of measuring derived responses with high-pass noise is probably the most frequency specific of the procedures that we have reviewed, its efficiency is low because of the increased electrical noise in the recording caused by the subtractions. Furthermore, the technique is limited at high intensities by the high levels of acoustic noise required. Our recommendation is the use of brief tones in notched noise. A 2–1–2 tone, a noise level 20 dB SPL below the peak equivalent SPL of the tone, and a notch with a width of one octave and a depth of at least 20 dB is preferrable. Since the efficiency of the measure is improved by recording responses of larger amplitude, notched noise rather than white noise is recommended. Furthermore, it is best to present the stimuli at a rate of about 40/s. At this rate wave V and the 40-Hz response are superimposed and the overall response is larger. The bandpass of the amplifier should therefore be approximately 20–2000 Hz to allow both wave V and the 40-Hz components to be recorded. Finally, we recommend that the click-evoked ABR be recorded prior to evaluating frequency-specific thresholds. The click responses provide necessary information about the general threshold of hearing and about the integrity of the auditory brainstem.

Some Final Thoughts

It is presently possible to measure frequency-specific thresholds in patients by means of the ABR. Certain caveats should be recognized. First, although it is reasonably objective, the technique will never be as accurate as pure tone audiometry. One should expect in most patients to have a range of accuracy of -10 to $+30$ dB with regard to the pure tone audiogram. Second, patients with brainstem disorders may not have measurable responses even though they still have sufficient auditory function to mediate hearing. If there is some suggestion of a discrepancy between ABR thresholds and auditory behavior, one should consider the use of electrocochleography to assess cochlear function. Third, the presence of ABRs does not necessarily indicate normal hearing. The auditory system may be able to generate brainstem EPs but not the more complex patterns that allow the full perception of speech and music. In audiology, the pure tone audiogram is helpful in the initial evaluation of the patient, but speech tests and other tests of suprathreshold audition are necessary when evaluating impairment or therapeutic improvement. At this time we should turn our research to designing objective electrophysiological tests of these suprathreshold hearing abilities. One must always fall asleep prepared to dream.

This research was supported by the Medical Research Council of Canada, the Ontario Deafness Research Foundation, and the United Nations Development Program.

REFERENCES

Alberti, P. W., Hyde, M. L., Riko, K., Corbin, H., & Abramovich, S. (1983). An evaluation of BERA for hearing screening to high-risk neonates. *Laryngoscope, 93,* 1115–1121.

American National Standards Institute (1973). Specifications for audiometers. ANSI S3.6—1969 (R1973), 1–22.

Békésy, G. von (1960). *Experiments in hearing.* New York: McGraw–Hill.

Berlin, C. I., & Shearer, P. D. (1981). Electrophysiological stimulation of tinnitus. In D. Evered & G. Lawrenson (Eds.), *Tinnitus.* Ciba Foundation Symposium 85. London: Pitman Books.

Brinkman, R. D., & Scherg, M. (1979). Human auditory on- and off-potentials of the brainstem. *Scandinavian Audiology, 8,* 27–32.

Burkard, R. (1984). Sound pressure level measurement and spectral analysis of brief acoustic transients. *Electroencephalography and Clinical Neurophysiology, 57,* 83–91.

Burkard, R., & Hecox, K. (1983a). The effect of broadband noise on the human brainstem auditory evoked response. I. Rate and intensity effects. *Journal of the Acoustical Society of America, 74,* 1204–1213.

Burkard, R., & Hecox, K. (1983b). The effect of broadband noise on the human brainstem auditory evoked response. II. Frequency specificity. *Journal of the Acoustical Society of America, 74,* 1214–1223.

Coats, A. C., & Martin, J. L. (1977). Human auditory nerve action potentials and brain stem evoked responses. *Archives of Otolaryngology, 103,* 605–622.

Coats, A. C., Martin, J. L., & Kidder, H. R. (1979). Normal short-latency electrophysiological filtered click responses recorded from vertex and external auditory meatus. *Journal of the Acoustical Society of America, 65,* 747–758.

Davis, H., & Hirsh, S. K. (1976). The audiometric utility of the brain stem response to low-frequency sounds. *Audiology, 15,* 181–195.

Davis, H., & Hirsh, S. K. (1979). A slow brain stem response for low frequency audiometry. *Audiology, 18,* 445–461.

Davis, H., Hirsh, S. K., Popelka, G. R., & Formby, C. (1984). Frequency selectivity and thresholds of brief stimuli suitable for electric response audiometry. *Audiology, 23,* 59–74.

Don, M., & Eggermont, J. J. (1978). Analysis of the click-evoked brainstem potentials in man using high-pass noise masking. *Journal of the Acoustical Society of America, 63,* 1084–1092.

Don, M., Eggermont, J. J., & Brackmann, D. E. (1979). Reconstruction of the audiogram using brainstem responses and high-pass noise masking. *Annals of Otology, Rhinology and Laryngology, Supplement 57,* 1–20.

Döring, W. H. (1983). *Recording superposed middle latency responses (SMLR) for an objective estimation of the hearing threshold at 500 Hz.* Paper presented at VIII Biennial Symposium of the International Evoked Response Audiometry Study Group, Ottawa, Canada, July.

Durrant, J. D. (1983). Fundamentals of sound generation. In E.J. Moore (Ed.), *Bases of auditory brain-stem evoked responses.* New York: Grune & Stratton.

Egan, J. P., & Hake, H. W. (1950). On the masking pattern of a simple auditory stimulus. *Journal of the Acoustical Society of America, 22,* 622–630.

Eggermont, J. J., & Don, M. (1980). Analysis of the click-evoked brainstem potentials in humans using high-pass noise masking. II. Effects of click intensity. *Journal of the Acoustical Society of America, 68,* 1671–1675.

Eggermont, J. J., & Odenthal, D. W. (1974). Frequency selective masking in electrocochleography. *Revue de Laryngologie, 95*(7–8), 489–496.

Elberling, C. (1974). Action potentials along the cochlear partition recorded from the ear canal in man. *Scandinavian Audiology, 3,* 13–19.

Elberling, C. (1976). Simulation of cochlear action potentials recorded from the ear canal in man. In R.J. Ruben, C. Elberling, & G. Salomon (Eds.), *Electrocochleography*. Baltimore: University Park Press.

Folsom, R. C. (1984). Frequency specificity of human auditory brainstem responses as revealed by pure-tone masking profiles. *Journal of the Acoustical Society of America, 75*, 919–924.

Gabor, D. (1947). Acoustical quanta and the theory of hearing. *Nature (London), 159*, 591–595.

Galambos, R., & Hecox, K. E. (1978). Clinical applications of the auditory brain stem response. *Otolaryngologic Clinics of North America, 11*, 709–722.

Galambos, R., Makeig, S., & Talmachoff, P. J. (1981). A 40-Hz auditory potential recorded from the human scalp. *Proceedings of the National Academy of Sciences of the United States of America, 78*, 2643–2647.

Geisler, C. D., & Sinex, D. G. (1980). Responses of primary auditory fibers to combined noise and tonal stimuli. *Hearing Research, 3*, 317–334.

Gorga, M. P., & Worthington, D. W. (1983). Some issues relevant to the measurement of frequency-specific auditory brainstem responses. *Seminars in Hearing, 4*, 353–362.

Gravendeel, D. W., & Plomp, R. (1960). Perceptive bass deafness. *Acta Otolaryngologica, 51*, 548–560.

Harris, F. J. (1978). On the use of windows for harmonic analysis with the discrete Fourier transform. *Proceedings of the Institute of Electrical & Electronic Engineers, 66*, 51–83.

Hecox, K., & Deegan, D. (1983). Rise–fall time effects on the brainstem auditory evoked response: Mechanisms. *Journal of the Acoustical Society of America, 73*, 2109–2116.

Hecox, K. E., Squires, N. K., & Galambos, R. (1976). Brainstem auditory evoked responses in man. I. Effect of stimulus rise–fall time and duration. *Journal of the Acoustical Society of America, 60*, 1187–1192.

Helfer, T. M., & Gerken, G. M. (1983). Frequency information in the auditory brainstem response evoked by tonal transients. *Journal of the Acoustical Society of America, 74*, 1747–1751.

Huis in't Veld, F., Osterhammel, P., & Terkildsen, K. (1977). The frequency selectivity of the 500 Hz frequency following response. *Scandinavian Audiology, 6*, 35–42.

Jacobson, J. T. (1983). Effects of rise time and noise masking on tone pip auditory brainstem responses. *Seminars in Hearing, 4*, 363–372.

Jerger, J., & Mauldin, L. (1978). Prediction of sensorineural hearing level from the brain stem evoked response. *Archives of Otolaryngology, 104*, 456–461.

Kileny, P. (1981). The frequency specificity of tone-pip evoked auditory brainstem responses. *Ear and Hearing, 2*, 270–275.

Klein, A. J. (1983a). Properties of the brain-stem response slow-wave component. I. Latency, amplitude, and threshold sensitivity. *Archives of Otolaryngology, 109*, 6–12.

Klein, A. J. (1983b). Properties of the brain-stem response slow-wave component. II. Frequency specificity. *Archives of Otolaryngology, 109*, 74–78.

Kodera, K., Marsh, R. R., Suzuki, M., & Suzuki, J. (1983). Portions of tone pips contributing to frequency-selective auditory brain stem responses. *Audiology, 22*, 209–218.

Kodera, K., Yamane, H., Yamada, O., & Suzuki, J. (1977). Brain stem response audiometry at speech frequencies. *Audiology, 16*, 469–479.

Laukli, E. (1983a). High-pass and notch noise masking in suprathreshold brainstem response audiometry. *Scandinavian Audiology, 12*, 109–115.

Laukli, E. (1983b). Stimulus waveforms used in brainstem response audiometry. *Scandinavian Audiology, 12*, 83–89.

Mauldin, L., & Jerger, J. (1979). Auditory brain stem evoked responses to bone-conducted signals. *Archives of Otolaryngology, 105*, 656–661.

McDonald, J. M., & Shimizu, H. (1981). Frequency specificity of the auditory brain stem response. *American Journal of Otolaryngology, 2*, 36–42.

Moore, E. J. (1983). Effects of stimulus parameters. In E. J. Moore (Ed.), *Bases of auditory brain-stem evoked responses*. New York: Grune & Stratton.

Moushegian, G., Rupert, A. L., & Stillman, R. D. (1978). Evaluation of frequency-following potentials in man: Masking and clinical studies. *Electroencephalography and Clinical Neurophysiology, 45,* 711–718.

Pantev, Ch., & Pantev, M. (1982). Derived brain stem responses by means of pure-tone masking. *Scandinavian Audiology, 11,* 15–22.

Parker, D. J., & Thornton, A. R. D. (1978a). Derived cochlear nerve and brainstem evoked responses of the human auditory system.*Scandinavian Audiology, 7,* 1–8.

Parker, D. J., & Thornton, A. R. D. (1978b). Frequency specific components of the cochlear nerve and brainstem evoked responses of the human auditory system. *Scandinavian Audiology, 7,* 53–60.

Parker, D. J., & Thornton, A. R. D. (1978c). The validity of the derived cochlear nerve and brainstem evoked responses of the human auditory system. *Scandinavian Audiology, 7,* 45–52.

Pfeiffer, R. R. (1974). Consideration of the acoustic stimulus. In W. D. Keidel & W. D. Neff (Eds.), *Handbook of sensory physiology, Vol. 1: Auditory system. Anatomy and physiology (ear).* New York: Springer-Verlag.

Pickles, J. O. (1982). *An introduction to the physiology of hearing.* New York: Academic Press.

Picton, T. W. (1978). The strategy of evoked potential audiometry. In S. E. Gerber & G. T. Mencher (Eds.), *Early diagnosis of hearing loss* (pp. 297–307). New York: Grune & Stratton.

Picton, T. W., Linden, R. D., Hamel, G., & Maru, J. T. (1983). Aspects of averaging. *Seminars in Hearing, 4,* 327–340.

Picton, T. W., Ouellette, J., Hamel, G., & Smith, A. D. (1979). Brainstem evoked potentials to tonepips in notched noise. *Journal of Otolaryngology, 8,* 289–314.

Picton, T. W., Stapells, D. R., & Campbell, K. B. (1981). Auditory evoked potentials from the human cochlea and brainstem. *Journal of Otolaryngology, 10,* 1–41.

Picton, T. W., Woods, D. L., Baribeau-Braun, J., & Healey, T. M. (1977). Evoked potential audiometry. *Journal of Otolaryngology, 6,* 90–119.

Pratt, H., Ben-Yitzhak, E., & Attias, J. (1984). Auditory brain stem potentials evoked by clicks in notch-filtered masking noise: Audiological relevance, *Audiology, 23,* 380–387.

Pratt, H., & Bleich, N. (1982). Auditory brain stem potentials evoked by clicks in notch-filtered noise. *Electroencephalography and Clinical Neurophysiology, 53,* 417–426.

Sachs, M. B., & Kiang, N. Y. S. (1968). Two-tone inhibition in auditory nerve fibers. *Journal of the Acoustical Society of America, 43,* 1120–1128.

Schuknecht, H. F. (1960). Neuroanatomical correlates of auditory sensitivity and pitch discrimination in the cat. In G. L. Rasmussen & W. F. Windle (Eds.), *Neural mechanisms of the auditory and vestibular systems.* Springfield, IL: Thomas.

Smith, R. L. (1979). Adaptation, saturation, and physiological masking in single auditory-nerve fibers. *Journal of the Acoustical Society of America, 65,* 166–178.

Stapells, D. R. (1984). *Studies in evoked potential audiometry.* Doctoral dissertation, University of Ottawa, Ontario, Canada.

Stapells, D. R., & Picton, T. W. (1981). Technical aspects of brainstem evoked potential audiometry using tones. *Ear and Hearing, 2,* 20–29.

Stapells, D. R., Picton, T. W., & Smith, A. D. (1982). Normal hearing thresholds for clicks. *Journal of the Acoustical Society of America, 72,* 74–79.

Starr, A., & Don, M. (in press). Brain potentials evoked by acoustic stimuli. In T. W. Picton (Ed.), *Human event-related potentials.* Amsterdam: Elsevier.

Stockard, J. E., Stockard, J. J., & Coen, R. W. (1983). Auditory brain stem response variability in infants. *Ear and Hearing, 4,* 11–23.

Suzuki, T., Hirai, Y., & Horiuchi, K. (1977). Auditory brainstem responses to pure tone stimuli. *Scandinavian Audiology, 6,* 51–56.

Suzuki, T., & Horiuchi, K. (1977). Effect of high-pass filter on auditory brainstem responses to tone pips. *Scandinavian Audiology, 6,* 123–126.

Suzuki, T., & Horiuchi, K. (1981). Rise time of pure-tone stimuli in brain stem response audiometry. *Audiology, 20,* 101–112.

Teas, D. C., Eldridge, D. H., & Davis, H. (1962). Cochlear responses to acoustic transients: An interpretation of whole-nerve action potentials. *Journal of the Acoustical Society of America, 34,* 1438–1459.

Terkildsen, K., Osterhammel, P., & Huis in't Veld, F. (1973). Electrocochleography with a far field technique. *Scandinavian Audiology, 2*(3), 141–148.

Terkildsen, K., Osterhammel, P., & Huis in't Veld, F. (1975). Far-field electrocochleography. Frequency specificity of the response. *Scandinavian Audiology, 4,* 167–172.

Thümmler, I., Tietze, G., & Matkei, P. (1981). Brain-stem responses when masking with wideband and high-pass filtered noise. *Scandinavian Audiology, 10,* 255–259.

Vanderbilt University Hereditary Deafness Study Group. (1968). Dominantly inherited low-frequency hearing loss. *Archives of Otolaryngology, 88,* 242–250.

Yamada, O., Kodera, K., & Yagi, T. (1979). Cochlear processes affecting wave V latency of the auditory evoked brain stem response. *Scandinavian Audiology, 8,* 67–70.

Yamada, O., Yagi, T., Yamane, H., & Suzuki, J.-I. (1975). Clinical evaluation of the auditory evoked brain stem response. *Auris–Nasus–Larynx, 2,* 97–105.

Zanten, G. A. van, & Brocaar, M. P. (1974). Frequency specific auditory brainstem responses to clicks masked by notch noise. *Audiology, 23,* 253–264.

SECTION III
NEUROLOGICAL DISORDERS

Chapter 10

ABR in Eighth Nerve and Low Brainstem Lesions

Frank E. Musiek
Karen M. Gollegly

INTRODUCTION

The auditory brainstem response (ABR) has been shown to have significant clinical value in the detection of eighth nerve and low brainstem lesions (Daly, Roeser, & Aung, 1977; Selters & Brackmann, 1977). A host of subsequent studies has corroborated the conclusions of these initial reports. Although ABR is a powerful tool in detecting eighth nerve disorders, it is not without limitations.

The focus of this chapter is to demonstrate both the strengths and weaknesses of ABR in evaluating eighth nerve and low brainstem lesions. Discussion includes only lesions of the auditory nerve, cerebellopontine angle (CPA), and the low to midpons (referred to subsequently as low brainstem). The most common lesion in this area is the acoustic schwannoma which, in the majority of cases, grows into the CPA and affects the lower brainstem (Rosenhall, Hedner, & Bjorkman, 1981). Though at times there can be subtle differences, ABR findings are often quite similar for lesions of the auditory nerve, CPA, and low brainstem. Therefore, we believe it appropriate to discuss lesions of these three close anatomical regions in one chapter.

The framework of this chapter includes brief comments on anatomical and pathophysiological aspects of eighth nerve and low brainstem lesions. This is followed by general data on the clinical value of ABR in eighth nerve and low brainstem lesion detection and considerations for the degree and type of hearing loss. The use of various ABR indices such as latency, wave morphology, amplitude ratio, and repetition rate is presented next. Also discussed are some unique ABR findings in reference to large acoustic tumors and lesions of the auditory nerve and low brainstem other than eighth nerve schwannomas. Finally, information on the use of ABR with other audiological tests in the identification of eighth nerve dysfunction is explored.

OVERVIEW OF ANATOMICAL AND PATHOPHYSIOLOGICAL ASPECTS

Auditory Pathway

The eighth nerve is composed of an auditory and vestibular portion. These nerves, along with the facial nerve, course through the internal auditory meatus (IAM) and connect the vestibular and auditory receptor organs to the brainstem. The auditory nerve has about 35,000 axons, which is approximately 10,000 more than the vestibular nerve has (Rasmussen, 1960). The spiral ganglion has large (90%) and small (10%) diameter neurons that make up the auditory nerve (Engstrom, 1958). As Spoendlin (1973) has shown, most auditory nerve fibers (95%) connect to the inner hair cells. It also seems the larger neurons are those that innervate the inner hair cells (Morest & Bohne, 1983).

The auditory nerve has a definite tonotopic arrangement with generally higher frequency fibers on the periphery and lower frequency fibers in the core (Portmann, Sterkers, Charachon, & Chouard, 1975). The auditory nerve projects to the lateral posterior aspect of the brainstem at the pontomedullary junction. In this area there is a recess formed by the anterior inferior aspect of the cerebellum and the pons termed the cerebellopontine angle. The auditory nerve, upon projecting to the brainstem, divides into three main branches leading to the dorsal cochlear nucleus (DCN), anterior ventral cochlear nucleus (AVCN), and posterior ventral cochlear nucleus (PVCN), all of which are located in the lateral caudal pons. The superior olivary complex (SOC) is also located in the caudal pons, but is more medial than the cochlear nuclei. Input from the cochlear nuclei to the five nuclei complexes of the SOC is primarily contralateral and follows three main routes: the trapezoid body tract, the dorsal stria, and the intermediate stria (Kiang, 1975). A definite tonotopic arrangement continues through the low brainstem. Nerve cells at the cochlear nuclei (CN) and SOC modify intensity representation in a variety of ways. Also, different types of cells in the CN or SOC yield varying discharge patterns for the same acoustic stimulus (Pfeiffer, 1966). These are all examples of physiological processes which code the acoustic stimulus for frequency, intensity, and temporal characteristics.

Of additional consideration is the vascular supply to the low brainstem/internal auditory canal area. The vertebral basilar system is the primary source of vascularization to this area. The vertebral arteries arise through the cervical vertebrae and enter the cranium. At the level of the low pons, these arteries join to form the basilar artery. The anterior inferior cerebellar artery (AICA) arises from the basilar artery and travels superiorly to the IAM. Mazzoni and Hansen (1970) have reported that the AICA may loop in or near the internal auditory canal or may lie in the adjoining cerebellopontine area. At this point, the AICA produces collaterals for the internal auditory and subarcuate arteries before continuing to the cerebellum. Some anatomical descriptions state that the internal auditory artery branches directly from the basilar artery (Chusid, 1979). The internal auditory artery divides into two or three branches consisting of the anterior vestibular, cochlear, and vestibulocochlear divisions. The course of this artery varies, buy may pass between the seventh and eighth nerve to reach the anterior superior or inferior posterior surface of the eighth nerve. Further branching occurs within the inner ear itself (Mazzoni & Hansen, 1970; Portmann et al., 1975).

A detailed account of the anatomy and physiology of the low brainstem and auditory nerve is beyond the scope of this chapter. For more information the reader is directed to the aforementioned references and Møller and Jannetta's chapter in this book (chapter 2), as well as Brugge and Geisler (1978) and Pickles (1982).

Pathophysiology

When one considers various pathologies of the eighth nerve and low brainstem, neoplasms, specifically the acoustic neuroma (schwannoma), head the list. In regard to tumors of the brainstem, there are two major classifications, termed *intra-* and *extraaxial* tumors. Simply stated, the intraaxial tumor is a neoplasm which originates from within the brainstem. The extraaxial tumor originates outside but close to the brainstem. However, tumors are not the only type of lesion which affect this anatomical region. Vascular disease is of great clinical significance and occurs more often than generally expected (Rosenhall et al., 1981). Therefore, in this segment, devoted to pathophysiology, the focus is on vascular lesions and neoplasms. However, it should be understood that a variety of lesions other than tumors and vascular insults may affect the eighth nerve and low brainstem. Some of these pathologies will be covered in other chapters; others we felt too rare to mention in an overview.

By far the most common tumor found in the CPA and low pontine area is the acoustic schwannoma, better known by the term "acoustic neuroma," although this latter term is incorrect. Tumors of the eighth nerve arise from the Schwann cells which form the nerve sheath, hence the more appropriate term "schwannoma." These tumors most often arise from the vestibular portion of the eighth nerve (Skinner, 1929). A good example of the incidence of acoustic schwannomas is related by Rosenhall et al. (1981), who in an ABR study examined 23 patients with extraaxial posterior fossa tumors. In this group, 16 had large acoustic schwannomas that compressed the brainstem. The remaining seven cases were represented by four different types of tumors.

Meningiomas and gliomas are probably a distant second and third most common type of extraaxial tumor found in the posterior fossa region (Huertas & Haymaker, 1969). The meningioma is a benign, slow-growing, primary tumor of the meninges of the brain. Gliomas are tumors that arise from the glial cells that make up the connective tissue of the brain. Probably the most common intraaxial tumor of the low brainstem is the glioma (Huertas & Haymaker, 1969).

The actual mechanism of a lesion of the eighth nerve or low brainstem resulting in an abnormal ABR is not clear. Certainly, a tumor may stretch or compress nerve fibers which may *slow the conduction velocity* of the nerve impulse. However, *desynchronization of the firing rate* of neurons as a result of a variety of pathologies may be a more plausible explanation (Eggermont, Don, & Brackmann, 1980). In addition, *selective action of a tumor on high and low frequency fibers of the auditory nerve* may be responsible for ABR wave V delays (Eggermont et al., 1980). Specifically, if the high-frequency fibers are selectively compromised by the eighth nerve tumor and the low-frequency fibers are not, then it may be the low-pitched fibers that yield the ABR waveform. Since low-frequency fibers (because of the traveling wave time) naturally yield more latent waves, the ABR is abnormal. Recall that high-frequency eighth nerve fibers are on the periphery and are more likely to be affected by a tumor than low-frequency fibers located in the middle of the nerve trunk.

Changes in the vascular supply to the IAM and low brainstem may also occur with resultant symptoms and clinical findings similar to space-occupying lesions (Møller & Møller, in press; Starr & Achor, 1975). Because the vertebrobasilar system is the origin for the AICA and its collaterals, including the internal auditory artery, deficiencies in this network may subsequently be noted in eighth nerve and other cranial nerve functions. The arteries may become restricted in diameter secondary to arteriosclerotic changes and compromise oxygenation in this area. These vessels may also compress the adjoining nerves, causing damage to the central myelin. In particular, the anterior inferior cerebellar arterial loop in the CPA may be compressed, with ensuing pressure on the cochlear and vestibular portions of the eighth nerve, which it may encircle. The pulsatile pressure of the artery on the nerve may create hyperfunction or total loss of function. These nerves then may be disrupted from their normal activity, resulting in tinnitus, hearing loss, and vestibular disorders (Møller & Møller, in press).

The eighth nerve is not the only nerve sensitive to vascular compression. The facial (VII) and trigeminal (V) nerves may also be damaged due to compression of a similar nature. As with the eighth nerve, the pulsatile pressure may create artificial stimulation or compression of the nerve, resulting in hemifacial spasm and trigeminal neuralgia. It is hypothesized that in cases of hemifacial spasm, the close proximity of the dysfunctioning nerve to the eighth nerve may result in disruption of auditory nerve function with subsequent changes in the ABR (Møller, Møller, & Jannetta, 1982). Møller and Møller (in press) suggest that trigeminal neuralgia may be associated with pressure from a loop of the anterior inferior cerebellar artery on the fifth nerve and low brainstem (in the area of the cochlear nucleus or trapezoid bodies), thereby creating delays in the ABR for both the ipsilateral and contralateral sides. They have also observed similar findings in a select group of patients in which a loop of the superior cerebellar artery, rather than the AICA, was observed in surgery. Finally, aneurysms in the vertebral basilar artery system are a less common phenomenon, but have been reported by several authors in recent years (Cler, 1975; Johnson & Kline, 1978; Mori, Miyazaki, & Ono, 1978; Porter & Eyster, 1973). Based on our own clinical experience with aneurysms of the CPA, symptoms are similar to most lesions of this area, but fluctuate in intensity.

GENERAL VALUE OF ABR IN THE DETECTION OF EIGHTH NERVE AND LOW BRAINSTEM LESIONS

The greatest otoneurological value of ABR is its high detection rate for eighth nerve and low brainstem lesions. A variety of studies have demonstrated a better than 90% hit rate for acoustic/CPA tumors (see Table 10-1) (Bauch, Rose, & Harner, 1982; Clemis & McGee, 1979; Eggermont et al., 1980; Glasscock, Jackson, Josey, Dickins, & Wiet, 1979; Harker, 1980; Selters & Brackmann, 1979; Terkildsen, Osterhammel, & Thomsen, 1981). This sensitivity is better than any other audiological test for the detection of eighth nerve and CPA tumors (Musiek, Mueller, Kibbe, & Rackliffe, 1983b). ABR has also been effective in detecting vascular lesions of the low brainstem. Rosenhall et al. (1981) reported abnormal ABR findings in 36 out of 48 patients with deficits in the vertebrobasilar system. Also, several articles have reported cases of vascular anomalies of the low brainstem that yielded either no response or latency delays of the ABR (Coats, 1978; Rowe 1981; Stockard, Stockard, & Sharbrough, 1980).

There is a fair degree of variance in false-positive rates among ABR studies in the detection of eighth nerve lesions. For example, Selters and Brackmann (1979), Glasscock et al. (1979), and Terkildsen et al. (1981) all report a false positive rate of approximately 10%. However, Clemis and McGee (1979) and Bauch et al. (1982) have reported false-positive rates of 33 and 25%, respectively. Reasons for this variance could be related to differing clinical populations, criteria for abnormality, procedural approaches, and even equipment (Musiek, Mueller, Kibbe, & Rackliffe, 1983b). Generally, when false-positive finds are noted, the patient has hearing loss, most often of a high-frequency nature (Musiek, Sachs, Geurkink, & Weider, 1980).

THE EFFECTS OF HEARING LOSS

Hearing loss may have a significant effect on ABR latencies. Thus, it is important to obtain at least basic audiological data on patients scheduled for ABR. The type, degree, and

TABLE 10-1.
Some Major Studies Indicating the Sensitivity of ABR for Confirmed Acoustic Tumors and False Positive Rate as Tested on Various Cochlear Lesions.

		Hit rate		False positive
Selters and Brackmann	1979	92.7%	$(n = 94)$	8%*$(n = 266)$
Clemis and McGee	1979	92.0%	$(n = 29)$	33% $(n = 115)$
Glasscock et al.	1979	98.0%	$(n = 49)$	7%* $(n = 399)$
Harker	1980	94.6%	$(n = 36)$	9% $(n = 111)$
Eggermont et al.	1980	95.0%	$(n = 36)$	
Terkildsen et al.	1981	96.0%	$(n = 56)$	9% $(n = 71)$
Bauch et al.	1982	96.0%	$(n = 26)$	25% $(n = 229)$

Note.
* = Approximated.
Taken from Musiek et al., 1983b.

configuration of hearing loss is critical in the otoneurological evaluation. Each may contribute differentially to the morphology, latency, and amplitude of individual wave components. Since cochlear and conductive loss can result in absolute latency shifts, it is difficult to determine if hearing loss or retrocochlear pathology is responsible for the delay. If wave I and wave V are obtained, the interwave interval (IWI) measure that often resolves this problem can be derived (Eggermont et al., 1980). However, in many cochlear and retrocochlear hearing losses, wave I cannot be identified; hence, IWIs cannot be used. For example, Eggermont et al. (1980) reported 30% of their patients with CPA lesions failed to yield a wave I. Bauch et al. (1980, 1982) commented that interwave latencies often cannot be used due to the absence of wave I in the hearing impaired and occasionally even in normal hearers.

Although an unidentified conductive loss can result in misinterpretation, it is not discussed here because there are many ways this problem can and should be delineated by tests other than ABR. The foremost consideration for hearing loss in ABR testing is the high-frequency deficit. High-frequency loss can result in delays of all ABR waves, poor waveform morphology, and even a flat ABR tracing (Jerger, Mauldin, & Anthony, 1978; Musiek, Sachs, Geurkink, & Weider, 1980; Rose, 1978; Rosenhamer, 1981). It seems the steeper the slope and the greater the loss, the more notable these effects (Jerger & Mauldin, 1978). In support of the existence of this phenomenon, Rosenhamer (1981) demonstrated a high correlation between the increase in absolute latency of wave V and the degree of hearing loss at 4000 Hz for 65 ears with high-frequency hearing loss. Given this problem, one should consider some manner of offsetting the effects of high-frequency hearing loss when using ABR for detection of retrocochlear lesions.

Jerger and Mauldin (1978) advocate a 0.2-ms offset for every 30 dB of threshold difference between 1000 and 4000 Hz (e.g., if the hearing was 0 dB HL at 1000 Hz and 60 dB HL at 4000 Hz, one should allow a 0.4-ms increase in wave V latency beyond the "acceptable" criterion). Selters and Brackmann (1977) advise adding 0.1 ms to wave V latency criteria for every 10 dB of hearing loss greater than 50 dB at 4000 Hz (e.g., an adjustment of 0.2 ms would be recommended if hearing loss at 4000 Hz was 70 dB HL). As previously stated, all ABR waves may be extended in latency in subjects with high-frequency sensorineural hearing loss of cochlear origin. However, in many of these cases the earlier waves (I, II, and III) cannot be seen. Hence, wave V must be used for interpretive purposes, and some method should be employed to compensate for the possible effects of the hearing loss.

Flat losses, especially when obtained from recruiting ears, generally do not present much of a problem. Often in these cases, clear waveforms can be obtained at a 10–20 dB SL (Jerger et al., 1978). However, if the hearing loss is severe to profound, regardless of the configuration, a reliable ABR may not be obtained. This type of result may be associated with either a cochlear or retrocochlear lesion.

SPECIFIC ABR INDICES AND EIGHTH NERVE AND LOW BRAINSTEM LESIONS

Latency Measures

There are three ABR latency measures of value in defining eighth nerve and low brainstem lesions. Absolute, interwave, and interaural latency differences (ILD) can all be of help in detecting retrocochlear involvement.

Interwave measure. The most powerful latency measure in the detection of otoneurological deficits is the *interwave measure*, specifically the I–V interval (Figure 10-2). A variety of studies have indicated that the "normal" I–V interval is approximately 4.0 ms with a standard deviation of about 0.2 ms (Chiappa, Gladstone, & Young, 1979; Eggermont et al., 1980; Musiek & Geurkink, 1982; Starr & Achor, 1975; Stockard, 1982). The I–V latency interval can be broken down into the I–III and the III–V intervals. Generally, the normal mean I–III latency is slightly greater than 2.0 ms, while the normal mean III–V latency is slightly less than 2.0 ms. Standard deviations for the I–III and III–V intervals range between 0.1 and 0.2 ms (Chiappa et al., 1979; Eggermont et al., 1980; Starr & Achor, 1975; Stockard, 1982). Interwave intervals do not appear affected by conductive or cochlear hearing loss (Eggermont et al., 1980).

Eggermont et al. (1980) reported a 95% hit rate and a 5% false-positive rate for 45 tumors of the CPA. The criterion that yielded these findings was a I–V interval which was greater than two standard deviations beyond their "normal" mean of 4.01 ms (SD was 0.16 ms). Other studies have also shown the value of the I–V abnormality in eighth nerve tumors (Glasscock et al., 1979; Musiek et al., 1980).

In studying the I–III and III–V intervals in acoustic tumors, there are several aspects requiring comment. First, in the majority of cases with acoustic tumors, the early waves may be undefinable. Hence, I–III or III–V intervals cannot be measured. However, in our own acoustic tumor cases where waves I, III, and V could be identified, the I–III interval was more affected than the III–V. Eggermont et al. (1980) have also shown examples of this pattern. However, tumors of the acoustic nerve and CPA can result in an increased III–V and a normal I–III (Harris & Almquist, 1981). This occurrence, however, seems much less common that the I–III interval increase.

In subjects with vertebral basilar disease, Ragazzoni, Amantine, Rossi, et al. (1982) reported increased IWIs. Rosenhall et al. (1981) noted abnormal I–V intervals in patients with vascular disease of the low brainstem region. Increased IWIs have also been observed in subjects with compression of the arterial loop in the CPA. Increased I–III and III–IV wave intervals have been reported for patients with hemifacial spasm secondary to vascular compression (Møller & Møller, in press). Patients with vascular compression in the brainstem resulting in trigeminal neuralgia have yielded an increased III–V interwave latency (Møller & Møller, in press).

Absolute latency

In cases where wave I is absent, one must employ some alternate measure to the interwave indices, such as absolute latencies, as a measure of neurological function. The measurement of absolute latency can be employed only if one has the proper normative data. These normative data should be acquired for selected stimuli, intensity levels, and repetition rates (see chapter 5). In patients with hearing loss, it is probably advantageous to use a high-intensity stimulus to permit optimal waveform morphology (Selters & Brackmann, 1977).

If the absolute latency of wave V is greater than two standard deviations beyond the mean for normal hearers, one should be concerned about a retrocochlear lesion (see Figure 10-6). However, as mentioned earlier, when there is hearing loss (especially high-frequency loss), this must be considered in determining abnormal absolute latencies (Jerger & Mauldin, 1978; Rosenhamer, 1981). Absolute latencies have been shown to be of value in detecting eighth nerve, CPA, and vertebrobasilar lesions in a number of studies, but are seldom used as the "only" latency measure (Bauch et al., 1982; Clemis & McGee, 1979; Glasscock et al., 1979; Rosenhall et al., 1981).

Interaural latency difference (ILD). The ILD is one of the most commonly used latency measures. It requires the comparison of wave V (absolute) latencies for each ear. Several reports have shown hit rates for acoustic tumors of 90% or better using the ILD (Bauch et al., 1982; Clemis & McGee, 1979; Selters & Brackmann, 1977, 1979; Terkildsen et al., 1981). There is general agreement that ILDs of greater than 0.3 ms are significant and may indicate a retrocochlear lesion (Clemis & McGee, 1979; Terkildsen et al., 1981; Thompsen, Terkildsen, & Osterhammel, 1978). Again, hearing loss must be taken into account. Clemis and McGee (1979) relate that when hearing loss is greater than 65 dB HL, a 0.4-ms ILD criterion should be employed to indicate retrocochlear involvement. Terkildsen et al. (1981) noted that several Meniere's patients with a unilateral loss of at least 60 dB HL showed an ILD greater than 0.3 ms, inferring the need for adjusting criteria when the loss is unilateral. Bauch et al. (1982) used an ILD of greater than 0.2 ms as a retrocochlear indicator which might have contributed to their relatively high false-positive rate (25%) in non-tumor patients with hearing loss. However, ILD must be cautiously interpreted since the degree of loss and auditory configuration between ears as well as the intensity presentation levels may significantly affect ILD results.

Waveform Morphology

The determination of abnormal waveform morphology is perhaps the most subjective index. This topic will be discussed in three categories: (1) totally absent (unreadable) waves, (2) absence of certain waves, and (3) noisy waveforms.

Total absence. The absence of all waves or unreadable waveforms is often noted in cases of acoustic neuromas (Figure 10-1). For example, Selters and Brackmann (1977, 1979) reported that approximately one-half of their acoustic neuroma subjects had no response for ABR. Harker (1980) reported 28% of his patients with acoustic tumors showed no ABR. Rosenhall et al. (1981) observed complete absence of waves in 2 of 36 ABRs recorded from patients with vertebrobasilar deficits. However, again it must be noted that if the hearing loss is severe enough, there may be an absent ABR without any retrocochlear involvement.

Total absence of ABR waves is even more likely to occur in an eighth nerve or low brainstem lesion if there is hearing loss. It appears relatively common to note only a wave I in eighth nerve or low brainstem lesions, especially if the hearing is good (House & Brackmann, 1979; Selters & Brackmann, 1977). One explanation for this is that wave I is generated at the more lateral aspect of the auditory nerve and most acoustic tumors arise more medially, close to the CPA. This rationale is even more logical for lesions of the CPA or low brainstem where the acoustic nerve segment responsible for generating wave I has a higher probability of being "intact. "

Partial absence. In addition to total wave absence or the presence of wave I only, eighth nerve or low brainstem lesions can yield a variety of other waveform abnormalities. For example, waves I and III may be present and wave V absent. Although this finding is more common in high brainstem lesions, it has been reported in lesions of the CPA region (Harris & Almquist, 1981; Rosenhall et al., 1981). An absent wave III with a normal I and V has also been reported (Møller, et al., 1982; Rowe, 1981). A physiologic or pathologic rationale is difficult to ascertain for these latter findings. Certainly there could be secondary effects of the lesion, individual patient differences, unusual hearing losses, or a variety of other entities that may result in these waveforms.

Noisy waveforms. The noisy-appearing waveform is a very subjective analysis, but does occur. If the patient is quiet during testing, has good hearing, and there are no technical problems (e.g., electrode contact), yet the waveform is noisy and poorly formed, retrocochlear involvement should be considered (Musiek, 1982). This must be viewed as a "soft" sign, but at times it can be of value if used within its obvious interpretative constraints.

To reiterate, interpretation of the noisy waveform and totally absent wave must be based on audiometric information. These situations can occur with cochlear involvement; therefore, this must be ruled out in order to use these indices appropriately.

Amplitude Ratio

Another index of possible value in detecting retrocochlear lesions with ABR is the amplitude ratio (Musiek, Kibbe, Rackliffe, & Weider, 1984; see Figure 10-3). Though more work needs to be done and there is some controversy surrounding this issue, it appears amplitude ratio can be of value in detecting eighth nerve and low brainstem lesions (Hecox, 1980; Musiek et al., 1984; Stockard & Rossiter, 1977).

Amplitude ratio is simply the amplitude of wave V compared to wave I. By dividing the amplitude of wave V by wave I a ratio is derived. In a recent study at our medical center, a ratio of less than 1.0 was considered abnormal in the adult population if it was repeatable (Musiek et al., in press). We found that of 25 ears with retrocochlear lesions where both waves I and V were present, 11 had an abnormal amplitude ratio. Additionally, it was noted that in 4 of these 25 retrocochlear ears, the only ABR abnormality was amplitude ratio. Stockard and Rossiter (1977), Rosenhall et al. (1981), and Musiek (1982) have also shown examples of abnormal amplitude ratios in patients with retrocochlear lesions.

Though these writers feel that amplitude ratio measurements are of value in detecting eighth nerve and brainstem lesions they must be used with caution. "Normal" criteria for amplitude ratios may vary according to instrumentation used, intensity level, repetition rate, and a host of other variables. Hence, an amplitude ratio of 1.0 may not be a universal criterion and normative data should be obtained for each clinic or laboratory.

Repetition Rate

There have been several case reports of eighth nerve or brainstem lesions that have shown significant wave V latency shifts or degradation of wave V morphology at high repetition rates (Paludetti, Maurizi, & Ottaviani 1983; Weber & Fuijikawa, 1977; Yagi & Kaga, 1979). It is believed that the use of high repetition rates stresses the auditory system and therefore in some cases can uncover an abnormality that may not be identified otherwise. The physiologic basis for repetition rate studies is the neural refractory period. The absolute refractory period is the time interval in which the nerve cell cannot respond. The length of the refractory period for a given nerve cell is dependent, among other things, upon the "health" of the cell. If the nerve cell or cells are not functioning properly, a longer refractory period is required. Neural delay or asynchrony resulting from a lengthened refractory period may be detected by employing a high repetition rate. Further examples of the effect of repetition rate on neurological disorders are illustrated in chapter 12.

To examine the repetition rate effect, one must compare the latency of wave V at high and low repetition rates (see Figure 10-4). In normal subjects there is an increase in wave V latency for the high repetition condition (Don, Allen, & Starr, 1977; Paludetti et al., 1983). The criteria for abnormality are not well published. At our center a 0.1-ms shift is allowed for every 10 clicks/s increase with a variance factor of 0.2 ms. For example, if a low repetition rate was 10/s and the high 50/s, the upper limit of normal for wave V latency shift would be 0.6 ms. Hecox (1980) employs another formula for the interpretation of wave V latency shifts for various repetition rates with adults. The upper limit of acceptable latency shift is determined by 0.006 ms multiplied by the difference between high and low repetition rates plus 0.4 ms. In the previous example: $50 - 10 = 40$; $40 \times 0.006 = 0.24$; $0.24 + 0.4 = 0.64$ ms maximum (normal) shift.

Those using ABR must await a major study on repetition rate and eighth nerve lesions to provide more definitive evidence for its use. However, given the short amount of time required and the value noted in several case reports, repetition rate functions should be included in an ABR workup for retrocochlear lesions.

OPPOSITE EAR EFFECTS IN CPA LESIONS

A large CPA tumor in an individual may displace or compress the brainstem enough to affect the ABR obtained from the ear opposite the lesion (Lynn & Gilroy, 1980; Musiek, 1982; Nodar & Kinney, 1980; Rosenhall et al., 1981). This finding has several important clinical implications. One of these is a rationale for performing an ABR on a patient with absent or very poor hearing in an ear which is suspected of having of an acoustic tumor. Since the hearing may be too poor for the ear in question to be tested by ABR, the opposite ear can be assessed for any ABR abnormality. If ABR results are abnormal in the ear opposite the suspected lesion, there may be brainstem involvement resulting from a large CPA tumor. This in turn may be important information to relay to the surgeon.

In some recent work we have noted a specific type of ABR abnormality in the ear opposite the CPA tumor in a series of patients. It seems that only the ABR waves IV and V are affected for the ear opposite the tumor (see Figure 10-5). Though this type of abnormality is not the only variation we have seen in this situation, it appears to be the most common in our series of patients (Musiek, Kibbe, & Strojny, 1983a).

Laterality Aspects

Excluding large CPA tumors, acoustic tumors typically affect the ipsilateral ABR. However, when there is a lesion of the low brainstem, the effects may not be as clear. When the lesion is in the brainstem, ipsilateral and bilateral findings are probably more common (Musiek & Geurkink, 1982; Oh, Kuba, Soyer, Choi, Bonikowski, & Vitek, 1981). However, to a lesser extent, contralateral abnormalities may also exist (Stockard, Stockard, & Sharbrough, 1977). Laterality findings depend on many factors such as ABR recording sites, and the level (rostral or caudal to the level of auditory decussation), size, and type of the lesion.

The rationale for using multiple ABR indices such as those just reviewed is a logical and important one. First, with a variety of measures, the probability of detecting a lesion in the eighth nerve or low brainstem is greater than if only one ABR measurement were employed. In addition, for a given patient, various ABR indices may not be applicable. As mentioned, if wave I cannot be obtained, the I–V interwave measure is not possible. However, if one has obtained good normative data for the other indices, these can be used to evaluate the ABR.

Finally, as alluded to earlier, not all the previously discussed indices should be viewed as having equal clinical value. The latency measures remain the most valid and reliable tool for ABR assessment. The other parameters can be useful but generally are not as robust as the various ABR latency measurements.

THE USE OF OTHER AUDIOLOGIC TESTS FOR EIGHTH NERVE AND LOW BRAINSTEM LESIONS

Although ABR measures have contributed greatly to the identification of eighth nerve and brainstem lesions, the need for and benefits of behavioral audiometric assessment cannot be overstated. These behavioral tests are often critical when the efficacy of the ABR is reduced due to confounding hearing loss. Numerous measures have evolved over the years and vary in their effectiveness and clinical feasibility (Musiek, Mueller, Kibbe, & Rackliffe, 1983b). These tests should provide a measure for adaptation, rollover, recruitment, binaural release of masking, and integrity of the reflex arc—phenomena often associated with eighth nerve and brainstem dysfunction. Time constraints may necessitate a selected sample of these procedures; however, one or more is advised when evaluating the suspect patient.

SUMMARY

This chapter has focused on the value, limitations, and precautions in the evaluation of eighth nerve and low brainstem lesions using ABR. Basic anatomical and pathophysiological data have been reviewed to provide a basis for correlation between various lesions of the posterior fossa and ABR results.

A review of major studies indicates a 90% or better detection rate for acoustic tumors using ABR. The detection rate may not be quite this high for other types of lesions affecting the eighth nerve or low brainstem, but it remains impressive.

The differentiation of eighth nerve and low brainstem lesions from more rostral brainstem lesions can be difficult because at times the ABR results may be similar. However, some differential ABR trends can be noted in comparing results from high and low brainstem lesions as noted below:

Low Brainstem

Earlier waves or entire waveform may be absent.

Most common interwave latency prolongation is between I-III.

Ipsilateral abnormalities are commonly observed (unless the lesion is large).

High Brainstem

Earlier waves are present; later waves may be absent.

Most common interwave latency prolongation is between III-V.

Bilateral, ipsilateral, and contralateral abnormalities may be present.

Needless to say, there are many exceptions to these trends. The type, size, and exact location of the lesion will directly affect the accuracy of predictions based on these trends. However, in clinical practice, knowledge of these trends may be of value. (A thorough discussion of ABR and high brainstem lesions follows this chapter.)

Optimal use of ABR in evaluating suspected lesions of the low brainstem and eighth nerve requires the use of several kinds of indices. ABR measures of absolute, interwave, and interaural latencies should be obtained whenever possible. Findings from these measures should be coupled with results from intensity and repetition rate functions, as well as observations of waveform morphology and V/I amplitude ratios. Proper use of almost all these indices is dependent on critical information from the basic audiogram. Without the consideration and quantification of hearing loss, ABR interpretation may become a tenuous and ambiguous matter.

Finally, although ABR is a powerful clinical procedure in the detection of eighth nerve and low brainstem disorders, it is not infallible. Therefore, employment of various other audiologic site of lesion tests remains necessary and clinically prudent.

CASE ILLUSTRATIONS

FIGURE 10–1.
Case One is a 60-year-old male who complained of a right-sided, progressive hearing loss, slight occasional dizziness, and high-pitched tinnitus on the right side for almost 1 year. He could not use the phone on the right ear. This patient had a normal neurological examination and the initial CT scan was normal. Repeat CT scan with enhancement and contrast studies revealed a small, mostly intracannicular acoustic tumor which was removed at surgery. The right ear ABR shows, in essence, no response at several intensities. Though this tumor was small, there was a moderately severe degree of hearing loss and extremely poor speech discrimination ability on the right. These latter findings, interestingly, are in contrast to Cases Two and Three, which profile much larger tumors.

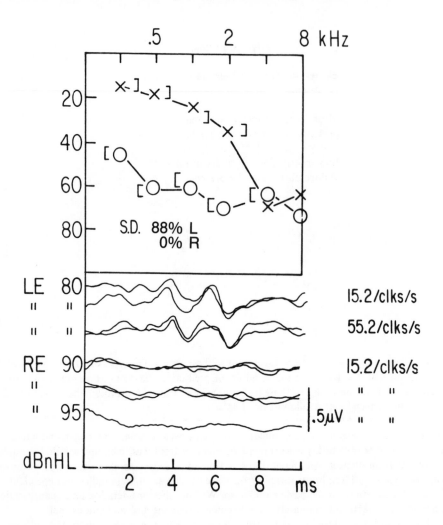

FIGURE 10–2a, b.

Case Two is a 36-year-old female who complained of left-sided numbness and tingling of the face, arm, and leg for about 6 months to 1 year. During this period she had occasional bilateral tinnitus and mild imbalance. Her main complaint, surprisingly, was a clicking noise in her left ear. She reported her hearing as being very good. Radiological and surgical findings revealed a large (4.0 cm) CPA tumor which was displacing the brainstem (Figure 2b). The left ear ABR shows wave V, by our interpretation, at about 7.3 ms (see arrow). Therefore, absolute and interwave latencies (I–V—5.7 ms) are abnormal for the left ear. In addition, the relatively "flat" response at 60 dB HL is inappropriate for a patient with a normal audiogram.

The right ear ABR is missing wave V, though waves I through IV (4.8 ms) seem robust. This absence of wave V is probably due to brainstem compression. A more specific case of this occurrence is shown later (Case Five).

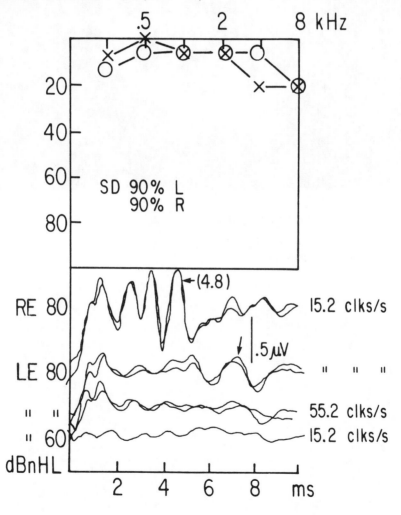

Figure 10–2a.

Illustration continued on following page.

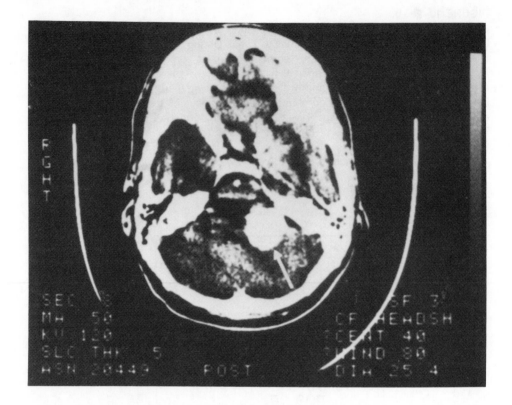

Figure 10–2b. See legend on preceding page.

FIGURE 10–3a, b, c.
Case Three is a women in her early thirties who 5 months prior to diagnosis reported a vague facial numbness along the right eye, nose, and lateral upper lip. A few months later she noted bilateral tinnitus and intolerance to loud sounds. Neurological examination revealed hyposensitivity of the second and third divisions of the fifth cranial nerve. Radiological and surgical findings documented a 4-cm, right-sided fifth nerve neuroma intimately attached to the low to midpons. The tumor was removed and the hearing preserved. (Figures 3a, 3b are pre- and post-operative audiograms; Figure 3c is the pre- and post-operative ABR.)

The right ear ABR shows an abnormal amplitude ratio and an abnormally "flat" waveform at 60 dB HL. However, latency measures are normal. Note that postoperatively the amplitude ratio is appropriate, and there is a much better waveform at 60 dB HL (taken in part from Musiek, Weider, & Mueller, 1983c).

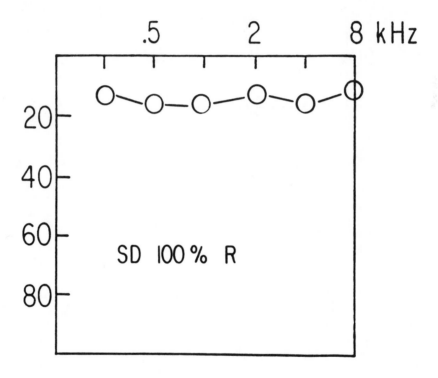

Figure 10–3a.   *Illustration continued on following page.*

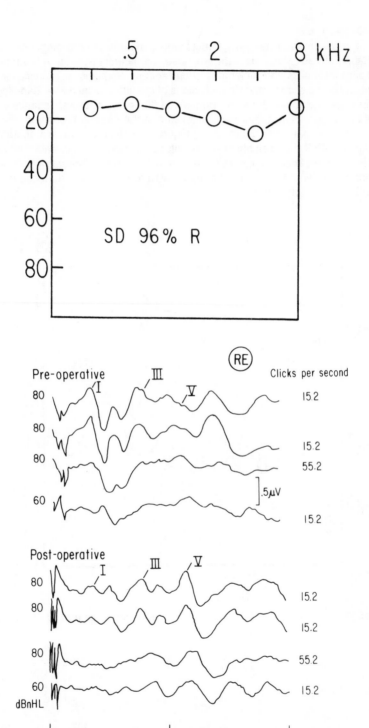

Figures 10–3b and c. See legend on preceding page.

FIGURE 10–4.
Case Four is a woman in her midfifties who incurred mild generalized trauma to the brainstem as a result of a car accident. Clinically, she demonstrated neuromotor deficits consistent with brainstem involvement. Given the patient's hearing loss, the ABR results for the low repetition rate are grossly consistent with a cochlear pathology. However, at the high repetition rate (55.3 clicks/s) the wave V latency shifts an abnormal amount (1.2 ms), indicating possible brainstem and/or auditory nerve involvement.

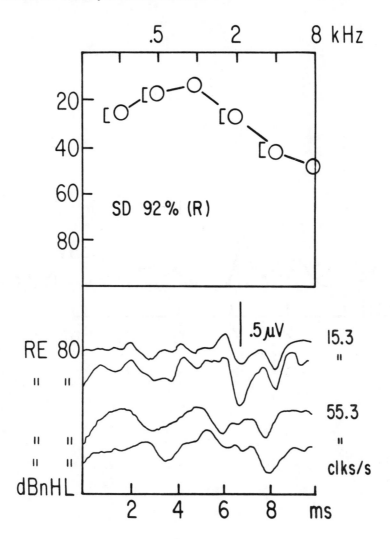

FIGURE 10–5.
Case Five is a woman in her midthirties who presented essentially classic symptoms of an acoustic neuroma on the left side. Audiologically, she demonstrated a profound hearing loss for the left side. Surgical findings revealed a large CPA tumor displacing the brainstem. The ABR shown is from the normal hearing ear opposite the CPA tumor. Note the ABR shows waves I through IV, but an absent V. As in Case Two, the absence of wave V is probably an effect of brainstem involvement related to a large mass lesion on the opposite side.

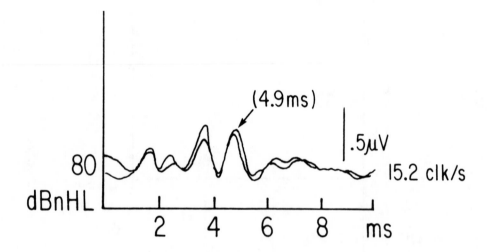

FIGURE 10–6.

Case Six is a woman in her midthirties who 1 year before diagnosis, had an acute attack of vertigo with tinnitus in the right ear. The dizziness subsided, but 2 months later she developed a twitching of the right eyelid and right side of the face (hemifacial spasm). At this time there was slight numbness of the right side of the face and occasional light-headedness. Over the next few months these symptoms worsened. Two months prior to being seen at our center, a CT scan and tomogram of the internal auditory canals were normal. The ABR demonstrates a delayed wave V (7.5 ms) with severely reduced amplitude for the right ear. Waveforms are practically flat on the right. The left ABR was essentially normal. Follow-up CT scan and subsequent surgery revealed a small acoustic tumor and an enlarged vascular loop in the right CPA.

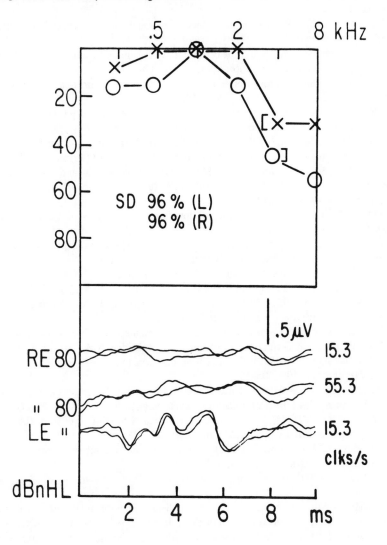

REFERENCES

Bauch, C., Rose, D., & Harner, S. (1980). Brainstem responses to tone, pip, and click stimuli. *Ear and Hearing, 1,* 181–184.

Bauch, C., Rose, D., & Harner, S. (1982). Auditory brainstem response results from 255 patients with suspected retrocochlear involvement. *Ear and Hearing, 3,* 83–86.

Brugge, J.F., & Geisler, C.D. (1978). Auditory mechanisms of the lower brainstem. *Annual Review of Neuroscience, 1,* 363–394.

Chiappa, K., Gladstone, K., & Young, R. (1979). Brainstem auditory evoked responses. Studies of waveform variations in 50 normal human subjects. *Archives of Neurology, 36,* 81–87.

Chusid, J. (1979). *Correlative neuroanatomy and functional neurology.* Los Altos, CA: Lange Medical Publications.

Clemis, J., & McGee, T. (1979). Brainstem electric response audiometry and the differential diagnosis of acoustic tumors. *Laryngoscope, 89,* 31–42.

Cler, J.M. (1975). Aneurysms of the middle cerebellar artery simulating a neuroma of the acoustic nerve. *Review of Otoneuro-ophthalmology, 47,* 339–344.

Coats, A. (1978). Human auditory nerve action potentials and brainstem evoked responses. *Archives of Otolaryngology, 104,* 709–717.

Daly, D., Roeser, R., & Aung, M. (1977). Early evoked potentials in patients with acoustic neuroma. *Electroencephalography and Clinical Neurophysiology, 43,* 151–159.

Don, N., Allen, A., & Starr, A. (1977). Effect of click rate on the latency of auditory brainstem response in humans. *Annals of Otolaryngology, Rhinology and Laryngology, 86,* 186–195.

Eggermont, J., Don, M., & Brackmann, D. (1980). Electrocochleography and auditory brainstem electric responses in patients with pontine angle tumors. *Annals of Otology, Rhinology and Laryngology, 89, Supplement 75.*

Engstrom, H., (1958). On the innervation of the sensory epithelium of the inner ear. *Acta Otolaryngology, 49,* 109–118.

Glasscock, M., Jackson, C., Josey, A., Dickins, J., & Wiet, R. (1979). Brainstem evoked response audiometry in clinical practice. *Laryngoscope, 89,* 1021–1034.

Harker, L. (1980). *ABR in cases of acoustic tumors.* Presented at a Symposium on Auditory Evoked Response in Otology and Audiology, Cambridge, MA, August 8–9.

Harris, J., & Almquist, B. (1981). ABR in operatively verified cerebello-pontine angle tumors. *Scandinavian Audiology, Supplement 13,* 113–114.

Hecox, K. (1980). *ABR and brainstem involvement.* Presented at a Symposium on Auditory Evoked Response in Otology and Audiology. Cambridge, MA, August 8–9.

House, J., & Brackmann, D. (1979). Brainstem audiometry in neurologic diagnosis. *Archives of Otolaryngology, 105,* 305–309.

Huertas, J., & Haymaker, W. (1969). Localization of lesions involving the statoacoustic nerve. In W. Haymaker (Ed.), *Bing's localization in neurological disease (ed. 15).* St. Louis: Mosby

Jerger, J., & Mauldin, L. (1978). Prediction of sensorineural hearing level from the brainstem evoked response. *Archives of Otolaryngology, 103,* 181–187.

Jerger, J., Mauldin, L., & Anthony, L. (1978). Brainstem evoked response audiometry. *Audiology and Hearing Education, 4,* 17–23, July/July.

Johnson, J.H., & Kline, D.G. (1978). Anterior inferior cerebellar artery aneurysms. *Neurosurgery, 48,* 455–460.

Kiang, N.Y.S.(1975). Stimulus representation in the discharge patterns of auditory neurons. In D.B. Tower (Ed.), *The nervous system* (Vol. 3, pp. 81–96). New York: Raven Press.

Lynn, G., & Gilroy, J. (1980). *Effects of auditory nerve lesions on the auditory evoked response.* Presented at the ASHA Conference, Detroit, Nov. 23.

Mazzoni, A., & Hansen, C. (1970). Surgical anatomy of the arteries of the internal auditory canal. *Archives of Otolaryngology, 91,* 128–135.

Møller, M., & Møller, A. (in press). Auditory brainstem evoked responses (ABR) in diagnosis of eighth nerve and brainstem lesions. In M. Pinheiro & F. Musiek (Eds.), *Assessment of central auditory dysfunction: Its foundations and clinical correlates.* Baltimore: Williams & Wilkins.

Møller, M., Møller, A., & Jannetta, P. (1982). BSER in patients with hemifacial spasm. *Laryngoscope, 92,* 848–852.

Morest, K., & Bohne, B. (1983). Noise induced degeneration in brain and representation of inner and outer hair cells. *Hearing Research, 9,* 145–151.

Mori, K., Miyazaki, H., & Ono, H. (1978). Aneurysm of the anterior inferior cerebellar artery at the internal auditory meatus. *Surgical Neurology, 10,* 297–304.

Musiek, F. (1982). ABR in eighth nerve and brainstem disorders. *American Journal of Otology, 3,* 243–248.

Musiek, F., & Geurkink, N. (1982). Auditory brainstem response and central auditory test findings for patients with brainstem lesions, a preliminary report. *Laryngoscope, 92,* 891–900.

Musiek, F., Kibbe, D., Rackliffe, L., & Weider, D. (1984). The ABR I–V amplitude ratio in normal cochlear and retrocochlear ears. *Ear and Hearing, 5,* 52–55.

Musiek, F., Kibbe, K., & Strojny, L. (1983a). *ABR results in the ear opposite large cerebellopontine angle lesions. A paper presented at the ASHA Convention, Cincinnati, Nov 22.*

Musiek, F., Mueller, R., Kibbe, K., & Rackliffe, L. (1983b). Audiologic test selection in the detection of eighth nerve disorders. *American Journal of Otology, 4,* 281–287.

Musiek, F., Sachs, E., Geurkink, N., & Weider, D. (1980). Auditory brainstem response and eighth nerve lesions: A review and presentation of cases. *Ear and Hearing, 1,* 279–301.

Musiek, F., Weider, D., & Mueller, R. (1983c). Reversible audiological results in a patient with an extra-axial brainstem tumor. *Ear and Hearing, 4,* 169–172.

Nodar, R., & Kinney, S. (1980). The contralateral effects of large tumors on brainstem auditory evoked potentials. *Laryngoscope, 90,* 1762–1768.

Oh, S., Kuba, T., Soyer, A., Choi, I., Bonikowski, F., & Vitek, J. (1981). Lateralization of brainstem lesions by brainstem auditory evoked potentials. *Neurology, 31,* 14–18.

Paludetti, G., Maurizi, M., & Ottaviani, F. (1983). Effects of stimulus repetition rate on the auditory brainstem response. *American Journal of Otolaryngology, 4,* 226–234.

Pfeiffer, R.R. (1966). Classification of response patterns of spike discharges for units in the cochlear nucleus: Tone-burst stimulation. *Experimental Brain Research, 1,* 220–235.

Pickles, J.O. (1982). *An introduction to the physiology of hearing.* New York: Academic Press.

Porter, R., & Eyster, E. (1973). Aneurysms in the anterior inferior cerebellar artery at the internal acoustic meatus. *Surgical Neurology, 1,* 27–28.

Portmann, M., Sterkers, J., Charachon, R., & Chouard, C. (1975). *The internal auditory meatus: Anatomy, pathology, and surgery.* New York: Churchill Livingstone.

Ragazzoni, A., Amantine, A., Rossi, L., Pagnine, P., Arnetoli, G., Marini, P., Nencioni, C., Versari, A., & Zappoli, R. (1982). Brainstem auditory evoked potentials and vertebral-basilar reversible ischemic attacks. *Advances in Neurology, 2,* 187–194.

Rasmussen, G. (1960). Efferent fibers of the cochlear nerve and cochlear nucleus. In G. Rasmussen and W. Windle (Eds.), *Neural mechanisms of the auditory and vestibular system.* Springfield, IL: Thomas.

Rose, D. (1978). Brainstem auditory responses 'letters'. *Mayo Clinic Proceedings, 53,* 132.

Rosenhall, U., Hedner, M., & Bjorkman, G. (1981). ABR and brainstem lesions. *Scandinavian Audiology (Supplement 13,* 117–123.

Rosenhamer, H. (1981). The auditory evoked brainstem electric response (ABR) in cochlear hearing loss. *Scandinavian Audiology (Supplement 13),* 83–93.

Rowe, M. (1981). Brainstem auditory evoked response in neurological disease: A review. *Ear and Hearing, 2,* 41–51.

Selters, W. A., & Brackmann, D. E. (1977). Acoustic tumor detection with brainstem electric response audiometry. *Archives of Otolaryngology, 103,* 181–187.

Selters, W. A., & Brackmann, D. E. (1979). Brainstem electric response audiometry acoustic tumor detection. In W. House & C. Luetje (Eds.), *Acoustic tumors* (Vol. 1). Baltimore: University Park Press.

Skinner, H. (1929). The origin of acoustic nerve tumors. *British Journal of Surgery, 16,* 440–463.

Spoendlin, H. (1973). The innervation of the cochlear receptor. In A. Møller (Ed.), *Basic mechanisms of hearing.* New York: Academic Press.

Starr, A., & Achor, J. (1975). Auditory brainstem responses in neurological disease. *Archives of Neurology, 32,* 761–768.

Stockard, J. J. (1982). Brainstem auditory evoked potentials in adult and infant-sleep apnea syndromes, including sudden infant death syndrome and near miss for sudden infant death. *Annals of the New York Academy of Sciences, 388,* 443–465.

Stockard, J. J., & Rossiter, V. G. (1977). Clinical and pathologic correlates of brainstem auditory response abnormalities. *Neurology, 27,* 316–325.

Stockard, J. J., Stockard J. E., & Sharbrough, F. W. (1977). Detection and localization of occult lesions with brainstem auditory responses. *Mayo Clinic Proceedings, 52,* 761–767.

Stockard, J. J., Stockard, J. E., & Sharbrough, F. W. (1980). Brainstem auditory evoked potentials in neurology: Methodology, interpretation, clinical application. In M. Aminoff (Ed.), *Electrodiagnosis in clinical neurology* (pp. 370–413). New York: Churchill Livingstone.

Terkildsen, K., Osterhammel, P., & Thomsen, J. (1981). The ABR and MLR in patients with acoustic neuromas. *Scandinavian Audiology (Supplement 13),* 103–108.

Thomsen, J., Terkildsen, K., & Osterhammel, P. (1978). Auditory brainstem responses in patients with acoustic neuromas. *Scandinavian Audiology, 7,* 179–184.

Weber, B., & Fuijikawa, S. (1977). Brainstem evoked response (BER) audiometry at various stimulus presentation rates. *Journal of the American Audiology Society, 3,* 59–62.

Yagi, T. & Kaga, K. (1979). The effect of the click repetition rate on the latency of the auditory evoked brainstem response and its clinical use for a neurological diagnosis. *Archives of Otorhinolaryngology, 222,* 91–97.

Chapter 11

ABR in Upper Brainstem Lesions

George E. Lynn
Narayan P. Verma

ANATOMICAL CONSIDERATIONS

This chapter focuses on alterations of the auditory brainstem response (ABR) in upper brainstem lesions.

The principal auditory centers and pathways of the upper brainstem that give rise to components of the ABR consist of (1) the rostral extension of the lateral lemniscus in the upper part of the pons, (2) the inferior colliculus located in the caudal region of the midbrain, and (3) the medial geniculate body of the caudal thalamus, the most rostral part of the auditory system in the brainstem.

The lateral lemniscus is the principal ascending auditory tract in the brainstem. Initially, this bundle lies lateral and rostral to the superior olivary nuclei in the lower pons and courses rostrally along the lateral edge of the pontine tegmentum to assume a more dorsal position as it approaches the inferior colliculus in the midbrain. Clumps of cells located among the fibers of this bundle constitute the ventral and dorsal nuclei of the lateral lemniscus. The inferior colliculus receives its major input from the contralateral cochlear nucleus, the ipsilateral and contralateral nuclei of the superior olivary complex, and the inferior colliculus of the opposite side via the commissure of the inferior colliculus. Afferent neurons of the lemniscal tract terminate almost entirely in the ventrolateral region of the central nucleus of the inferior colliculus and from here project to the medial geniculate body via the brachium of the inferior colliculus. The ventral portion of the parvocellular region constitutes the auditory part of the medial geniculate body. Extraaxial structures, namely the cerebellum, blood vessels, tentorium, and pineal gland, are relevant to this system because extrinsic pressure from mass lesions arising from these extraaxial sites may affect upper brainstem auditory functions.

EFFECTS OF UPPER BRAINSTEM LESIONS ON ABR COMPONENTS

Since the first description of scalp-recorded auditory evoked brainstem potentials (Jewett, Romano, & Williston, 1970), the consensus has been that the human ABR waves IV, V, and possibly VI, and animal ABR waves 4 and 5 reflect electrical activity occurring primarily from auditory centers and pathways in the upper brainstem. This generally accepted belief stems from the results of numerous experimental studies in animals and clinical reports in humans correlating activity recorded with surface and indwelling electrodes and changes in ABR components associated with lesions localized to the upper brainstem.

The effects of upper brainstem lesions on the ABR are varied; changes in latency, amplitude, and waveform, alone or in combination and on one or both sides, have been described in experimental animal and clinical (human) studies. Theoretically, because of the predominance of the contralateral pathway of the auditory system in the brainstem, ABRs in unilateral upper brainstem lesions should be expected to reflect abnormalities when the ear opposite the involved side is stimulated. However, there is not complete agreement in the literature on this point. Some authors believe that the abnormal ABR features occur on stimulating the ear ipsilateral to the lesion (Chiappa, 1983; Oh, Kuba, Soyer, Choi, Bonikowski, & Vitek, 1981) while others have noted (Chiappa & Ropper, 1982; Epstein, Stappenbeck, & Karp, 1980) that ABR abnormalities may occur in rostral brainstem lesions when the stimulus is presented to the contralateral ear. In the following sections of this chapter, relevant findings from specific experimental and clinical upper brainstem lesion studies are reviewed and discussed.

Experimental Studies

Lev and Sohmer (1972) found that lesions in the brainstem of anesthetized cats just caudal to the inferior colliculus caused a greater reduction in amplitude of waves 4 and 5 compared to other ABR components.

Similar observations were made by Buchwald and Huang (1975) in cats and Henry (1979) in mice. Buchwald and Huang demonstrated a loss of wave 5 in the cat's ABR following bilateral aspiration or undercutting of the inferior colliculus. Moreover, they also reported that sagittal section of almost all of the crossed auditory pathways of the brainstem, from the level of the cochlear nuclei to the inferior colliculus, resulted in loss of wave 5 contralateral to the stimulated ear and about 50% reduction in amplitude of wave 4. Buchwald and Huang concluded from their experiments that, in the cat, wave 5 depended on the integrity of the crossed auditory projections, and that wave 4 was equally dependent on both ipsilateral and contralateral pathways relative to the stimulated ear.

Henry (1979) found that all components after wave 4 disappeared in the mouse when a lesion was made to include the nuclei of the medial geniculate bodies, the brachia of the inferior colliculus, the nuclei externalis, the interstitialis brachii, the parabrachialis, and the extreme lateral portion of the central nucleus of the inferior colliculus. Even when the lesion involved the medial 90% of the central nucleus of the inferior colliculus, wave 5 was not abolished if the nuclei externalis, interstitialis brachii, and parabrachialis were spared. When the inferior colliculus and dorsal nucleus of the lateral lemniscus were removed on the side contralateral to the stimulated ear (sparing all ipsilateral structures above and below the contralateral dorsal midbrain), wave 5 disappeared. In another experiment, Henry removed afferent pathways to the contralateral inferior colliculus by midsagittal collicular transection and a contralateral coronal section just posterior to the inferior colliculus and found a loss of wave 5 as well as local activity recorded with an indwelling electrode from the contralateral inferior colliculus. A small wave 5 amplitude could still be recorded from the ipsilateral inferior colliculus. Henry concluded that ABR components in the mouse have the same origin as found by Jewett (1970) and Buchwald and Huang (1975) in the cat. Wave 4 appears to correlate with bilateral activity in the region between the cochlear nuclei and the inferior colliculi, presumably at the lateral lemniscal level. Wave 5 amplitude was larger when recorded from the contralateral inferior colliculus than from the ipsilateral and there was a loss of wave 5 following a lesion of the lateral portion of the contralateral inferior colliculus.

Jones, Stockard, Rossiter, and Bickford (1976) described the results of unilateral and bilateral cooling of the rostrolateral regions of the pons and the lateral aspects of the inferior colliculus in the cat. During unilateral cooling on the side of the brainstem opposite the stimulated ear (contralateral cooling), amplitude of wave 4 was significantly reduced to monaural stimulation. There was no noticeable change in wave 4 latency compared to the pre- and post-cooling conditions; however, wave 5 latency was delayed. During bilateral cooling, there was no significant reduction in wave 4 amplitude to monaural stimulation; however, latencies of waves 4 and 5 were prolonged. Jones et al. speculated that unilateral cooling delays conduction time along the crossed pathways, sparing the ipsilateral, uncrossed conduction velocities, and thus desynchronizing to some extent the ipsilateral and contralateral events responsible for wave 4. In other words, the activity along the ipsilateral and contralateral pathways contributing to wave 4 gets out of phase, creating a cancellation effect and reducing wave 4 amplitude. Bilateral cooling slows latencies along both the ipsilateral and contralateral pathways equally with preserved phase relationships. Thus, the latencies of waves 4 and 5 are prolonged but not reduced in amplitude.

Achor and Starr (1980) studied the effects of discrete lesions of the lateral lemniscus and inferior colliculus in three cats. Destruction of a large portion of the central nucleus of the inferior colliculus on one or both sides had no immediate (acute) effect (within 30 min) on the ABR of 2 cats; however, in one animal there was a 50% reduction in the amplitude of wave 5 to contralateral stimulation, but no effect during ipsilateral stimulation. The effect diminished to insignificant proportions in chronic, 3- to 4-week preparations. Lesions limited to the posterior portion of the lateral lemniscus had either no effect on the ABR or only a short temporary effect (less than 20 min) on amplitudes of the negative ABR components before and after the peak of wave 4 (N3 and N4). However, a decrease in the amplitude of wave N3 to contralateral stimulation was found to be associated with the acute lesions of the anterior portion of the lateral lemniscus. In chronic lesions, N3 was either diminished or completely abolished. Similar findings were observed by Wada and Starr (1983) in the guinea pig. Unilateral lemniscal lesions reduced amplitudes of the negative components of waves 3 and 4 (N3 and N4) only during stimulation of the contralateral ear, whereas in bilateral lesions, these components were affected with stimulation of either ear. Aspiration or undercutting of the inferior colliculus had no consistent effect on any ABR components, waves 1 through 5.

Buchwald, Hinman, Norman, Huang, and Brown (1981) found that wave 6 in the unanesthetized cat (presumably corresponding to wave VII in man) occurred at the same time as activity in pars principalis of the medial geniculate body recorded with indwelling electrodes and was abolished following complete transection of the brainstem just rostral to the inferior colliculus.

The results of these studies in the cat, mouse, and guinea pig showed that the major effect of various types of lesions on auditory structures of the upper brainstem was a reduction in amplitude of ABR components after wave 3 with little or no significant change in latency of response. Lesions of the inferior colliculus had no effect on wave 4 and on wave 5 the effect was inconsistent. No experimental evidence is available on the effects of lesions of the medial geniculate body.

Clinical Studies

Intrinsic or intraaxial lesions originate within the substance of the brainstem. Examples of such lesions include a mass, such as a tumor infiltrating brain tissue, a plaque resulting from a demyelinating process like multiple sclerosis, an infarction resulting from insufficient blood supply to a particular region resulting from stenosis or occlusion of a blood vessel, or a hemorrhage resulting from rupture of a blood vessel. Extrinsic or extraaxial lesions originate outside the brainstem. Although they affect primarily structures outside the brainstem, such as cranial nerves, blood vessels, tentorium, cerebellum, or pineal gland, they may affect the brainstem secondarily by pressure, distortion, local extension into the substance of the brainstem, or by compromising the brainstem's blood supply. These secondary factors alter the ABRs only if generators and/or pathways in the auditory system are involved.

At least four mechanisms may account for ABR alterations in brainstem lesions (Achor & Starr, 1980): (1) the lesion may involve generators directly, (2) fibers which course through the area of the lesion to terminate in remote generators may be damaged, (3) the secondary effects of lesions remote from the primary site may affect the ABRs, and (4) the function of uninvolved generators may be affected by lesions located elsewhere. Thus, ABRs reflect functional changes (evoked electrical activity) of the auditory system at or above the level of the lesion or at some distance remote from the primary site of involvement. It is important to remember that abnormal ABRs do not reveal the nature of the lesion, but merely reflect functional alterations, if any, related to the location of the lesion. It is in this regard that ABR data contribute to an anatomical localization of a lesion. Furthermore, it is not possible to differentiate between primary and secondary effects of a lesion on the basis of the ABR alone.

These points are illustrated by the following case material taken from the published literature and our laboratory.

Starr and Hamilton (1976) reported findings from two patients with upper brainstem lesions confirmed at autopsy. In one case (Figure 11-1), a hemorrhagic tumor (germinoma of the pineal gland) obliterated most of the midbrain and a portion of the rostral pontine tegmentum. The cochlear nuclei, trapezoid bodies, and superior olives in the caudal brainstem were grossly spared. ABR waves IV through VII were absent bilaterally to monaural stimulation and waves II and III were slightly prolonged in latency, presumably due to secondary effects of pressure from the tumor. Starr and Hamilton concluded that intact midbrain auditory structures are essential for detection of components after wave III. In the second case (Figure 11-2), gemistocytic tumor astrocytes involved the left inferior colliculus and lateral lemniscus, the periaquaductal gray matter, the floor of the fourth ventricle and the left cochlear nuclei. ABR responses to left ear stimulation showed only wave I with all subsequent components absent, a condition which is to be expected with involvement of the medullopontine region on the left side. Responses to stimulation of the right ear revealed preservation of all ABR components, including waves IV and V. However, amplitudes of waves IV and V were reduced approximately 50% of wave I amplitude. This case demonstrates that unilateral upper brainstem lesions involving the lateral lemniscus in the rostral pons and the inferior colliculus in the midbrain can reduce the amplitude of the IV–V wave complex when recorded during stimulation of the ear opposite the involved side of the upper brainstem.

Similar findings were reported by Epstein et al. (1980) in a patient with palatal myoclonus. There was vertical diplopia, left-sided hemisensory loss, and right-sided incoordination. Clinically, the lesion localized to the right side of the brainstem with definite involvement of the midbrain on that side. The ABR showed a delayed wave V latency with significant amplitude reduction only when stimulating the left or contralateral ear. Waves IV and V were normal in latency and amplitude when stimulating the right or ipsilateral ear. ABR abnormalities involving waves IV and V in patients with upper brainstem lesions have also been reported by Stockard and Rossiter (1977), Starr (1977), and Chiappa and Ropper (1982).

Three examples of intrinsic lesions are illustrated by the following cases from our laboratory.

Case one. A 12-year-old female with an upper brainstem tumor had a 2-month history of ataxia, vertigo, and difficulty in swallowing. Physical examination revealed decreased sensation over the left two-thirds of the tongue, impaired gag reflex, scanning speech, mild bilateral incoordination, and marked hearing loss thought to be congenital. Computed tomographic

FIGURE 11–1.
Distribution of neuropathology in the upper brainstem (stippled areas) of a patient with a germinoma and ABRs compared to a normal response. R and L refer to stimulated ear: right (R) or left (L). IC, inferior colliculus; LL, lateral lemniscus; PCN, posterior cochlear nucleus; ACN, anterior cochlear nucleus; SO, superior olive; VIII N, eighth cranial nerve. Reproduced with permission from Starr and Hamilton (1976).

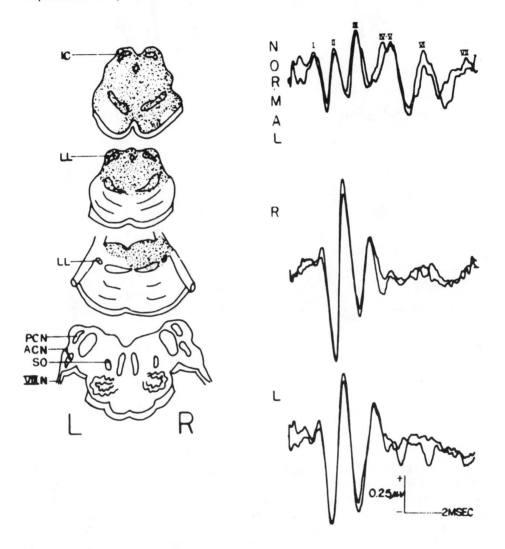

(CT) scan (Figure 11-3) revealed expansion of the midbrain at the collicular level, especially in the inferior half, and of the entire pons along with obliteration of the prepontine cistern (arrows).

Arteriography confirmed the midbrain and pontine location of the lesion. Thus, this patient had definite evidence of a mass lesion in the pontomesencephalic region of the brainstem, most

FIGURE 11-2.
Distribution of neuropathology on the left side of the brainstem (stippled areas) of a patient with tuberous sclerosis with gemistocytic astrocytoma and ABRs compared to a normal response. Abbreviations are the same as in Figure 11-1. Reproduced with permission from Starr and Hamilton (1976).

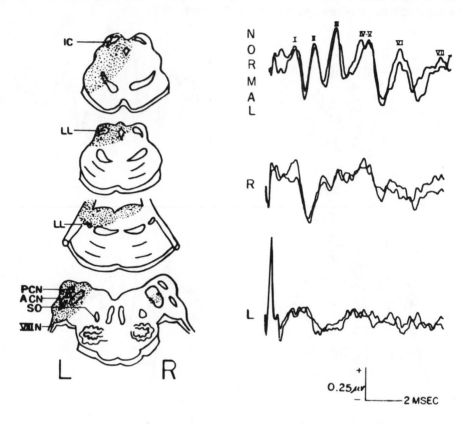

likely a glioma. The audiogram (Figure 11-3) confirmed the presence of a severe, bilateral sensorineural hearing loss, which, according to the parents, was discovered during early infancy. ABRs (Figure 11-3) demonstrated bilateral amplitude reduction and distorted morphology of waves V, VI, and VII. Wave V could not be identified with certainty, especially when stimulating the right ear. Latencies for all components after wave III were significantly delayed on both sides. The I–III interpeak latency (2.6 ms) on the left side reached +3.0 standard deviations (SD) and suggested a caudal extension of the abnormality on the left side of the pons by infiltration of tumor or secondary pressure effects.

This case demonstrated a bilateral slowing of conduction velocity and reduced voltage on later components of the ABR (waves IV and V) associated with an intrinsic tumor of the upper brainstem. In addition, there was ABR evidence of some slowing of neural conduction involving more caudal auditory structures of the brainstem on just the left side. Thus, the ABRs identified multiple level involvement.

Case two. This was a 50-year-old male with an upper brainstem infarction with a history of hypertension, sudden onset of occipital headaches, light-headedness, slurring of speech, and bilateral incoordination (greater on the left side than the right). The CT scan (Figure 11-4) revealed a lucency in the midbrain and pontine area with effacement of the prepontine and ambient cisterns due to associated edema (arrows). An angiogram revealed impaired blood flow in the region of the brainstem supplied by the superior cerebellar artery, especially on the left side. The audiogram and ABRs are shown in Figure 11-4. Threshold sensitivity for pure tones was normal bilaterally although sensitivity at 8000 Hz was slightly elevated on the left side. The ABRs revealed a significant increase in the III–V interpeak latency to 2.5 and 2.6 ms on stimulating right and left ears, respectively, without change in amplitude. These latency values exceeded $+3.0$ SD and were considered abnormal. All components of the response on the left side showed smaller amplitudes than on the right side with waveform distortion that may have been a reflection of some degree of auditory nerve involvement on the left side.

In this case, an infarction was located in the region of the upper brainstem supplied by branches of the superior cerebellar artery, namely the tectum (superior and inferior colliculus) and the tegmentum of the midbrain and rostral pons. Thus, the rostral portion of the lateral lemniscus and auditory areas of the inferior colliculus, located in this region, would have been vulnerable. The ABRs in this case, demonstrating prolonged III to V interval latency bilaterally, were consistent with involvement in this region of the brainstem.

Case three. This is a 34-year-old woman with multiple sclerosis, who, when she became symptomatic for the first time, had weakness of the left lower extremity, twitching of the left eyelid, and severe emotional depression. Cerebral spinal fluid (CSF) protein at that time was normal. She was diagnosed as having possible multiple sclerosis. ABRs at that time were normal. Two years later, she developed severe depression and right-sided weakness. The EEG, ABR, and CT scans were normal. A year later there was another episode of nervousness, right-sided weakness as before, and unsteadiness of gait. Although the EEG, ABR, CT scans and routine laboratory studies continued to be normal, in a few months she suddenly developed titubation of the head and marked violent intention tremor, suggesting midbrain involvement. At this time, CSF protein was more characteristic of multiple sclerosis. Although CT scans were still normal, ABRs changed to definitely abnormal (Figure 11-5) revealing a marked prolongation of the III to V interwave interval to 2.35 and 2.3 ms for the right and left ears, respectively. These latencies exceeded $+3.0$ SD and were abnormal. Significant amplitude reduction of the IV/V complex with loss of definition of waves VI and VII during stimulation of each ear was also seen. The audiogram showed normal hearing sensitivity for pure tones bilaterally.

The ABRs in this case of multiple sclerosis localized an abnormality affecting auditory centers and pathways above the level of the superior olivary nuclei on both sides of the brainstem. The abnormal waves IV and V suggested involvement of the ascending fiber tracts of the lateral lemniscus at mid or rostral pontine levels.

Extrinsic lesions of the brainstem are illustrated in the following two cases.

Case four. This is a 36-year-old male with a tumor of the pineal gland. When first seen, the major clinical finding was vertical diplopia, especially on downward gaze, followed later by a similar complaint noticed during lateral gaze, expecially to the left. The rest of the physical examination was essentially negative. CT scan (Figure 11-6) revealed a tumor mass in the region of the quadrigeminal plate. At this time, the ABRs (Figure 11-6) showed a significant prolongation (more than $+3.0$ SD) of the III to V interval latency (2.3 ms) on each side, with reduced wave V amplitude. There was slight distortion in wave V morphology. Hearing sensitivity for pure tones remained normal. During the course of his illness, the patient deteriorated clinically, showing increased diplopia, dysarthria, dysphagia, and quadriparesis. The physical examination revealed vertical and horizontal diplopia, asymmetry of pupils (left larger than the right), and marked weakness of all four limbs. A repeat CT scan showed extension of the tumor mass in the region of the splenium of the corpus callosum along with hydrocephalus. The audiogram

FIGURE 11–3.
Case one: 12-year-old female with an upper brainstem tumor. CT scan shows enlargement of the midbrain with involvement of the pons (arrows). The audiogram reveals a severe, bilateral sensorineural hearing loss, congenital in origin. ABRs show abnormal waves IV through VII bilaterally with abnormal I–III interpeak latency on the left side.

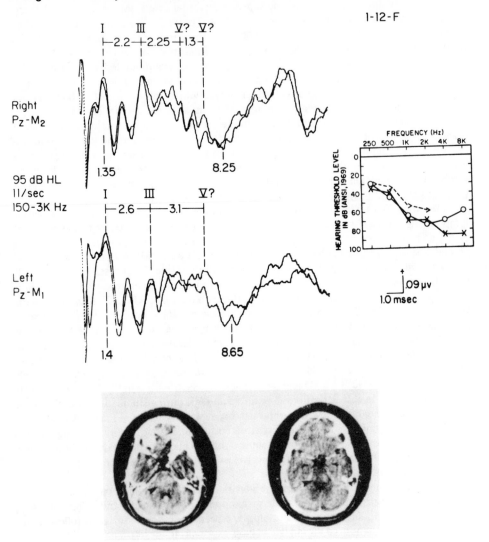

and ABRs were repeated with no significant changes relative to the first tests. The patient continued to deteriorate after initial transitory improvement following the insertion of a shunt for the hydrocephalus. A year later the patient died. An autopsy revealed a pinealoblastoma which had replaced the pineal gland and had metastisized to the cerebellum, splenium of the corpus callosum, spinal cord, and leptomeninges with pressure on the quadrigeminal plate of the midbrain.

FIGURE 11–4.
Case two: 50-year-old male with an upper brainstem infarction. CT scan shows a lucency in the midbrain and pontine areas (arrows). The audiogram reveals normal hearing bilaterally. ABRs show bilaterally prolonged III–V and I–V interpeak latencies with reduced amplitudes on the left side compared to the right.

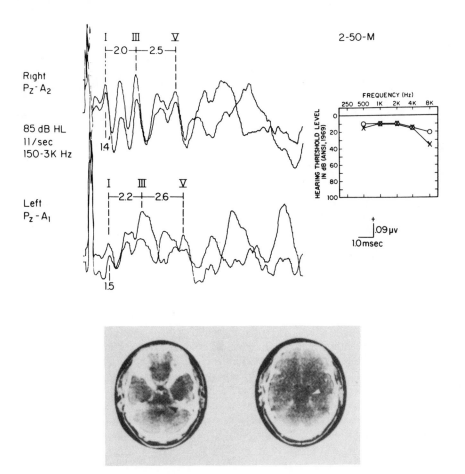

The clinical findings and CT scans were clearly indicative of a tumor mass in the region of the inferior and superior colliculi of the midbrain. The CT localized the lesion to the midline region with no apparent evidence that one side may have been more involved than the other. The bilateral delay in wave V latency with reduced amplitude was thus consistent with the clinical, radiological, and autopsy findings.

Case five. An 11-year-old boy with a cerebellar astrocytoma was first seen following a 2-week history of headaches, located primarily in the occipital area, and intermittent vomiting. Physical examination revealed truncal ataxia and bilaterally impaired finger-to-nose coordination. CT scan (Figure 11-7) demonstrated a large cystic astrocytoma of the cerebellum (arrows) with its major bulk located in the midline but eccentric to the left. The upper brainstem showed significant shift from left to right. Preoperatively (Figure 11-7), hearing levels were normal bilaterally and

FIGURE 11–5.

Case three: 34-year-old female with multiple sclerosis. The audiogram shows normal hearing sensitivity, bilaterally. ABRs demonstrate bilaterally prolonged III–V and I–V interpeak latencies with reduced amplitudes for the IV–V wave complex and waveform distortion.

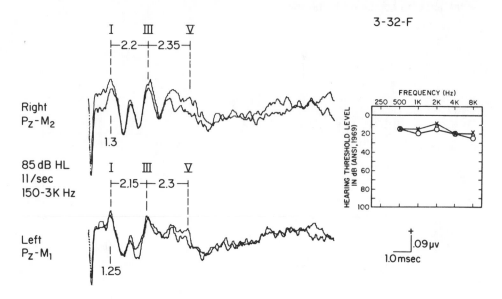

the ABR, when stimulating the right ear, revealed prolonged III to V latency (2.2 ms) of +3.0 SD with normal amplitudes and waveform. Earlier components of the right ABR were normal. On the left side, although the I to III interpeak latency was slightly increased (2.4 ms), it did not reach statistical significance to be classed as abnormal. Postoperative studies (Figure 11-8) obtained 15 days after successful removal of the cystic tumor and decompression of the cerebellum showed a significant reduction in tumor size on the CT scan and a normal III to V latency (1.85 ms) during right ear stimulation. A slight decrease (0.2 ms) in I–III interpeak latency on the left side was also demonstrated after surgery.

The major portion of this patient's tumor was located in the left cerebellar hemisphere, causing significant secondary pressure effects on the left side of the upper brainstem. The ABRs revealed a definite increase in the III to V interval latency when stimulating the right or contralateral ear, but not when the left or ipsilateral ear was stimulated. This contralateral effect can be explained on the basis of either (1) involvement of auditory projections from the right ear after crossing to the left side at upper brainstem levels, or (2) contralateral pressure effects associated with shift of the brainstem from left to right. Moreover, the slightly longer I–III interpeak latency on the left side as compared to the right also could be due to secondary pressure effects on the left side of the brainstem in the caudal region. These interpretations are supported by the postoperative improvements in the III to V latency following stimulation of the right ear and the I to III latency following stimulation of the left. These findings offer clinical evidence in support of the hypothesis that unilateral upper brainstem lesions may cause a III to V latency abnormality or reduced amplitude for waves IV or V when stimulating the ear contralateral to the lesion.

FIGURE 11–6.
Case four: 36-year-old male with a pineal gland tumor. CT scan shows a tumor mass (arrows) in the region of the quadrigeminal plate. The audiogram is normal bilaterally. ABRs reveal bilaterally prolonged III–V and I–V interpeak latencies with reduced wave V amplitudes. Waves I through IV are normal bilaterally.

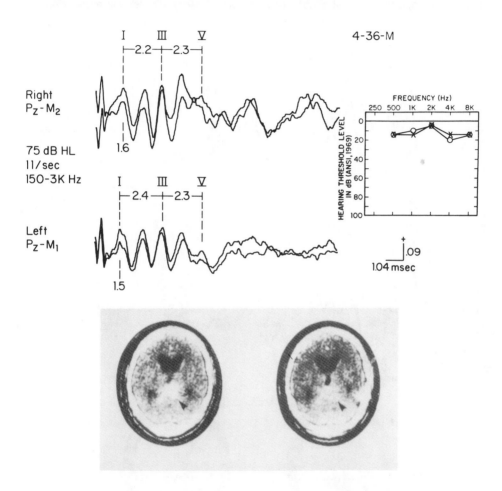

COMMENT

Even though there may be a lack of general agreement regarding the sources or generators of ABR components IV, V, and VI in man, evidence from experimental and clinical lesion studies demonstrates that alterations of these ABR components are associated with upper brainstem lesions. In man, waves IV and V are affected by abnormalities involving the lateral lemniscus in its rostral region (mid and upper pons) and the inferior colliculus (caudal midbrain), respectively. Alterations in wave VI may reflect abnormalities in the region of the inferior colliculus and at the level of the medial geniculate body. This interpretation has important

FIGURE 11-7.
Case five: 11-year-old male with a cerebellar astrocytoma. Preoperative findings. CT shows a large midline cystic astrocytoma of the cerebellum eccentric to the left (arrows) with displacement of the upper brainstem from left to right. The audiogram is normal bilaterally. ABRs reveal prolonged III–V and I–V interpeak latencies when stimulating the right ear and slightly prolonged, but not abnormal, I–III interwave latency with left ear stimulation.

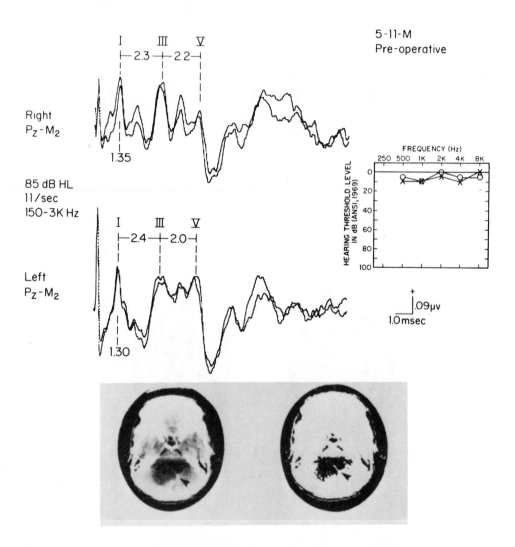

implications in the clinical evaluation when one attempts to differentiate between lower and upper brainstem involvement. Related to this is the matter of identifying which side of the brainstem is primarily involved in cases with unilateral abnormalities. In this regard, the literature seems to be less definite, although, in our opinion, evidence has been presented to suggest that unilateral upper brainstem lesions are manifest in the altered ABR when recorded during contralateral stimulation. This is not to say that the generators for these components are

FIGURE 11–8.
Case five: Postoperative findings (15 days) from same patient shown in Figure 11–7. CT scan shows significantly reduced tumor size compared to preoperative CT. Normal audiogram and ABRs bilaterally.

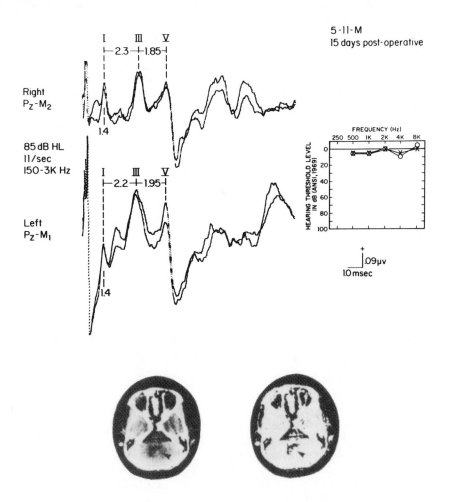

contralateral to the stimulated ear; in fact, the evidence is quite clear that electrical activity on both sides of the upper brainstem contribute to these later ABR wave components. Based on the known anatomical organization of the afferent auditory system in the brainstem and the literature and cases cited in this chapter, upper brainstem lesions involving the auditory system can be expected to alter the normal configurations of waves IV, V, and VI on one or both sides. Further, in the case of a unilateral lesion of the upper brainstem, the effect on the ABR is demonstrated in the recordings made during stimulation of the contralateral ear. This "contralateral effect" for upper brainstem lesions stands in contrast to the "ipsilateral effect" associated with unilateral peripheral and lower brainstem abnormalities. For an account of the latter relationships, see chapter 10.

Alterations in ABRs help the clinician in locating the abnormality to an approximate anatomical site, without revealing whether it is a primary or secondary effect on that site, let alone the nature of the abnormality. History and physical examination coupled with other data help to determine the nature of the lesion. ABRs are of value to the clinician in identifying clinically unsuspected or asymptomatic lesions. This is especially true in the diagnosis of multiple sclerosis, one of the most common neurologic diseases, whose documentation requires showing lesions affecting different parts of the nervous system, (a detailed account of MS may be found in chapter 12). Moreover, ABRs help to confirm the clinical suspicion of brainstem involvement in situations such as brainstem infarction, hemorrhage, glioma, and encephalitis. Serial ABRs in follow-up studies of patients over a period of time aid in correlating clinical improvement, stability, or deterioration. Having thus established rather solid electroanatomical correlations, it is possible to clinically assess, or study from a research point of view, patients with more subtle "lesions" (at biochemical or physiological level) such as metabolic coma, drug-induced coma, or hypothermia.

REFERENCES

Achor, L.J., & Starr, A. (1980). Auditory brain stem responses in the cat. II. Effects of lesions. *Electroencephalography and Clinical Neurophysiology, 48,* 174–190.

Buchwald, J.S., Hinman, C., Norman, R.J., Huang, C.M., & Brown, K.A. (1981). Middle- and long-latency auditory evoked responses recorded from the vertex of normal and chronically lesioned cats. *Brain Research, 205,* 91–109.

Buchwald, J.S., & Huang, C.M. (1975). Far-field acoustic response: Origins in the cat. *Science, 189,* 382–384.

Chiappa, K.H. (1983). *Evoked potentials in clinical medicine: Pattern shift visual, brainstem auditory and short-latency somatosensory: Techniques, correlations and interpretations.* New York: Raven Press.

Chiappa, K.H., & Ropper, A.H. (1982). Evoked potentials in clinical medicine. *The New England Journal of Medicine, 306,* 1140–1150.

Epstein, C.M., Stappenbeck, R., & Karp, H.R. (1980). Brainstem auditory evoked responses in palatal myoclonus. *Annals of Neurology, 7,* 592.

Henry, K.R. (1979). Auditory brainstem volume-conducted responses: Origins in the laboratory mouse. *Journal of the American Auditory Society, 4,* 173–178.

Jewett, D.L. (1970). Volume-conducted potentials in response to auditory stimuli as detected by averaging in the cat. *Electroencephalography and Clinical Neurophysiology, 28,* 609–618.

Jewett, D.L., Romano, M.N., & Williston, J.S. (1970). Human auditory evoked potentials: Possible brain-stem components detected on the scalp. *Science, 167,* 1517–1518.

Jones, T.A., Stockard, J.J., Rossiter, V.S., & Bickford, R.G. (1976). Application of cryogenic techniques in the evaluation of afferent pathways and coma mechanisms. *Proceedings of the San Diego Biomedical Symposium, 15,* 249–255.

Lev, A., & Sohmer, H. (1972). Sources of averaged neural responses recorded in animal and human subjects during cochlear audiometry (Electrocochleogram). *Arch Klin Exp Ohren, Nasen Kehlkopfheilk, 201,* 79–90.

Oh, S. J., Kuba, T., Soyer, A., Choi, I. S., Bonikowski, F. P., & Vitek, J. (1981). Lateralization of brainstem lesions by brainstem auditory evoked potentials. *Neurology, 31,* 14–18.

Starr, A. (1977). Clinical relevance of brainstem auditory evoked potentials in brain-stem disorders in man. In J.E. Desmedt (Ed.), *Progress in clinical neurophysiology. Vol. 2. Auditory evoked potentials in man. Psychopharmacology correlates of EPs.* Basel: Karger.

Starr, A., & Hamilton, A.E. (1976). Correlation between confirmed sites of neurological lesions and abnormalities of far-field auditory brainstem responses. *Electroencephalography and Clinical Neurophysiology, 41,* 595–608.

Stockard, J.J., & Rossiter, V.S. (1977). Clinical and pathologic correlates of brainstem auditory response abnormalities. *Neurology, 27,* 316–325.

Wada, S., & Starr, A. (1983). Generation of auditory brainstem responses (ABRs). III. Effects of lesions of the superior olive, lateral lemniscus and inferior colliculus on the ABR in guinea pig. *Electroencephalography and Clinical Neurophysiology, 56,* 352–366.

Chapter 12

Physiological Responses in Multiple Sclerosis and Other Demyelinating Diseases

Robert W. Keith
John T. Jacobson

INTRODUCTION

The auditory brainstem response (ABR) has been increasingly used as a noninvasive electrophysiological procedure in the detection and diagnosis of neurological disorders. The clinical utility of ABR has been demonstrated with a variety of neurological diseases. ABR wave components show minimal subject variability, are easily replicated, and appear insensitive to attention, sleep, sedation, or general anesthesia. Specific response parameters such as the relative latency difference between peak components and the amplitude ratio have proven invaluable as measures of neuropathology.

The ABR has recently surfaced as a valuable procedure in the identification of demyelinating lesions in the central nervous system (CNS). Demyelinating diseases such as multiple sclerosis (MS) are often diagnosed according to clinical symptomatology and the time course of the disease process, frequently resulting in an illusive diagnosis. The value of brainstem response measurement lies in its ability to monitor neural conduction within the auditory mechanism and, perhaps more important, objectively demonstrate subclinical lesions. Therefore, the intent of this chapter is to examine the relevant clinical applications of ABR and other physiological responses in the assessment of demyelinating lesions, and, in particular, those of MS.

BACKGROUND

Demyelinating Disease

The term demyelinating disease refers to a group of related neurological disorders characterized by a breakdown in myelin. Criteria used to delineate demyelinating disease normally include destruction of the nerve fiber myelin sheath, the relative sparing of associated axons, nerve cells, and supporting structures, and perivenous distribution of lesions throughout the brain and spinal cord (Adams & Kubik, 1952). In a less restrictive sense, Posner (1969) urged that any definition of demyelinating disease be considered not in terms of myelin as an isolated tissue, but rather as a complex, integrated functional system comprising the neuron, axon, myelin formation, and the spiral wrapping of the myelin sheath.

Myelin diseases may be divided into two major categories: those that disrupt the normal formation of myelin and those disorders, known as leukodystrophies, which result in abnormally formed myelin as a result of oligodendrocyte destruction (Pryse-Phillips & Murray, 1982). Specific myelin disorders will be discussed in relation to ABR results in following sections.

Though speculative, etiological agents implicated in myelin loss include those immune (allergic), virally induced, and inherited (leukodystrophies) diseases, toxic diseases, and those associated with physical and traumatic demyelination. Regardless of the inferred cause, demyelination adversely affects nerve transmission by either total conduction block, a reduction in conduction velocity, and/or an impairment in the ability to transmit trains of impulses (Sears, Bostock, & Sherratt, 1978).

Neural Conduction

To appreciate the complexity and impact of demyelinating diseases on neural conduction, a brief review of neural properties and function follows. Nerve cells are encapsulated by a semipermeable membrane that regulates the exchange of potassium and organic anions found in relatively high concentrations within the axoplasmic cell interior with surrounding interstitial fluid rich in sodium and chloride. Transmembrane ionic concentration differences maintain the cell interior at about -70 mV at rest. During excitation, the cell membrane experiences a transient electrochemical disturbance whereby an influx of positive sodium ions enters the cell cytoplasm. This transient voltage reversal is known as a spike or action potential.

Depolarization is immediately followed by a reversal in membrane permeability in which the cell returns to its resting state following a spontaneous disruption in the sodium current and a delayed outward flow of potassium, a process called repolarization. During repolarization, regardless of excitation intensity, a second action potential cannot be evoked, and the neuron is said to be in an absolute refractory state. This period is immediately followed by a relatively refractory period during which the initiation of an impulse is possible but the threshold is elevated. The propagation of a nerve impulse results from sodium ions flowing down their electrochemical gradient, exciting adjacent areas of resting cell membrane.

In the CNS, myelin, which serves as an electrical insulator, is manufactured and maintained by specialized glial cells (oligodendroglia). The myelin sheath consists of a lamellar structure of protein and lipids that concentrically wraps the axon. At regular intervals, the sheath is interrupted by gaps known as the nodes of Ranvier. These sites are characteristically devoid of myelin and as such exhibit a pronounced decrease in electrical resistance. During neural propagation, impulses tend to jump between these internodes, an activity called saltatory conduction. This process increases the speed of neural conduction in myelin fibers to an extent predicated on axon diameter, internode length, and myelin efficiency. As indicated, myelin destruction will either reduce the speed of or block signal transmission, resulting in abnormal electrophysiological measures.

Multiple Sclerosis

Multiple sclerosis is a primary human demyelinating disease of the CNS, characterized by exacerbations and remissions of symptoms. Although a number of tests help confirm the diagnosis in a majority of the patients, no pathognomonic laboratory tests have been found to confirm the disease process. Epidemiologic findings suggest that MS is acquired early in life, with a peak risk age of 15, but onset of symptoms is usually in the third or fourth decade. During the early stages of the disease, clinical diagnosis is sometimes difficult since it requires the objective demonstration and involvement of at least two distinct sites within the CNS over a long duration or on a number of occasions. The clinical diagnosis of MS normally requires evidence of fluctuations in the course of the disease and symptoms and signs indicating scattered lesions in the white matter of the CNS (Schumacher, 1971). While symptoms vary in degree, duration, and character, they usually involve, in isolation or combination, impairment of the sensory and motor systems.

Pathophysiology. In demyelination, plaque formation usually begins with perivenular infiltration of lymphocytes and monocytes, most often in the optic tract, the lateral and posterior columns of the spinal cord, the brainstem, and the cerebellum. The loss of myelin is characterized by glial cell proliferation, perivascular edema, inflammation, and gliosis (scarring). As the disease progresses, plaques increase in number and size, dependent on the manifestation of pathological interstitial space. Plaques frequently remit; and, while segmented remyelination is predictable, in the CNS it is usually restricted to a few layers of new myelin. Thus, normal function in the fiber tract is rare and conduction is slower.

Classification. Through the years, there have been numerous criteria proposed for the classification of MS (Schumacher, Beebe, Kibler, & Kurkland, et al., 1968). Recently, Bauer (1980) reported the results of a survey which established four categories into which all MS patients could be clinically diagnosed. They were (1) MS proven by autopsy, (2) "definite," (3) "probable," and (4) "possible" MS. While specific criteria varied among the latter three categories, those listed in the diagnosis of "definite" MS included a relapsing and remitting course, a slow or stepwise progression, documented neurological signs of predominantly CNS white matter pathology, characteristic cerebrospinal fluid findings, symptom onset between 10 and 50 years, and "no better" neurological explanation.

Epidemiology. Numerous epidemiological studies have been undertaken in an attempt to uncover possible etiologies and risk factors and the pathogenesis of MS (Alter, 1980). The results of such investigations indicate a unique geographic distribution. The prevalence of MS is substantially greater at higher latitudes in both hemispheres. For example, in North America, the prevalence is approximately 50/100,000 between 40° and 50° latitude compared to 6 to 14/100,000 between 25° and 30° latitude (Kurkland & Reed, 1964). In comparison, geographic regions with the highest reported prevalence rate per 100,000 are the Orkney and Shetland Islands with 258 and 152/100,000, respectively (Poskanzer, Walker, Yokondz, & Sheridan, 1976).

Although no direct link exists between latitude and etiology, epidemiological evidence indicates that genetic factors may be active in MS susceptibility, residence in low-prevalence areas during early life ensures long-term immunity, and migration to a low-prevalence area may modify the risk of clinical MS (Detels, Visscher, Coulson, Malmgren & Dudley, 1974).

Further inspection of epidemiological evidence shows that MS is more common in females (McAlpine, Lumsden, & Acheson, 1972), approximately two-thirds of all MS patients experience initial onset between ages 20 and 40 (Leibowitz, Alter, & Halpern, 1964), and familial incidence is higher than that in the general public (McAlpine et al., 1972). According to Pryse-Phillips and Murray (1982), about 10% of all MS patients have a positive family history, suggesting to them that inherited immune factors, which are seen in myelin destruction, may play an etiologic role. In part, epidemiological studies have accounted for the unique effects of environmental, genetic, and infectious conditions associated with geographic distribution.

The search for a causative agent continues. To date, serious consideration has been given to a slow-virus infection, which may explain the unusual dormant period between the early risk age and the later symptom onset. The finding of increased levels of measles virus antibody in the serum and cerebrospinal fluid (CSF) in MS patients has made the measles virus one of the viruses under suspicion, although many viruses can produce the same disorder.

Another theory supported by the presence of increased concentrations of myelin basic protein in the CSF has led to a possible immunological basis for MS (Cohen, Herndon, & McKhann, 1976). About two-thirds of all active, clinically diagnosed MS patients have increased IgG in the CSF, whereas 90% of all cases show the presence of oligoclonal IgG bands on CSF immunoelectrophoresis (Johnson & Nelson, 1977). Myelin basic protein has also been found in patients with metrachromatic leukodystrophy and central pontine myelinolysis (Cohen, Brune, Herndon, & McKhann, 1980). Thus, the excessive synthesis of immunoglobulin may produce antibodies responsible for destruction of myelin in MS and other demyelinating diseases.

AUDIOLOGICAL FINDINGS

The reported degree and incidence of peripheral auditory impairment varies widely in MS patients. In a comprehensive review, Noffsinger, Olsen, Carhart, Hart, and Sahgal (1972) found the incidence of pure tone deficits to range from 1 to 86%. Though the most frequently observed peripheral abnormality was a mild high-frequency cochlear hearing loss, a diversity of audiometric configurations and aberrations has been described (Dayal & Swisher, 1967; LeZak & Selhub, 1966; Rose & Daly, 1964; Simpkins, 1961). Speech reception and discrimination scores are usually normal and in good agreement with pure tone sensitivity (Parker, Decker, & Richards, 1968), although reduced discrimination scores have been reported in the presence of competing noise (Daughtery, Lederman, Nodar, & Conomy, 1983; Dayal, Tarantino, & Swisher, 1966).

Pure Tone Tests

Traditional site-of-lesion tests have been unpredictable in their ability to diagnose hearing loss or correlate clinical severity in MS patients (Daughtery et al., 1983). Abnormal adaptation scores have been reported (Daughtery et al., 1983; Noffsinger et al., 1972) with some evidence of fluctuation and a return to normal during remission (Rose & Daly, 1964). The presence of recruitment is not common (Dix, 1965; Noffsinger et al., 1972), nor have any conclusive diagnostic results generated from the Short Increment Sensitivity Index (SISI) test (LeZak & Selhub, 1966; Noffsinger et al., 1972). These findings and those from conventional pure tone and speech audiometry have not contributed significantly toward the diagnosis of auditory deficits in MS patients. To date, any postulation of a causal relationship between MS and hearing loss is purely speculative, lacking correlating neurological evidence (Antonelli & DeMitri, 1963; Citron, Dix, Hallpike, & Hood, 1963; Parker et al., 1968; Rose & Daly, 1964).

Sensitized Speech Tests

Acoustically modified linguistic stimuli have gained a prominent role in the diagnosis of central auditory nervous system dysfunction. Unfortunately, sensitized speech materials are infrequently employed in MS patients (Antonelli & DeMitri, 1963; Noffsinger et al., 1972; Stephens & Thornton, 1976). Factors that contribute to the lack of test information include the often distant relationship between the audiology community and the neurologist and the fact that traditional audiological test results rarely provide abnormal findings, a fact that may discourage further investigative evaluation.

The results of sensitized speech tests appear related to the degree of extrinsic redundancy found in the speech material, the intrinsic redundancy of the auditory system, and the nature, site, and size of the neurological lesion. In MS, test results vary depending on the specific test

and the status (classification, remission, exacerbation, etc.) of the patient. In a study by Jacobson, Deppe, and Murray (1983), a series of dichotic speech paradigms was compared in a group of 20 "definite" MS patients. The results suggested that a dichotic consonant–vowel nonsense-syllable and synthetic sentence identification (SSI) test proved clinically useful in the overall diagnosis of central auditory deficits in MS patients. The SSI results have been similarly confirmed in other test observations (Hannley, Jerger, & Rivera, 1983; Russolo & Poli, 1983). Binaural fusion and dichotic sentence tests have also demonstrated abnormal findings in varying classifications of MS patients (Daughtery et al., 1983).

PHYSIOLOGICAL RESPONSES

Acoustic Reflex (AR)

One physiological response that can be used in conjunction with ABR in the evaluation of patients with possible MS is the acoustic reflex. The acoustic reflex refers to the involuntary contraction of the stapedius muscle in response to a sufficiently intense auditory stimulus. Measurements of the acoustic reflex response can include response threshold, latency of onset, rise time, time to maximum contraction, amplitude of response, offset, and adaptation to sustained stimulus presentation. Acoustic reflex testing has been shown to be useful in detecting eighth nerve pathology. In these disorders, common findings include elevated or absent reflexes, or abnormal adaptation to sustained tones.

Similarly, abnormalities in the acoustic reflex response have been observed in patients with MS. Acoustic reflex abnormalities in this disease include prolongation of reflex onset latency (Bosatra, 1977; Hess, 1979) and increases in the rise time (Colletti, 1975; Hess, 1979). In addition, patients with MS have aberrations in acoustic response amplitude, with many patients showing reduced amplitude (Bosatra, Russolo, & Poli, 1976; Colletti, 1975), while others show enhanced response amplitude (Bosatra et al., 1976).

In a study reported by Garza, Keith, and Barajas (1982), of 23 normal hearing subjects with definite or probable MS, according to McAlpine's (1972) classification, five had absent acoustic reflexes. The other 18 subjects showed no significant difference compared to normal subjects in acoustic reflex onset latency or amplitude. There was a significant group difference in acoustic reflex amplitude, especially at 1000 and 2000 Hz.

Evaluation of studies of acoustic reflex dynamics completed on MS subjects indicates that abnormalities occur in a substantial number, though not a majority, of persons. When acoustic reflex abnormalities occur in the presence of normal peripheral hearing, they are a sensitive measure of a lesion involving the brainstem reflex arc. In this regard, acoustic reflex testing continues to be an important and integral part of the diagnostic evaluation of patients with a possible neurologic disorder.

Electronystagmography (ENG)

Approximately 50% of patients with MS report vertigo at some time during the course of the disease. Pathologic nystagmus has been observed at one time or another in approximately 90% of MS patients (Baloh & Honrubia, 1979). According to these authors, ENG recordings of patients suspected of having MS are valuable in detecting smooth pursuit, saccadic, and optokinetic nystagmus abnormalities that are not apparent on visual inspection of eye movements. In addition, MS produces every other variety of abnormality, including gaze and positional nystagmus, unilateral or bilateral caloric weakness, and directional preponderance. These ENG findings are found with both CNS and peripheral vestibular abnormalities as a result of plaques within the nerve root where peripheral nerves contain CNS myelin (Baloh & Honrubia, 1979). Thus, the ENG is not particularly helpful in differentiating MS from many other disease processes.

Somatosensory and Visual Evoked Potentials

Somatosensory evoked potentials (SEP) can be elicited from multiple peripheral nerve sites. Clinical studies often stimulate mixed nerves containing both sensory and motor fibers because the motor response assures proper electrode placement and adequate stimulus levels. Nerves that are commonly stimulated include the median nerve at the wrist, the posterior tibial nerve at the ankle, and the personeal nerve at the knee. A constant current stimulus is applied at these sites using durations of 0.1 to 0.5 ms at presentation rates of one to five per second.

A response can theoretically be recorded from any place along the nerve pathway, although some sites offer such a low-voltage response that they offer little clinical utility (e.g., the cervical spine). Cortical evoked potentials are larger voltage, and are usually easy to record in a cooperative, unanesthetized patient. The cortical response is best recorded from the midparietal scalp over the posterior portion of the fissure of Rolando. Filter settings of 1 to 250 Hz optimize SEP response using an analysis time window of approximately 40 ms for the median nerve and 100 ms for posterior tibial nerve stimulation. The cortical evoked potential consists of a biphasic wave with Pa, Pb response at 16 and 24 ms for median nerve stimulation and 40 and 60 ms for the posterior tibial nerve.

Similarly, visual evoked potentials (VEP) can be recorded from the visual cortex in response to the flash of a strobe light or a pattern reversing checkerboard design on a television screen. The VEP response of primary interest occurs at approximately P 100 ms. According to Chiappa and Ropper (1982) both the absolute latency of P 100 and the difference in latency between the two eyes are very sensitive indicators of disease. Amplitude measurements are more variable than latency and have less clinical utility.

In the evaluation of patients suspected of having demyelinating disease, Matthews, Wattam-Bell, and Pountney (1982) comment that visual evoked potentials have "the greatest predictive value" over other evoked potential measurements. However, by comparison, Matthews et al. measured only the latency and amplitude of wave V of the ABR. Their criteria utilized +3 SD of their normal population mean, calling all wave V responses of 6.7 ms or amplitudes lower than 0.5 μV abnormal. Recent studies that use more sophisticated ABR data analysis result in a higher percentage of identification of MS patients. The question raised by Matthews et al. of whether SEP, VEP, or ABR is more predictive remains to be answered. In fact, the question may forever remain moot since test battery approaches are always more fruitful than single test approaches.

Auditory Brainstem Responses

Prevalence of abnormalities. The development of techniques used to record and measure short-latency electrical events generated along the auditory pathway of the brainstem resulted in a dramatic change in the approach to differential diagnosis in patients with various eighth nerve and brainstem lesions, including MS.

Early studies by Robinson and Rudge (1975, 1977), Shanon, Gold, Himmelfarb, and Carasso (1979), Starr and Achor (1975), and Lynn, Taylor, and Gilroy (1980) indicated that a substantial number of patients with MS showed ABR abnormalities. Estimates of abnormalities ranged from 34% (Chiappa & Norwood, 1977) to 73% (Robinson & Rudge, 1975) of all patients tested. The overall percentage of abnormalities is the summation of patient subgroups classified as definite, probable, or possible MS. Lynn et al. (1979), for example, found 75% of definite, 33% of probable, and 29% of possible MS patients with ABR abnormalities. Similarly, patients with clinical evidence of brainstem involvement show a higher rate of ABR abnormalities than patients who show no evidence of brainstem disorder. For example, 79% of Robinson and Rudge's (1977) patients with definite evidence of brainstem lesion and 51% of those without clinical sign of brainstem involvement had ABR abnormalities. Manifestations of brainstem abnormalities include internuclear ophthalmoplegia, sixth or seventh nerve palsy, horizontal or vertical gaze nystagmus (Robinson & Rudge, 1977), dizziness, gait disturbance, cerebellar signs, and sensory or motor abnormalities (Chiappa, Harrison, Brooks, & Young, 1980). Other studies have shown evidence of ABR abnormalities in an even higher percentage of patients with definite clinical brainstem involvement with estimates as high as 93% (Stockard & Rossiter, 1977). It should be noted that these results are reported in the absence of symptomatic hearing impairment, although many investigators are vague about procedures used in assessing peripheral hearing levels. Since ABR results are dependent upon middle ear and cochlear function, the technique should be used in conjunction with standard audiometry.

Types of ABR abnormalities. There is considerable variability in ABR abnormalities observed in MS patients. The findings include abnormality of symmetry, delay in latency, fragmented response, decreased amplitude or absence of peaks, poor response reliability, abnormal responses to changes in rate, and abnormal latency–intensity function.

Latency and amplitude. Chiappa, Young, and Goldie (1979) report that 13% of 202 patients had abnormal I–V separation, 55% had only wave V amplitude abnormalities, and 33% had both abnormalities. Stockard & Rossiter (1977) reported that 69% of abnormalities were related to latency, while 31% were amplitude related. Robinson and Rudge (1977) also reported that latency was a more reliable discriminator than amplitude, with wave V the single most important component. For example, wave V was the only abnormality in 71% of patients reported by Robinson and Rudge (1977) who had abnormal ABRs. These authors and others (Hausler & Levine, 1980) report normal wave I responses in all of their subjects.

The most common interwave interval (IWI) latency abnormality appears to occur in the III–V separation (Chiappa, 1980; Lynn et al., 1980; Shanon, Gold, & Himmelfarb, 1981), although Shanon et al. (1981) found the I–III interval to be prolonged more than the III–V interval. Barajas (1982) reported 25% of ABR abnormalities were related to IWI alone, 45% to wave V amplitude, and 30% had both abnormalities.

While absolute and relative latency has been shown to be a sensitive indicator of brainstem dysfunction associated with MS, Robinson and Rudge (1975) found that in patients with normal brainstem latencies, 50% showed a decrease in response amplitude. Starr and Achor (1975) report that with the exception of wave I all of their MS patients showed reduced amplitude. Chiappa et al. (1980) reported that 87% of MS patients show absent or abnormally low wave V amplitude.

Peripheral nerve involvement. Until recently, the effects of MS were thought to be restricted to the CNS. However, new evidence has shown segmental demyelination (Pollack, Calder, & Allpress, 1977) and abnormal refractory periods (Hopf & Eysholdt, 1978) in the peripheral nerves of MS patients. Using ABR and electrocochleography to confirm wave I presence, Hopf and Maurer (1983) tested 71 MS patients. Eight (11%) exhibited prolonged wave I latencies (>3 SD). They attributed peripheral involvement to segmental demyelination of the distal part of the acoustic nerve. There appears to be anatomical support for their conclusions. The neuroglial-neurolemmal junction of the acoustic nerve is located 7 to 13 mm distal to the brainstem near the fundus of the internal meatus (Nager, 1969). This junction may prove to be the functional site of peripheral demyelination, although further study will be necessary to confirm such an hypothesis.

Figure 12-1 illustrates some of the ABR abnormalities previously described. These results were obtained from patients with definite MS who were in a state of remission. All persons had normal hearing sensitivity. The responses were obtained using alternating click polarity presented monaurally at 80 dB nHL at a rate of 21.1 per second. The data were obtained by Garza (1981) and presented in part by Garza et al. (1982).

Tracing A is a response obtained from a normal subject; tracing B has a normal I and III with delayed wave V, resulting in a prolonged III–V interval. Tracing C has an absent wave I and delayed latency to wave III with a normal III–V interval. Tracing D has waves I and V present at normal latencies with an absent wave III. In fact, it is not possible to determine if the response at 5.92 ms is wave V or a delayed wave III with normal III–V conduction between the responses at 5.92 and 7.98 ms. Tracing E shows two trials from the same subject with a normal wave I response and nonrepeatable waves III and V. Tracing F has responses with normal latencies but abnormally large amplitude of waves I and V.

Repeatability. Test–retest repeatability in normal subjects is excellent with highly reproducible waveform morphology and latency. In contrast, a common finding in MS patients is poor repeatability of ABR results with investigators reporting poor agreement on retest in as many as 80% of MS patients (Garza et al., 1982; Nodar, 1978: Prasher & Gibson, 1980; Robinson & Rudge, 1980). Lacquaniti, Benna, Gillis, Trone, & Bergamasco (1979) report that response variability is independent of stimulus intensity. This finding supports the common clinical practice of repeated measurements at each stimulus intensity and repetition rate.

Rate effects. The effects of increased repetition rate on the ABR have been documented in normal (Don, Allen, & Starr, 1977; Hyde, Stephens, & Thornton, 1976; Pratt & Sohmer, 1976; Weber & Fujikawa, 1977) and neurologically impaired human subjects (Hecox, Cone, & Blaw, 1981; Pratt, Ben-David, Peled, Podoshin, & Scharf, 1981; Stockard, Stockard, & Sharbrough, 1977; Yagi & Kaga, 1979). Generally, an increase in repetition rate will differentially prolong wave latency while decreasing wave amplitude. The more rostral the response, the greater the latency shift. A number of investigators have shown small but consistent wave I latency increases (Terkildsen, Osterhammel, & Huis in't Veld, 1975; Thornton & Coleman, 1975; Yagi & Kaga, 1979; Zollner, Karnahl, & Stange, 1976), whereas wave V latency increases at about 0.06/10 Hz (Hecox, Lastimosa, Mokotoff, & Sandlin, in press).

Despite the evidence that rate effects are clinically useful in the identification of neurological disorders, little information exists with regard to demyelinating diseases and those results are conflicting. Chiappa et al. (1980) confirmed earlier work (Chiappa & Norwood, 1977) that rate effects did not alter the incidence of MS abnormality. Using a constant click stimulus polarity and an abnormality criterion of 3 SD above the normal mean, they found no significant difference in relative latency values in 57 MS patients tested at 10 and 70/s. In comparison, Shanon et al. (1981) employed alternating click polarity at three rates of 10, 50, and 100/s in 10 MS patients. Brainstem results produced greater wave variability, amplitude alterations, and increases in latency (N_1–P_4) of 0.66 ms between rates of 10 and 100/s. Increases in the identification of MS abnormality associated with higher rates have been reported by Robinson and Rudge (1977), Stockard and Rossiter (1977), and Stockard, Stockard, and Sharbrough (1978).

It is well known that response variabilitiy increases with rate; the MS population is no exception. Brainstem responses alter wave morphology, response replicability on consecutive runs (see Figure 12-2), and wave amplitude. Figure 12-2 illustrates wave aberrations from one MS patient as a function of rate increase.

Recently, Jacobson (1983) reported the results of rate effects on 20 MS patients diagnosed with "definite" MS. Patients exhibited normal peripheral hearing sensitivity, absent middle ear

FIGURE 12-1.
ABR responses obtained on a normal and several MS subjects. Responses were obtained and are displayed under identical conditions. See text for description of results.

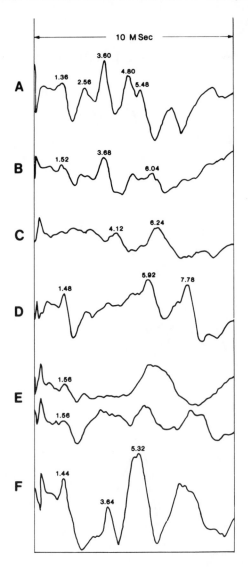

pathology, and positive neurological evidence of brainstem abnormality. A 70-dB SL alternating click stimulus was used to measure absolute and relative response latency at four rates of 10, 33, 67, and 80/s. Latency values exceeding the 95% confidence interval were considered abnormal. The results indicate that the incidence of abnormality was dependent on the rate of presentation. Abnormal IWI (I–V) increased from 52.5% at 10/s to 65% at 67 and 80/s. In these patients, rate effects produced latency abnormalities at the higher presentation rates not evident at 10 and 33/s (see Figure 12-3). Latency shifts have been attributed to adaptation or fatigue (Don et al., 1977), reduced refractory period, and decreased synaptic efficiency (Pratt & Sohmer, 1976).

FIGURE 12–2.
ABR responses obtained from a patient with MS using click rates from 10 to 80/s. Note the
abnormal change in response morphology that results from an increase in click rate.

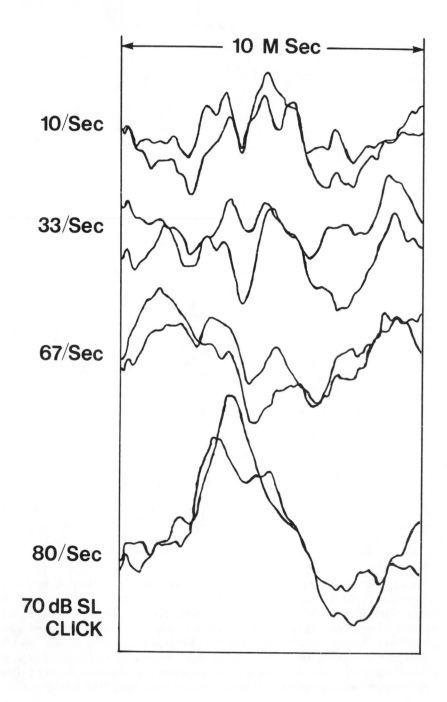

Latency–intensity effects. Parving, Elberling, and Smith, (1981) studied 15 patients with "definite" MS using electrocochleography (ECochG), ABR, and an objective technique of analyzing electrophysiological data. Stimulus intensities of 35–115 dB peSPL were used to obtain latency–intensity functions. Results of ECochG yielded a normal cochlear action potential. However, the latency–intensity function was abnormal for both latency and amplitude at low stimulus intensities despite normal hearing sensitivity at 2000 Hz. These investigators also found normal wave I–V intervals in all subjects. Parving et al. interpret the differences between their results and others as following from (1) difficulties in the ability to assign values to ABR components, (2) influences on the ABR from cochlear dysfunction, and (3) data interpretation. It would appear that based on the results of the latency–intensity function on MS patients further research is required before it can be used with diagnostic confidence.

Ipsilateral versus contralateral stimulation. Some early investigators used binaural stimulus presentation in obtaining ABR, obscuring a lateralized abnormality because of the normal response from the contralateral site. Several investigators have since documented the need for using monaural stimulation to identify patients with lateralized lesions (Barajas, 1982; Prasher & Gibson, 1980; Rowe, 1981).

In addition, two publications (Barajas, 1982; Prasher & Gibson, 1980) suggest that occasionally only contralateral stimulation results in an abnormally late response in MS subjects. Their data are vague regarding specific abnormalities, however, and further investigations are required that compare ipsilateral and contralateral recordings in this patient population.

ABR related to psychophysical data. There is presently a lack of sufficient published information relating ABR findings to results of psychoacoustic studies. Clinically, the authors have observed patients for whom no repeatable ABR could be recorded who had normal hearing sensitivity with 100% word discrimination scores in quiet. One study by Hausler and Levine (1980) attempted to relate estimates of the just-noticeable difference (JND) for intra-aural time and intensity in patients with MS. In general, their results showed that patients with abnormal time JNDs had abnormal ABRs on at least one side, while those with normal time JNDs tended to yield normal ABRs. The authors suggest that these results indicate that the same auditory structure of the brainstem subserves intraural time discrimination and short-latency, click-evoked potentials. While the data available on relationship between psychophysical testing and evoked potentials are scant, the study by Hausler and Levine suggests further avenues of exploration to better understand auditory function in normal and disordered populations.

Effects of warming on ABR. An increase in body temperature can provoke a transitory worsening of clinical symptoms of MS, and has been used in the past to help diagnose MS (Guthrie, 1951). Geraund, Coll, Arne-Bes, Arbus, Lacomme, and Bes, (1982) have reported on ABR changes observed following warming MS subjects by an average of 0.7° C. Of 18 MS subjects studied, there was no change of wave V latency or amplitude in 10 cases, while eight patients showed either a significant increase or a decrease in the response. The result is due to a slight increase in conduction velocity with increased temperature until a blocking temperature is reached, at which time conduction velocity slows (Geraund et al., 1982). The authors consider ABR testing after warming to have possible diagnostic advantages.

Comment. There are a wide variety of ABR results possible in multiple sclerosis, with disseminated lesions possible at all levels of the brainstem. While data remain inconclusive, the normal wave I data reported in two studies are consistent with the report that MS does not usually affect the peripheral portion of the auditory nerve where the myelin sheath is formed by Schwann cells rather than glial cells (Hausler & Levine, 1980). The III–V interval is likely to be prolonged since the area between the superior olivary complex and the inferior colliculus

FIGURE 12–3.
ABR responses obtained from a patient with MS using click rates from 10 to 80/s. Note the abnormal increase in I–V central conduction time at the faster click rates.

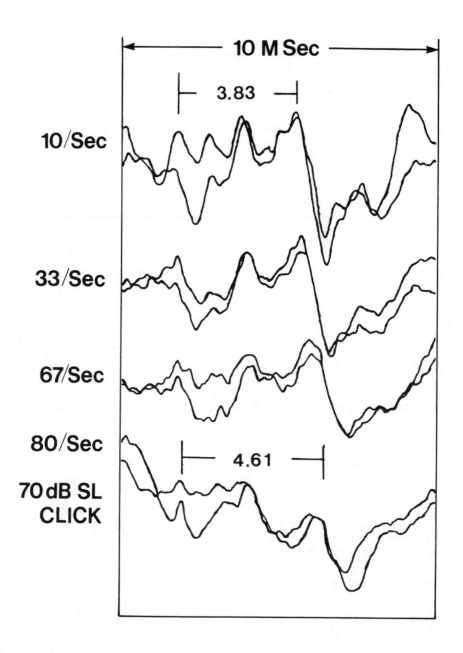

is "the longest tract of white matter in the CNS, and therefore the most susceptible to the effects of demyelinating disease" (Shanon et al., 1979). Also, demyelinization results in increased refraction period of transmission of the axons with reduced conduction velocity along the central auditory pathways, yielding delays in latency of progressive waves of the auditory evoked potential (Lacquaniti et al., 1979; Thornton & Hawkes, 1976). In the final analysis, however, clinicians should not expect to find a homogeneous pattern of results in a patient population with so many possibilities for distribution of lesions. Also, the clinician should always keep in mind that ABR abnormalities are not specific to identification of multiple sclerosis. Robinson and Rudge (1980) note that the ABR is like many tests of the CNS in that it merely indicates an abnormality of the system.

Acoustic neuromas, covered elsewhere in the book (chapter 10), are known to have profound effects on ABR response. Other degenerative diseases have been shown to have similar effects on ABR results. They include, for example, Charcot–Marie–Tooth disease (Musiek, Weider, & Mueller, 1982), adrenoleukodystrophy (Gang, Markland, DeMyer, & Warren, 1983), metachromatic leukodystrophy (Skomer, Stears, & Austin, 1983), olivopontocerebellar atrophy (Hammond & Wilder, 1983), sarcoidosis, Jamaican neuropathy, and vascular disease (Robinson & Rudge, 1980), among others. The point is that, as with all other audiologic procedures, the ABR identifies site, not type of lesion.

ROLE OF ABR IN NEUROLOGICAL DIAGNOSIS

Evoked potentials measurements have come to play an extremely important role in the diagnosis of patients who present with symptoms suggesting possible MS. According to Maurer and Lowitzsch (1982), the diagnosis of MS is based on three main criteria including the clinical course of the disease, the dissemination of the demyelinating process, and characteristic changes in cerebrospinal fluid. The notion of dissemination of lesions in the CNS means that the diagnosis of MS is dependent upon fulfilling a diagnostic requirement of a second nervous system lesion. For many patients who present with symptoms indicating a single lesion, evoked potential measurements can demonstrate clinically silent disease. The significance of increasing the sensitivity of diagnostic tests for multiple sclerosis lies in the fact that a great deal of time and effort is required in ruling out other disease processes. For many of these patients, evoked potentials may demonstrate subclinical abnormalities in areas other than the presenting symptoms. Demonstrating the presence of separate lesions in the CNS can, therefore, speed the diagnosis and remove the need for invasive tests that may have been required to rule out other pathology (Kjaer, 1980; Picton, Suranyi, Smith, & Picton, 1981; Tackmann, Strenge, & Barth, 1980). Chiappa and Ropper (1982) note that brainstem responses identify clinically silent lesions in MS less frequently than VEP and SEP, because of the pathoanatomy of the disease. However, they state that 20–50% of MS patients without brainstem symptoms will have abnormal ABRs. Since even small MS plaques produce marked ABR abnormality, the test has substantial clinical utility. Other important uses for ABR in MS include possible assistance in evaluating effectiveness of therapeutic measures (Stockard & Rossiter, 1977) and the "apparent ability" of ABR to predict the course of MS (Robinson & Rudge, 1980).

The authors would like to thank T. J. Murray, MD, for his critique and valuable suggestions on sections of this chapter.

REFERENCES

Adams, R., & Kubik, C. (1952). Morbid anatomy of the demyelinative diseases. *American Journal of Medicine, 12,* 510.

Alter, M. (1980). The geographic distribution of multiple sclerosis: New concepts. In H.J. Bauer, S. Poser, & G. Ritter (Eds.), *Progress in multiple sclerosis research* (pp. 495–502). Berlin: Springer-Verlag.

Antonelli, A., & DeMitri, T. (1963). Reperti audiometrici nella sclerosi a placche. *Sistema Nervosa, 15,* 138–145.

Baloh, R., & Honrubia, V. (1979). *Clinical neurophysiology of the vestibular system.* Philadephia: Davis.

Barajas, J.J. (1982). Evaluation of ipsilateral and contralateral brainstem auditory evoked potentials in multiple sclerosis patients. *Journal of Neurological Sciences, 54,* 69–78.

Bauer, H.J. (1980). IMAB-enquete concerning the diagnostic criteria for MS. In H.J. Bauer, S. Poser, & G. Ritter (Eds.), *Progress in multiple sclerosis research* (pp. 555–563). Berlin: Springer-Verlag.

Bosatra, A. (1977). Pathology of the nervous arc of the acoustic reflexes. *Audiology, 16,* 307–317.

Bosatra, A., Russolo, M., & Poli, P. (1976). Oscilloscope analysis of stapedial muscle reflex in brainstem lesions. *Archives of Otolaryngology, 102,* 284–285.

Chiappa, K.H. (1980). Pattern shift visual, brainstem auditory and short latency somatosensory evoked potentials in multiple sclerosis. *Neurology, 30,* 110–123.

Chiappa, K.H., Harrison, J.L., Brooks, E.B., & Young, R.R. (1980). Brainstem auditory evoked responses in 200 patients with multiple sclerosis. *Annals of Neurology, 7,* 135–143.

Chiappa, K.H., & Norwood, A.E. (1977). Brainstem auditory evoked responses in clinical neurology: Utility and neuropathological correlates. *Electroencephalography and Clinical Neurophysiology, 43,* 518–527.

Chiappa, K.H., & Ropper, A.H. (1982). Evoked potentials in clinical medicine: Part I. *New England Journal of Medicine, 306,* 1140–1210.

Chiappa, K.H., Young, R.R., & Goldie, W.D. (1979). Origins of the components of human short latency somatosensory evoked responses. *Neurology, 29,* 598.

Citron, L., Dix, M., Hallpike, C., & Hood, J. (1963). A recent clinicopathologic study of cochlear nerve degeneration resulting from tumor pressure from particular reference to the finding of normal threshold sensitivity for pure tones. *Acta Otolaryngologica, 56,* 330–337.

Cohen, S.R., Brune, M.J., Herndon, R.M., & McKhann, G.M. (1980). Diagnostic value of myelin basic protein in cerebrospinal fluid. In H.J. Bauer, S. Poser, & G. Ritter (Eds.), *Progress in multiple sclerosis research* (pp. 161–168). Berlin: Springer-Verlag.

Cohen, S.R., Herndon, R.M., & McKhann, G.M. (1976). Radioimmunoassay of myelin basic protein in spinal fluid: An index of active demyelination. *New England Journal of Medicine, 295,* 1455–1457.

Colletti, V. (1975). Stapedius reflex abnormalities in multiple sclerosis. *Audiology, 14,* 63–69.

Daughtery, W.T., Lederman, R.J., Nodar, R.H., & Conomy, J.P. (1983). Hearing loss in multiple sclerosis. *Archives of Neurology, 40,* 33–35.

Dayal, V., & Swisher, L. (1967). Pure tone thresholds in multiple sclerosis. *Laryngoscope, 77,* 2169–2177.

Dayal, V., Tarantino, L., & Swisher, L. (1966). Neurotologic studies in multiple sclerosis. *Laryngoscope, 76,* 1798–1809.

Detels, R., Visscher, B., Coulson, A., Malmgren, R., & Dudley, J. (1974). Multiple sclerosis in Japanese-Americans. A preliminary report. *International Journal of Epidemiology, 3,* 341–345.

Dix, M.R. (1965). Observations upon the nerve fiber deafness of multiple sclerosis with particular reference to the phenomenon of loudness recruitment. *Journal of Laryngology and Otology, 79,* 695–706.

Don, M., Allen, A.R., & Starr, A. (1977). The effect of click rate on the latency of auditory brainstem responses in humans. *Annals of Otology, Rhinology, and Laryngology, 86,* 186–196.

Gang, B.P., Markland, O.W., DeMyer, W.E., & Warren, C., Jr. (1983) Evoked response studies in patients with adrenoleukodystrophy and heterozygous relatives. *Archives of Neurology, 40,* 356–359.

Garza, Y.A. (1981). *Acoustic reflex dynamics and auditory brainstem responses in normal and multiple sclerosis subjects.* Unpublished master's thesis. University of Cincinnati, Cincinnati.

Garza, Y.A., Keith, R.W., & Barajas, J. (1982). *Acoustic reflex latency and auditory brainstem response in multiple sclerosis.* Presented at the International Symposium on Evoked Potentials, Cleveland, Ohio, October 16–18.

Geraund, G., Coll, J., Arne-Bes, C., Arbus, L., Lacomme, Y., & Bes, A. (1982). Brainstem auditory evoked potentials in multiple sclerosis: Influence of body temperature increase. *Advances in Neurology, 32,* 501–505.

Guthrie, T.C. (1951). Visual and motor changes in patients with multiple sclerosis. *Archives of Neurology and Psychiatry, 65,* 437–451.

Hammond, E.J., & Wilder, B.J. (1983). Evoked potentials in olivopontocerebellar artrophy. *Archives of Neurology, 40,* 366–369.

Hannley, M., Jerger, J., & Rivera, M. (1983). Relationships among auditory brainstem responses, masking level differences and the acoustic reflex in multiple sclerosis. *Audiology, 22,* 20–33.

Hausler, R., & Levine, R. (1980). Brainstem auditory evoked potentials are related to interaural time discrimination in patients with multiple sclerosis. *Brain Research, 191,* 589–594.

Hecox, K., Cone, B., & Blaw, M.E. (1981). Brainstem auditory evoked response in the diagnosis of pediatric neurological diseases. *Neurology, 31,* 832–839.

Hecox, K., Lastimosa, A.C.B., Mokotoff, B., & Sandlin,R. (in press). Human brainstem auditory evoked potentials: Rate effects, 1984.

Hess, K. (1979). Stapedius reflex in multiple sclerosis. *Journal of Neurology, Neurosurgery, and Psychiatry, 42,* 331–337.

Hopf, H.C., & Eysholdt, M. (1978). Impaired refractory periods of peripheral sensory nerves in multiple sclerosis. *Annals of Neurology, 4,* 499–501.

Hopf, H.C., & Maurer, K. (1983). Wave I of early auditory evoked potentials in multiple sclerosis. *Electroencephalography and Clinical Neurophysiology, 56,* 31–37.

Hyde, M.L., Stephens, S.D.G., & Thornton, A.R.D. (1976). Stimulus repetition rate and the early brainstem responses. *British Journal of Audiology, 10,* 41–50.

Jacobson, J.T. (1983). Auditory and electrophysiological effects in multiple sclerosis. Paper presented at the 17th Colorado Otology-Audiology Workshop, Aspen, Colorado.

Jacobson, J.T., Deppe, U., & Murray, T.J. (1983). Dichotic paradigms in multiple sclerosis. *Ear and Hearing, 4,* 311–317.

Johnson, K.P., & Nelson, B.J. (1977). Multiple sclerosis: Diagnostic usefulness of cerebrospinal fluid. *Annals of Neurology, 2,* 425–531.

Kjaer, M. (1980). Variations of brainstem auditory evoked potentials correlated to duration and severity of multiple sclerosis. *Acta Neurologica Scandinavica, 61,* 157–166.

Kurkland, L., & Reed, D. (1964). Geographic and climatic aspects of multiple sclerosis: A review of current hypotheses. *American Journal of Public Health, 54,* 588–597.

Lacquaniti, F., Benna, P., Gillis, M., Trone, W., & Bergamasco, B. (1979). Brainstem auditory evoked potentials and blink reflexes in quiescent multiple sclerosis. *Electroencephalography and Clinical Neurophysiology, 47,* 607–610.

Leibowitz, V., Alter, M., & Halpern L. (1964). Clinical studies of multiple sclerosis in Israel: III. Clinical course and prognosis related to age of onset. *Neurology, 14,* 926.

LeZak, R., & Selhub, S. (1966). On hearing in multiple sclerosis. *Annals of Otology, Rhinology and Laryngology, 75,* 1102–1110.

Lynn, G., Taylor, P., & Gilroy, J. (1980). Auditory evoked potentials in multiple sclerosis. *Electroencephalography and Clinical Neurophysiology, 50,* 167 (Abstract).

Matthews, W.B., Wattam-Bell, J.R.R., & Pountney, E. (1982). Evoked potentials in the diagnosis of multiple sclerosis. A follow-up study. *Journal of Neurology, Neurosurgery, and Psychiatry, 45,* 303–307.

Maurer, K., & Lowitzsch, K. (1982). Brainstem auditory evoked potentials in reclassification of 143 multiple sclerosis patients. *Advances in Neurology, 32,* 481–486.

McAlpine, D., Lumsden, C.E., & Acheson, E.D. (1972). *Multiple sclerosis: A reappraisal.* Baltimore: Williams & Wilkins.

Musiek, F.E., Weider, D.J., & Mueller, R.J. (1982). Audiologic findings in Charcot-Marie-Tooth disease. *Archives of Otolaryngology, 108,* 595–599.

Nager, G.T. (1969). Acoustic neurinomas. *Archives of Otolaryngology, 89,* 252–280.

Nodar, R.H. (1978). *The effects of MS on brainstem auditory evoked potentials.* Presented at the Annual Convention of the American Speech–Language–Hearing Association, San Francisco, Nov. 18–21.

Noffsinger, D., Olsen, W., Carhart, R., Hart, C., & Sahgal, V. (1972). Auditory and vestibular aberrations in multiple sclerosis. *Acta Otolaryngologica Supplement, 202.*

Parker, W., Decker, R., & Richards, N. (1968). Auditory function and lesions on the pons. *Archives of Otolaryngology, 87,* 26–38.

Parving, A., Elberling, C., & Smith, T. (1981). Auditory electrophysiology: Findings in multiple sclerosis. *Audiology, 20,* 123–142.

Picton, T.W., Suranyi, L., Smith, A., & Picton, N. (1981). General principles: Proceedings from the First International Workshop and Symposium on Evoked Potentials, Milan, April 9–12, 1980. Published in *Sensus/1, I,* (1), July–December, 1981.

Pollack, M., Calder, C., & Allpress, S. (1977). Peripheral nerve abnormalities in multiple sclerosis. *Annals of Neurology, 2,* 41–48.

Poskanzer, D.C., Walker, A.M., Yokondz, J., & Sheridan, J.L. (1976). Studies in the epidemiology of multiple sclerosis in the Orkney and Shetland Islands. *Neurology, 26,* 14–17.

Posner, C.M. (1969). Disseminated vasculomyelinopathy: A review of the clinical and pathologic reactions of the nervous system in hypergic diseases. *Acta Neurologica Scandinavica, 45, Supplement 37,* 3–44.

Prasher, D.K., & Gibson, W.P.R. (1980). Brainstem auditory evoked potentials: A comparative study of monaural vs. binaural stimulation in the detection of multiple sclerosis. *Electroencephalography and Clinical Neurophysiology, 50,* 247–253.

Pratt, H., Ben-David, Y., Peled, R., Podoshin, L., & Scharf, B. (1981). Auditory brainstem evoked potentials: Clinical promise of increasing stimulus rate. *Electroencephalography and Clinical Neurophysiology, 51,* 80–90.

Pratt, H., & Sohmer, H. (1976). Intensity and rate functions of cochlear and brainstem evoked responses to click stimuli in man. *Archives of Otology, Rhinology, and Laryngology, 212,* 85–92.

Pryse-Phillips, W., & Murray, T.J. (1982). *Essential neurology.* Garden City, NY: Medical Examination Publishing Co.

Robinson, K.H., & Rudge, P. (1975). Auditory evoked responses in multiple sclerosis. *Lancet,* May 24, 1164–1166.

Robinson, K.H., & Rudge, P. (1977). Abnormalities of the auditory evoked potentials in patients with multiple sclerosis. *Brain, 100,* 19–40.

Robinson, K.H., & Rudge, P. (1980). The use of the auditory evoked potential in the diagnosis of multiple sclerosis. *Journal of Neurological Science, 45,* 235–244.

Rose, R., & Daly, J. (1964). Reversible temporary threshold shift in multiple sclerosis. *Laryngoscope, 74,* 424–432.

Rowe, J. (1981). The brainstem auditory evoked response in neurologic disease. A review. *Ear and Hearing, 2,* 41–49.

Russolo, M., & Poli, P. (1983). Lateralization, impedance, auditory brainstem response, and synthetic sentence audiometry in brainstem disorders. *Audiology, 22,* 50–62.

Schumacher, G.A., (1971). Demyelinating diseases. In A.G. Baker & L.H. Baker (Eds.), *Clinical neurology* (pp. 1–92). New York: Harper & Row.

Schumacher, G.A., Beebe, G., Kibler, R.F., Kurkland, L.T., et al. (1968). Problems of experimental trials of therapy in multiple sclerosis: Report by the panel on the evaluation of experimental trial of therapy in multiple sclerosis. *Annals of the New York Academy of Science, 122,* 552–568.

Sears, T.A., Bostock, H., & Sherratt, M. (1978). The pathophysiology of demyelination and its implication for the symptomatic treatment of multiple sclerosis. *Neurology, 28,* 21–26.

Shanon, E., Gold, S., & Himmelfarb, M. (1981). Assessment of functional integrity of brainstem auditory pathways of stimulus stress. *Audiology, 20,* 65–71.

Shanon, E., Gold, S., Himmelfarb, Z., Carasso, R. (1979). Auditory potentials of cochlear nerve & brainstem in multiple sclerosis. *Archives of Otolaryngology, 105,* 505–508.

Simpkins, W. (1961). Audiometric profile in multiple sclerosis. *Archives of Otolaryngology, 73,* 557–564.

Skomer, C., Stears, J., & Austin, J. (1983). Metachromatic leukodystrophy adults MLD with focal lesions by computed tomography. *Archives of Neurology, 40,* 354–355.

Starr, A., & Achor, J. (1975). Auditory brainstem responses in neurological disease. *Archives of Neurology, 32,* 761–768.

Stephens, S., & Thornton, A. (1976). Subjective and electrophysiologic tests in brainstem lesions. *Archives of Otolaryngology, 102,* 608–613.

Stockard, J.J., & Rossiter, V.S. (1977). Clinical and pathological correlates of brainstem auditory response abnormalities. *Neurology, 27,* 316–325.

Stockard, J.J., Stockard, J.E., & Sharbrough, F.W. (1977). Detection and localization of occult lesions with brainstem auditory responses. *Proceedings of the Mayo Clinic, 52,* 761–770.

Stockard, J. J., Stockard, J. E., & Sharbrough, F. W. (1978). Nonpathologic factors influencing brainstem auditory evoked potentials. *American Journal of EEG Technology, 18,* 177–209.

Tackmann, W., Strenge, H., & Barth, S. (1980). Auditory brainstem evoked potentials in patients with multiple sclerosis. *European Neurology, 19,* 396–401.

Terkildsen, K., Osterhammel, P., & Huis in't Veld (1975). Far-field electrocochleography adaptation. *Scandinavian Audiology, 4,* 215–220.

Thornton, A.R.D., & Coleman, M.J. (1975). The adaptation of cochlear brainstem auditory evoked potentials in humans. *Electroencephalography and Clinical Neurophysiology, 39,* 399–406.

Thornton, A.R.D., & Hawkes, C.H. (1976). *Cochlear and brainstem evoked responses in multiple sclerosis.* Read before the 13th International Congress of Audiology, Jerusalem, August.

Weber, B. A., & Fujikawa, S. M. (1977). Brainstem evoked response (BER) audiology at various stimulus presentation rates. *Journal of American Audiology Society, 3,* 59–62.

Yagi, T., & Kaga, K. (1979). The effect of the click repetition rate on the latency of the auditory evoked brainstem response and its clinical use for a neurological diagnosis. *Archives of Otology, Rhinology, and Laryngology, 222,* 91–97.

Zollner, C., Karnahl, T., & Stange, G. (1976). Input–output functions and adaptation behavior on the five early potentials registered with the earlobe-vertex pickup. *Archives of Otology, Rhinology, and Laryngology, 212,* 23–33.

Chapter 13

The ABR in Intraoperative Monitoring

Paul Kileny
J. W. R. McIntyre

INTRODUCTION

Scalp recorded sensory evoked potentials (EP) are small alterations in the ongoing electrical activity of the central nervous system (CNS) following sensory stimulation that depend on the activation of specific sensory pathways in the CNS. Sensory EPs provide us with a noninvasive means to determine the functional integrity of selected neural pathways from periphery to cortex. Thus EP tests are an extension of a clinical neurological examination and are used for diagnostic and prognostic purposes (Chiappa & Ropper, 1982a, b). Advances in engineering have facilitated such testing in the operating room where space is at a premium and where for electrical and other reasons the environment is hostile. In these situations the test can supply immediate information regarding a threat to the patient's outcome that has been produced by anesthesia or by surgery. The intraoperative monitoring of sensory evoked potentials is becoming an essential part of patient care in the operating room (Grundy, 1983) though its precise role under all circumstances has yet to be determined.

Middle and Late Components of the Auditory Evoked Response

Cortical sensory evoked potentials recorded within the latency range associated with the middle latency auditory components have been considered to be mediated by the specific thalamic sensory pathways and nuclei (hence, specific responses) (Brazier, 1972). Responses recorded from the exposed human cortex within this latency range were described as two positive deflections elicited within 50 ms from stimulus onset by ipsilateral and contralateral stimuli. These components have been considered to be primary auditory responses with a cortical distribution limited to the posterior part of the superior temporal gyrus and the parietal and frontal operculum. They were minimally affected by anesthesia and were not susceptible to changes following repeated stimulation (habituation) (Celesia, Broughton, Rasmussen, & Branch, 1968; Heath & Galbraith, 1966; Puletti & Celesia, 1970). In a recent study, Kraus, Ozdamar, Hier, and Stein (1982) presented evidence suggesting that the vertex-recorded middle latency auditory evoked response components are generated by symmetrical bilateral generators. They also demonstrated that unilateral temporal lobe lesions primarily affect the integrity of components recorded over the involved hemisphere. These results infer temporal lobe cortex contribution to the scalp-recorded auditory MLR and coincide with earlier statements made by Picton, Hillyard, Kraus, and Galambos (1974), who considered the middle latency responses to originate from thalamus and/or primary auditory cortex.

The late components of the auditory evoked response are considered to be nonspecific components mediated by the reticular formation. The cortex- and scalp-recorded components occurring within this time frame correlate quite well and are diffusely distributed. Unlike the specific components, the nonspecific components are significantly affected by general anesthesia and habituate with repeated stimulation (Celesia et al., 1968; Davis, Mast, Yoshie, & Zerlin, 1966).

PHYSIOLOGICAL AND PHARMACOLOGICAL FACTORS INFLUENCING THE INTERPRETATION OF EVOKED POTENTIALS DURING ANESTHESIA AND SURGERY

If auditory evoked potentials are to be used effectively for intraoperative monitoring strict attention must be paid to certain details. Among these are the physiological and pharmacological factors that influence response configurations and characteristics in addition to the specific anesthetic and surgical events whose effects are being monitored. These factors are many and varied (Table 13-1). However, effects on different components of the responses vary and so some components may be better suited for intraoperative monitoring than others. Certain of these merit special comment.

TABLE 13–1. Physiological and Pharmacological Factors that May Affect Evoked Potentials

Anesthetic agents
Other CNS acting drugs
Temperature
Arterial blood pressure
Tensions of respiratory gases
Hematocrit
Electrolyte balance
Neuromuscular blocking agents
Repetitive stimulation

Pharmacologic Agents

All anesthetics depress the activity of the CNS; however, they differ in their mode of action. The understanding of how anesthetics work is incomplete, because of an unresolved appreciation of the physiological events associated with the anesthetic state. Thus, the effects of anesthetic drugs on various evoked potentials cannot be predicted with certainty because their exact mechanism and site of action have yet to be precisely defined (Koblin & Eger, 1981). Anesthetics almost certainly exert their effects by interacting with neural membranes and disrupting transmission in many parts of the CNS. Recent studies have provided the following information. Anesthetics depress the activity of excitatory synapses by reducing the magnitude of postsynaptic depolarization caused by the release of acetylcholine. Anesthetics may also block axonal conduction; however, that action necessitates higher doses than needed to depress synaptic transmission. There is evidence that certain anesthetics potentiate inhibitory synapses. For instance, barbiturates potentiate GABA (gamma aminobutyric acid)–mediated postsynaptic inhibition (Gage & Hamill, 1981).

The brainstem reticular formation is considered to be one of the prime sites of action of narcotic agents at anesthetic doses. As wakefulness and cortical activation depend upon impulses traveling via the extralemniscal brainstem reticular system, a reduction of its activity will coincide with a reduction of cortical activation (Moruzzi & Magoun, 1949). Afferent impulses mediated via lemniscal sensory pathways and the specific nuclei of the thalamus remain relatively unaffected even during deep anesthesia (Brazier, 1972). However, the brainstem reticular formation is not the only site of anesthetic drug action. Anesthetic drugs interrupt transmission in many areas of the CNS and anesthesia may not involve selectively one specific system.

Several reports dealt with the effects of pentobarbital on various components of the auditory evoked response. Kiang, Neame, and Clark (1961) found that the earlier positive peak of the auditory evoked response in cats was not affected; however, the later peaks disappeared following the administration of pentobarbital. Pradhan and Galambos (1963), on the other hand, documented some changes in the configuration of the early cortical response in cats following administration of pentobarbital. These investigators showed that the two early positive peaks blended into a single one. Borbely and Hall (1970) studied the effects of chlorpromazine and pentobarbital on auditory evoked responses recorded from cortex, hippocampus, and the medial geniculate body in rats. They documented increases in latencies and amplitudes of cortical and hippocampal auditory evoked response components. They also found slight increases in the latencies of components recorded from the medial geniculate body, as well as biphasic changes of cortical component amplitudes and latencies.

General anesthetic agents have been studied extensively. Lader and Norris (1969) found that the early scalp-recorded components of the auditory evoked response (latency range 18–37 ms) were not affected significantly by administration of nitrous oxide; the later components (beyond 50 ms latency), however, were most significantly affected.

Mori, Winters, and Spooner (1968) studied the effects of ether, pentobarbital, halothane, and nitrous oxide on auditory evoked responses recorded from cats at the anterior suprasylvian gyrus, dorsal cochlear nucleus, and reticular formation. They found that cochlear nucleus responses remained intact even under deep anesthesia. The amplitude of the earlier portion of the cortical auditory evoked response diminished significantly under deep ether- or pentobarbital-induced anesthesia but did not disappear. The later components (latencies beyond 50 ms) disappeared.

The picture that emerges from the above is one characterized by lack of consistency among reports dealing with effects of anesthetics on the later components of the auditory evoked response. While it is clear that the activity of auditory centers persists even under deep anesthesia, the nature of the effects reported by various investigators differ.

There is less variability among sources of information dealing with effects of pharmacologic agents on the auditory brainstem responses (ABR). Duncan, Sanders, and McCullough (1979) investigated the effects of nitrous oxide, halothane, and thiopentone on ABRs recorded from adult patients prepared for elective surgery. Following induction of anesthesia with 50% nitrous oxide and halothane, patients were exposed to several concentrations of halothane in oxygen (2–0.25%). Neither the amplitude nor the latency of wave V was affected by the above. Thiopentone (4 mg/kg–1) did not affect the ABRs either.

Bobbin, May, and Lemoine (1979) investigated the effects of ketamine hydrochloride (100 mg/kg) and pentobarbital (50 mg/kg) on latency-intensity functions and amplitude-latency functions of two auditory brainstem response peaks as well as their interpeak intervals in rats (component peaks I and IV). Changes in these components found in this study (which occurred both in the drug-treated group and in a control group injected with normal saline) were attributed to decrements in body temperature.

Some pharmacologic agents do affect the ABR; however, the effects are by and large minimal. Stockard, Stockard, and Sharbrough (1978b) and Stockard and Sharbrough (1980) documented changes in auditory brainstem responses recorded from cats and humans with two inhalational anesthetics, isoflurene and enflurene. They reported slightly reduced amplitudes of waves IV and V in cats with unaltered peak and interpeak latencies with isoflurene-induced anesthesia. They also documented increased interpeak latencies in ABRs recorded from humans and cats recovering from enflurene anesthesia.

Shea and Harell (1978) administered 100 mg lidocaine (commonly used as a local anesthetic) in 5 cc water intravenously over 30 s to patients in an attempt to alleviate their tinnitus and reported a reduction in the amplitude of wave I of the ABR. Javel, Mouney, McGee, and Walsh (1982) confirmed the adverse effects of lidocaine infusion upon the ABR elicited from cats. They found infusion rate-dependent delays in ABR peak and interpeak intervals as well as changes in response configuration in the form of peak splitting. The effect was greatest for the I–II interval.

Another pharmacologic agent that alters the ABR is phenytoin, an anticonvulsant known to selectively affect brainstem and cerebellar function. Green, Walcoff, and Lucke (1982) found that the administration of phenytoin at either subtherapeutic, therapeutic, or toxic levels significantly prolonged the interpeak latencies of the ABR.

Finally, cholinergic drugs may also be included among the group of pharmacological agents that alter the ABR. These are substances that affect the release of acetylcholine, a neurotransmitter believed to be active in the mammalian auditory pathway. Bhargava, Salamy, and McKean (1978) studied the effects of various cholinergic substances (physostigmine, carbachol, etc.) administered in various doses and in combinations on the ABR elicited from rats. They observed both increases and decreases in ABR component amplitudes. The direction of the amplitude change depended upon the dose of the cholinergic drugs as well as on the additional administration of an antagonist substance (i.e., osotremorine, a muscarinic agonist, and scopalamine, a muscarinic antagonist). None of cholinergic agents investigated by Bhargava et al. (1978) affected ABR peak latencies with the exception of carbachol when administered at a dose of 1 mg/kg or higher.

Neuromuscular blocking agents are routinely administered to patients prior to surgery in preparation for intubation. Contrary to earlier beliefs (Bickford, Jacobson, & Cody, 1964) Pa component of the MLR remains intact and unaltered following the administration of succinylcholine (Harker, Hosick, Voots, & Mendel, 1977) or pancuronium bromide (Kileny, Dobson, & Gelfand, 1983). The ABR is also unaffected by neuromuscular blocking agents. Figure 13-1 illustrates the absence of effects of general anesthesia and neuromuscular blocking agents on the ABR. These responses were elicited from an 8-month-old patient prior to open-heart surgery. The top trace was obtained prior to the induction of anesthesia and the administration of a muscle relaxant. The second trace was elicited following the induction of anesthesia (nitrous oxide–oxygen and halothane) and the administration of a neuromuscular blocking agent (pancuronium). Its configuration is essentially unaltered save for a "smoother" look, reflecting the absence of muscle artifacts.

While it is important to note the existence of pharmacological agents that do affect the configuration of the ABR, it is also important to realize that their effects are relatively minor when compared to the effects of pharmacological agents on the later components of the auditory evoked response.

Hypoxia

There is evidence that the endocochlear potential declines with anoxia. This coincides with a decrease in K^+ (potassium) concentration and an increase of Na^+ (sodium) concentration in the endolymph (Konishi, 1979). The endocochlear potential is considered to originate in the stria vascularis of the cochlea (Tasaki & Spiropoulos, 1959) and to interact with the intracellular potentials of the organ of Corti. Together they create a potential gradient across the reticular membrane of the cochlea that acts as an amplifier. Thus, a decline of the endocochlear potential may result in decreased output from the cochlea that may affect all subsequent auditory electrophysiological responses.

FIGURE 13–1.
Auditory brainstem responses elicited by 60 dB HL clicks from an 8-month-old female patient before and after the induction of anesthesia and muscle relaxation.

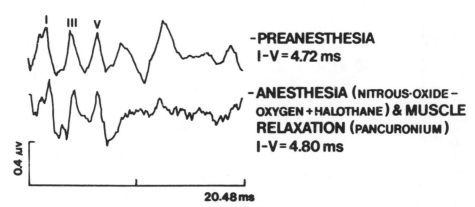

In a recent study, however (Sohmer, Gafni, & Chisin, 1982), the ABR proved to be resistant to both hypoxia and hypercapnia at levels that depress both the EEG and cortical evoked potentials. During inhalation of 5.5% of oxygen in inspired gases for 4 min or longer, the ABR disappeared. Sohmer et al. (1982) concluded that the brainstem abnormalities associated with hypoxia may be due to ischemia that follows depressed systemic circulation, rather than to a decrease of oxygen concentration in the circulating blood.

Temperature Effects

Both the middle latency response (MLR) and the ABR are sensitive to changes in body temperature. Some of the neurophysiological sequelae of reducing body temperature are increases in the duration of action potentials (Klee, Pierau, & Faber, 1974), slower nerve conduction velocity (Kraft, 1972), and an impairment of transmitter release across the synapse (Weight & Erulkar, 1976). With progressive reductions of body temperature, latencies of both auditory MLR and ABR become prolonged (Kaga, Takiguchi, Myokai, & Shiode, 1979; Kileny et al., 1983; Stockard, Sharbrough, & Tinker, 1978a). Both the MLR and the ABR disappeared at 20-23 °C, nasopharyngeal temperature. Figure 13-2 is a graph illustrating the differential effects of temperature on the components of the ABR. Temperature reduction brings about delays in all three major ABR components, waves I, III, and V. However, the effect is cumulative: in relative terms, the later components are delayed to a greater extent than the preceding components.

Repetitive Stimulation

Intraoperative monitoring with auditory (or any other sensory) evoked potentials involves repeated presentations of the same stimulus. Successive blocks of stimuli are needed to elicit consecutive samples of evoked potentials. Many behavioral and physiological responses exhibit a progressive decline in their magnitude during repeated and consecutive presentations of the same stimulus (Kileny, Ryu, McCabe, & Abbas, 1980). Response habituation may affect peripheral neuronal structures such as second-order neurons in vestibular nuclei of the cat, as well as cortical structures. To select an auditory evoked potential for intraoperative applications,

FIGURE 13–2.
The relationship between body temperature and auditory brainstem response components.

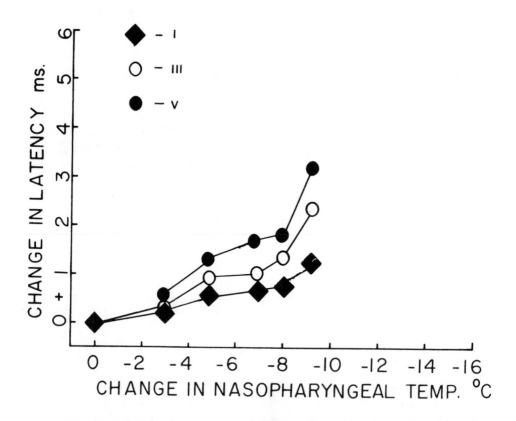

it is important to become familiar with the behavior of various components under repeated stimulation conditions. Picton, Hillyard, and Galambos (1976) have investigated the effects of repeated stimulation on the various components of the auditory evoked response. These investigators compared averaged auditory evoked responses elicited by consecutive blocks of auditory stimuli. They demonstrated that the N1 and P2 components of the late cortical auditory vertex potential decline in a progressive fashion with repeated stimulation. Thus, when comparing responses elicited by the nth block of stimuli to the first block of stimuli it was evident that there was a reduction in the amplitudes of N1 and P2 elicited by the latter. The middle latency of the brainstem components did not decline with repeated stimulation. These latter components would be the ones of choice for intraoperative monitoring, as one would not have to separate the effects of repeated stimulation and the potential effects of anesthesia and surgery.

INTRAOPERATIVE APPLICATIONS OF THE ABR

Several features make the ABR an adequate tool for utilization in intraoperative monitoring. As shown earlier in the chapter, the ABR is not altered appreciably by pharmacological agents commonly used prior to and during surgery. Intraoperative monitoring implies repeated elicitation of the response and the possibility of habituation. However, the ABR does not habituate with repetitive stimulation. Another advantage of the ABR is that in man the neural generators of some of the peaks are known (Møller & Jannetta, 1982; Møller, Jannetta, Bennett, & Møller, 1981).

Intraoperatively the ABR may have several applications. First and foremost, the ABR is a sensitive measure of the condition of the lower auditory pathway. Therefore it may be used to monitor the integrity of the lower auditory pathway and changes in hearing sensitivity during operations that may threaten the inner ear, the auditory nerve, or the auditory centers in the brainstem. The ABR is also a sensitive indicator of the condition of the brainstem in general. Thus, one may use the ABR to make inferences on the neurological status of the brainstem during operations that may compromise it directly or indirectly.

Intraoperative ABR may be interpreted on a moment-to-moment basis and may be followed by corrective action. The anesthetist, the surgeon, and the clinician performing the monitoring (if other than the anesthetist) must collaborate closely in this regard. Before attributing an ABR change to a surgical maneuver, possible changes produced by pharmacological or physiological factors must be ruled out. If the functional integrity of the auditory pathway deteriorates, then under certain circumstances it may be reasonable to conclude that the brainstem and possibly more extensive areas of the central nervous system are at risk. The circumstances in the operating room when this may be particularly valuable are (i) when the perfusion of areas of the brain is threatened by pharmacological or physiological interventions by the anesthetist, (ii) during the positioning of patients with cerebral perfusion problems, (iii) when brain perfusion is threatened by surgical maneuvers.

In the remainder of this chapter we attempt to review the specific intraoperative applications of the ABR and provide some examples.

Operations of the Posterior Cranial Fossa

Grundy, Jannetta, Procopio, Lina, Boston, and Doyle (1982) reviewed 54 neurosurgical operations of the cerebellopontine angle monitored with ABR. They found unaltered ABRs throughout the operation in only 11 cases. In 32 patients they observed reversible changes. In five cases the ABR changes observed during operation were irreversible. Six cases were discarded from this series due to significant preoperative hearing loss or technical problems arising during monitoring. Wave V latency was extremely stable following induction of anesthesia, and prior to the opening of the dura. Retraction of the cerebellum or the brainstem brought about reversible alterations in 22 cases. These alterations consisted of progressive delays in wave V latencies up to a complete loss of the ABR. Figure 13-3 (reproduced from Grundy et al., 1982, with permission) illustrates the effects of the retraction of the eighth cranial nerve on the ABR during posterior fossa surgery (microvascular decompression of the seventh cranial nerve for the relief of hemifacial spasm). This manipulation resulted initially in a delayed wave V and an increase in the I–V interpeak interval. With continued retraction (see Figure 13-3) the response disappeared. With a readjustment of the retractor, the response reappeared (waves I, III, and V), albeit with a prolonged I–V interpeak interval. A repositioning of the retractor or a brief cessation of the operation were as a rule successful in restoring a lost ABR; however, the I–V interpeak interval remained prolonged while in the operating room (Grundy, Jannetta, Procopio, Lina, Boston, & Doyle, 1982; Grundy, Lina, Procopio, & Jannetta, 1981). Audiometric and ABR follow-up done 4 days following surgery in one such case indicated a slight hearing impairment at 2000 Hz (otherwise normal, unchanged hearing), normal wave V latency but increased latencies for peaks II and III (Grundy et al., 1981). In two cases the amplitude of the ABR was significantly depressed as a result of mild arterial hypotension and hypocarbia, previously considered acceptable. The ABR recovered following the correction of these conditions. In most cases, changes in the configuration of the ABR were followed by various interventions performed

FIGURE 13-3.
(Reproduced from Grundy et al., 1982, with permission). Effects of the retraction of the eighth cranial nerve during posterior fossa surgery on the auditory brainstem response.

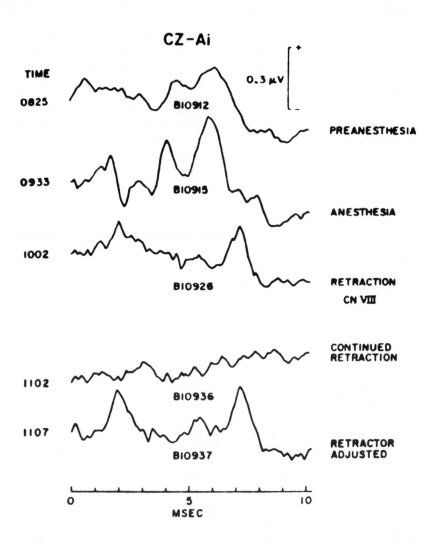

by the surgeon (i.e., repositioning retractors) or the anesthesiologist (i.e., adjusting ventilation) and resulted in an improvement of the ABR waveform. Hearing was preserved in all cases where these interventions were successful in restoring the ABR. Irreversible changes were observed only in cases where the eighth cranial nerve had to be sacrificed. Criteria of significant intraoperative ABR changes necessitating the implementation of corrective interventions were also developed by Grundy et al. (1982). They suggested that because at the time of the operation some patients may present with auditory brainstem responses considered abnormal according to accepted clinical criteria, each patient should act as his or her own control. They further suggested that intraoperative warning should be given if wave V latency increases at a rate exceeding 0.07 ms/min or if there is an absolute prolongation of wave V latency exceeding 1.5 ms.

Levine (1979) summarized six cases monitored during acoustic neurinoma surgery. The auditory nerve action potential was monitored in the ear canal simultaneously with the scalp-recorded auditory brainstem responses. Response configuration was most significantly affected during dissection and manipulation of the auditory nerve (i.e., tugging). In three patients, there was an abrupt disruption of the auditory brainstem response including the auditory nerve potential during tumor dissection. There was no recovery of the response in these patients during or following the operation and they all presented with a complete postoperative loss of hearing documented audiometrically. Hearing was preserved in the three remaining cases: two subtotal intracapsular removals of an acoustic neurinoma and one complete removal of a 1.4-cm tumor. In all three, the auditory brainstem response fluctuated during the course of tumor dissection; however, intraoperative manipulations were interrupted to allow for the recovery of the response. Levine cautioned that not all intraoperative manipulations result in immediate effects on the ABR. Indeed, some seemingly "spontaneous" subsequent alterations may result from an intervention. Similarly, the responses may take several days to fully recover, as indicated by Grundy and co-workers. Levine made the assumption that some of the ABR changes seen during manipulation of the eighth cranial nerve may be due to vascular effects. He also observed that "tugging" the auditory nerve medially (away from the cochlea) may have more significant effects on auditory function than tugging laterally. Medial "tugging" may sever the fibers from the sensory cells of the cochlea.

Factors other than intracranial manipulations or hypotension may also affect the ABR. Thus, in another report, Grundy, Procopio, Jannetta, Lina, and Doyle (1982) described ABR alterations unexpectedly brought about by positioning the patient for retromastoid craniectomy. The patient was placed in a lateral position with the head flexed on the neck, turned approximately 20° toward the site of the craniotomy, and secured in a head holder. The cervical column and cord were under mild traction in this position. The ABRs elicited by stimulating the ear ipsilateral to the operative site and the ear contralateral to the operative site were within normal limits prior to placing the patient in the position described above. The ipsilateral ABR was lost following positioning. The contralateral ABR was not affected. At operation, it was found that a loop of the posterior inferior cerebellar artery was compressing both the seventh and the eighth cranial nerves. The authors speculated that positioning the patient may have brought about an increase in the compression of the eighth cranial nerve. This in turn may have contributed to the loss of the brainstem response, including wave I. The ipsilateral ABR recovered after the patient was placed in the supine position, following the closure of the incision. There were no permanent effects on this patient's hearing, as documented by an audiological evaluation performed several days following the operation.

Cardiovascular Surgery

Surgical procedures for the correction of cardiac defects requiring cardiopulmonary bypass or total circulatory arrest are as a rule performed under hypothermia. While this measure is taken in order to protect the CNS from ischemic damage, it is also a potentially threatening condition. Therefore, it is desirable to monitor brain function during surgical procedures requiring hypothermia in order to ensure that no irreversible changes will occur as a result. Both EEG and evoked potentials have been used for this purpose (Kaga et al., 1979, Kileny et al., 1983; Wolin, Massopust, & Meder, 1964; Reilly, Kondo, Brunberg, & Doty, 1978). As shown earlier in the chapter (see Temperature Effects), the ABR exhibits predictable and orderly changes induced by reductions of body temperature. This property was found to be useful for monitoring purposes (Kaga et al., 1979; Stockard et al., 1978a).

Figure 13-4 illustrates sequences of auditory brainstem responses recorded during open-heart surgical procedures for an 18-month-old female patient (A) and a 56-year-old male patient

FIGURE 13–4A
Auditory brainstem responses recorded during open-heart surgery with hypothermia from an 18-month-old female patient (A) and a 56-year-old male patient (B). Both sets of responses were elicited by 60 dB HL clicks.

Illustration continued on following page.

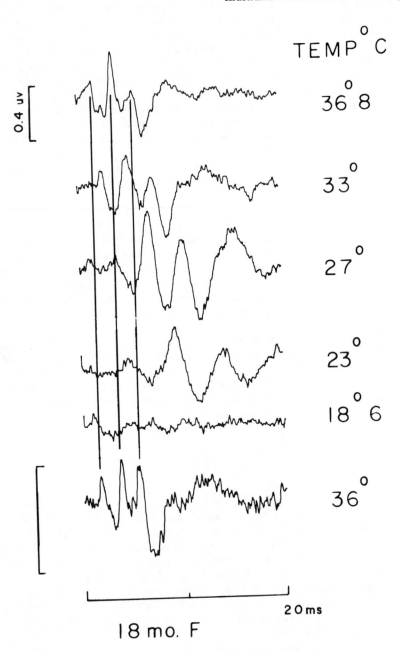

18 mo. F

FIGURE 13–4B (continued). See legend on preceding page.

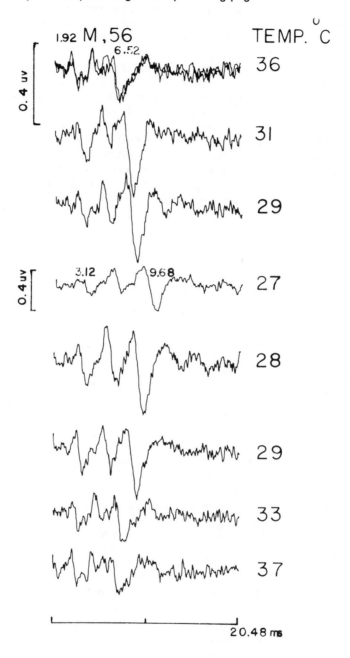

(B). In both cases peak latencies and interpeak intervals became progressively prolonged as nasopharyngeal temperatures decreased. Similarly, a restoration of normal temperature brought about a return to normal ABR peak latencies and interpeak interval values. As indicated by the data displayed in Figure 13-4A, the ABR was lost within the 23–18 °C temperature range.

It is also significant that the patient whose ABRs are displayed in Figure 13-4A was operated on under total circulatory arrest established when nasopharyngeal temperature reached 15° C and maintained for approximately 60 min. Following the reestablishment of circulation and rewarming, the ABR was restored to its normal preoperative configuration. Both patients illustrated in Figure 13-4 were neurologically normal postoperatively. Thus, the ABR may be used successfully to monitor brainstem function during open-heart operations requiring hypothermia and/or total circulatory arrest. As indicated by Kaga et al. (1979) it has only two limitations: a significant hearing impairment would preclude its use as a reliable indicator of brainstem function (this limitation applies to the ABR in general regardless of the specific application). The other limitation is inherent in the fact that the ABR disappears at approximately 20–23 °C nasopharyngeal temperature and therefore below that temperature range it is no longer possible to monitor brainstem function. This second limitation is not specific to the ABR; it affects other neurophysiological functions as well. ABR monitoring during open-heart operations will help to detect any changes in brainstem function beyond the changes induced by reduced body temperatures and to confirm the restoration of normal function with the resumption of normal temperature.

Practical Considerations

The minimum requirement to establish a patient's hearing sensitivity before deciding whether auditory EP monitoring would be appropriate is a pure tone audiogram. A hearing loss does not rule out the utilization of auditory evoked responses for intraoperative monitoring, but the effects that a hearing loss may have on the configuration of the response must be taken into account. A baseline auditory evoked response prior to anesthesia is particularly desirable under these circumstances. The purpose of utilizing auditory evoked responses during various operative procedures is to detect certain threats to patient outcome so that they can be countered as soon as possible. This cannot be done effectively if the audiologic status of the patient has not been previously established. Just as impairment of hearing sensitivity causes a distortion of auditory evoked potentials, so will a neurological impairment that may or may not be specific to the auditory pathway. For example, an acoustic neuroma will prolong ABR interpeak intervals or even abolish all peaks beyond wave I. Under such circumstances, auditory brainstem responses can be used to help protect the auditory nerve on the tumor side during surgery. Auditory evoked responses elicited from the contralateral side can be employed to monitor the neurological condition of the brainstem in general.

Once the patient reaches the operating room, technical management of the monitoring must be meticulous and interpretation of the EPs must be skilled. During each monitoring session stimulus and recording parameters must be as constant as possible. In most cases, for monitoring purposes auditory evoked responses are elicited by suprathreshold stimuli. To have a stimulus intensity reference under those circumstances, a physiological calibration of stimuli used during a specific procedure must be done by the operator and if possible using additional personnel with known normal hearing sensitivity. If that cannot be arranged, the normal hearing operator should use his own hearing to establish a reference for every situation. A monitoring earphone identical to the one attached to the patient set up in parallel for the operator can be employed for this purpose. If that is available, the operator may readjust stimulus intensity during the procedure as may be necessitated by changes in background noise. Purists might frown upon such a subjective method to establish stimulus intensity calibration; however, it is one that is practical, easy to do, and does not seem to be associated with clinically significant problems. An alternative is to monitor sound pressure level in the patient's ear canal by means of a probe microphone. Problems associated with this are as follows:

(i) There may not be an appreciable change of stimulus SPL with changes in background noise that will create subjective changes.

(ii) In a small ear canal of infants and young children it may be impossible to accommodate a probe microphone as well as an insert earphone commonly used in surgical monitoring.

(iii) The placement of a probe microphone may increase preparation time and thus interfere with operating room schedules.

When utilizing evoked potentials for intraoperative monitoring it is critical to follow procedures meant to minimize the likelihood of interference with the recording process. The operating room is an environment containing many possible sources of electrical artifact. To reduce their effects and to avoid the introduction of other sources of artifact, the following general guidelines should be taken into consideration:

(i) Do not use electrodes made of different metals on the same patient, in order to avoid or minimize electrode offset potential.

(ii) Use electrodes with "fast" discharge characteristics (avoid stainless steel).

(iii) If possible, use polarized electrodes (i.e., AgCl) in order to avoid the formation of electrode–electrolyte double layer.

(iv) Electrodes should make good contact and have low impedance; remember, you may not be able to have access to these recording electrodes during the operative procedure.

(v) In the presence of a periodic electrical interference, avoid averaging at rates which are integral multiples or divisibles of noise periodicity; twisting the electrode leads together may also help reduce the effects of this interference.

(vi) Avoid sharing an electrical outlet with other instrumentation.

(vii) Avoid recording during use of electrocautery; in fact, it is desirable to disconnect the patient electrode cable from the amplifier to avoid its possible damage.

It is important to realize that access to the patient during surgery will be limited. One potential problem source is poor coupling of the earphone transducer. To minimize the surface area involved, it is desirable to use hearing aid-type insert earphones. The operator must make sure that the earphone is adequately placed and that the earmold or tubing leading to the ear canal is clear and unobstructed. Failure to do so may abort monitoring. And finally, the surgical team must be aware of the nature of the monitoring process, just as the clinician responsible for monitoring must become familiar with the surgical procedure and the risks it imposes. The efficacy of ABR monitoring depends to a great extent upon cooperation between surgeon and the clinician responsible for monitoring.

The authors thank Mrs. Sandy Busse for her valuable help with this manuscript.

REFERENCES

Bhargava, V. K., Salamy, A., & McKean, C. M. (1978). Effect of cholinergic drugs on the brainstem auditory evoked response (far-field) in rats. *Neuroscience, 3,* 821–826.

Bickford, R. G., Jacobson, J. L., & Cody, D. T. (1964). Nature of average evoked potentials to sound and other stimuli in man. *Annals of the New York Academy of Sciences, 112,* 204–223.

Bobbin, R. P., May, J. G., & Lemoine, R. L. (1979). Effects of pentobarbital and ketamine on brain stem auditory potentials. *Archives of Otolaryngology, 105,* 467–470.

Borbely, A. A., & Hall, R. D. (1970). Effects of pentobarbitone and chlorpromazine on acoustically evoked potentials in the rat. *Neuropharmacology, 9,* 575–586.

Brazier, M. A. B. (1972). *The neurophysiological background of anesthesia.* Springfield, IL: Thomas.

Celesia, G. G., Broughton, R. J., Rasmussen, T. H., & Branch, C. (1968). Auditory evoked responses from the exposed human cortex. *Electroencephalography and Clinical Neurophysiology, 24,* 458–466.

Chiappa, K. H., & Ropper, A. H. (1982a). Evoked potentials in clinical medicine (first of two parts). *The New England Journal of Medicine, 306(19),* 1140–1150.

Chiappa, K. H., & Ropper, A. H. (1982b). Evoked potentials in clinical medicine. *The New England Journal of Medicine, 306(20),* 1205–1210.

Davis, H., Mast, T., Yoshie, N., & Zerlin, S. (1966). The slow response of the human cortex to auditory stimuli: Recovery process. *Electroencephalography and Clinical Neurophysiology, 21,* 105–113.

Duncan, P. G., Sanders, R. A., & McCullough, D. W. (1979). Preservation of auditory-evoked brainstem responses in anaesthetized children. *Canadian Anaesthesiology Society Journal, 26(6),* 492–495.

Gage, P. W., & Hamill, O. P. (1981). Effects of anesthetics on ion channels in synapses. In R. Porter (Ed.), *International review of physiology Vol. 25—Neurophysiology IV.* Baltimore: University Park Press.

Green, J. B., Walcoff, M., & Lucke, J. F. (1982). Phenytoin prolongs far-field somatosensory and auditory evoked potential interpeak latencies. *Neurology, 32,* 85–88.

Grundy, B. L. (1983). Intraoperative monitoring of sensory-evoked potentials. *Anesthesiology, 58,* 72–87.

Grundy, B. L., Jannetta, P. J., Procopio, P. T., Lina, A., Boston, R., & Doyle, E. (1982). Intraoperative monitoring of brain-stem auditory evoked potentials. *Journal of Neurosurgery, 57,* 674–681.

Grundy, B. L., Lina, A., Procopio, P. T., & Jannetta, P. J. (1981). Reversible evoked potential changes with retraction of the eighth cranial nerve. *Anesthesia and Analgesia, 60,* 835–838.

Grundy, B. L., Procopio, P. T., Jannetta, P. J., Lina, A., & Doyle, E. (1982). Evoked potential changes produced by positioning for retromastoid craniectomy. *Neurosurgery, 10,(1),* 766–770.

Harker, L. A., Hosick, E., Voots, R. J., & Mendel, M. I. (1977). Influence of succinylcholine on middle-component auditory evoked potentials. *Archives of Otolaryngology, 103,* 133–137.

Heath, R. G., & Galbraith, G. C. (1966). Sensory evoked responses recorded simultaneously from human cortex and scalp. *Nature, (London), 212,* 1535–1537.

Javel, E., Mouney, D. F., McGee, J., & Walsh, E. J. (1982). Auditory brainstem responses during systemic infusion of lidocaine. *Archives of Otolaryngology, 108,* 71–76.

Kaga, K., Takiguchi, T., Myokai, K., & Shiode, A. (1979). Effects of deep hypothermia and circulatory arrest on the auditory brain stem responses. *Archives of Otology, Rhinology, & Laryngology, 225,* 199–205.

Kiang, N. Y. S., Neame, J. H., & Clark, L. F. (1961). Evoked cortical activity from auditory cortex in anesthetized and unanesthetized cats. *Science, 13,* 1927–1928.

Kileny, P., Dobson, D., & Gelfand, E. T. (1983). Middle-latency auditory evoked responses during open-heart surgery with hypothermia. *Electroencephalography and Clinical Neurophysiology, 55,* 268–276.

Kileny, P., Ryu, J. H., McCabe, B. F., & Abbas, P. J. (1980). Neuronal habituation in the vestibular nuclei of the cat. *Acta Otolaryngology, 90,* 175–183.

Klee, M. R., Pierau, F. K., & Faber, D. S. (1974). Temperature effects on resting potential and spike parameters of cat motoneurons. *Experimental Brain Research, 19,* 789–792.

Koblin, D. D., & Eger, E. (1981). How anesthetics work. In R. A. Miller (Ed.), *Anesthesia* (2 vols.). New York: Churchill Livingstone.

Konishi, T. (1979). Some observations on negative endocochlear potential during anoxia. *Acta Otolaryngology, 87,* 506–516.

Kraft, H. (1972). Effects of temperature and age on nerve conduction velocity in the guinea pig. *Archives of Physical Medicine and Rehabilitation, 53,* 328–332.

Kraus, N. Ozdamar, O., Hier, D., & Stein, L. (1982). Auditory middle latency response (MLRs) in patients with cortical lesions. *Electroencephalography and Clinical Neurophysiology, 54,* 275–287.

Lader, M., & Norris, H. (1969). The effects of nitrous oxide on the human auditory evoked response. *Psychopharmacologia (Berlin), 16,* 115–127.

Levine, R. A. (1979). Monitoring auditory evoked potentials during acoustic neuroma surgery. In H. Silverstein and H. Norell (Eds.), *Neurological surgery of the ear, Vol. II (pp. 287–293).*Birmingham: Aesculapius.

Møller, A. R., & Jannetta, P. J. (1982). Evoked potentials from the inferior colliculus in man. *Electroencephalography and Clinical Neurophysiology, 53,* 612–620.

Møller, A. R., Jannetta, P. J., Bennett, M., & Møller, M. B. (1981). Intracranially recorded responses from human auditory nerve: New insights into the origin of brain stem evoked potentials (BSEPs). *Electroencephalography and Clinical Neurophysiology, 52,* 18–27.

Mori, K., Winters, W. D., & Spooner, C. E. (1968). Comparison of reticular and cochlear multiple unit activity with auditory evoked responses during various stages induced by anesthetic agents. II. *Electroencephalography and Clinical Neurophysiology, 24,* 242–248.

Moruzzi, G., & Magoun, H. W. (1949). Brain stem reticular formation and activation of the EEG. *Electroencephalography and Clinical Neurophysiology, 1,* 455–473.

Picton, T. W., Hillyard, S. A., & Galambos, R. (1976). Habituation and attention in the auditory system. In W. D. Keidel & W. D. Neff (Eds.), *Handbook of sensory physiology* (Vol. 5, No.3). New York: Springer-Verlag.

Picton, T. W., Hillyard, S. A., Kraus, H. I., & Galambos, R. (1974). Human auditory evoked potentials. I: Evaluation of components. *Electroencephalography and Clinical Neurophysiology, 36,* 179–190.

Pradhan, S. N., & Galambos, R. (1963). Some effects of anesthetics on the evoked responses in the auditory cortex of cats. *Journal of Pharmacology and Experimental Therapy, 139,* 97–106.

Puletti, F., & Celesia, G. G. (1970). Functional properties of primary cortical auditory area in man. *Journal of Neurosurgery, 32,* 244–247.

Reilly, E. L., Kondo, C., Brunberg, J. A., & Doty, D. B. (1978). Visual evoked potentials during hypothermia and prolonged circulatory arrest. *Electroencephalography and Clinical Neurophysiology, 45,* 100–106.

Shea, J. J., & Harell, M. (1978). Management of tinnitus aurium with lidocaine and carbamazepine. *Laryngoscope, 88,* 1477–1484.

Sohmer, H., Gafni, M., & Chisin, R. (1982). Auditory nerve–brain stem potentials in man and cat under hypoxic and hypercapnic condition. *Electroencephalography and Clinical Neurophysiology, 53,* 506–512.

Stockard, J., & Sharbrough, F. W. (1980). Unique contributions of short-latency auditory and somatosensory evoked potentials to neurologic diagnosis. *Progress in Clinical Neurophysiology, 7,* 231–263.

Stockard, J. J., Sharbrough, F. W., & Tinker, J. A. (1978a). Effects of hypothermia on the human brainstem auditory response. *Annals of Neurology, 3,* 368–370.

Stockard, J. J., Stockard, J. E., & Sharbrough, F. W. (1978b). Nonpathologic factors influencing brain-stem auditory evoked potentials. *American Journal of EEG Technology, 18,* 177–209.

Tasaki, I., & Spiropoulos, C. S. (1959). Stria vascularis as a source of endocochlear potential. *Journal of Neurophysiology, 22,* 149–155.

Weight, F., & Erulkar, S. D. (1976). Synaptic transmission and effects of temperature at the squid giant synapse. *Nature (London), 261,* 720–722.

Wolin, L. R., Massopust, L. C., & Meder, R. N. (1964). Electroretinogram and cortical evoked potentials under hypothermia. *Archives of Opthalmology, 72,* 521–524.

Chapter 14

Monitoring Neurologic Status of Comatose Patients in the Intensive Care Unit

James W. Hall III
Judy Mackey-Hargadine
Steven J. Allen

There is an important need for a clinical method of objectively monitoring neurologic status in patients comatose as a result of severe brain injury. Ideally, the method must meet at least 10 criteria for clinical utility and feasibility: (1) Noninvasiveness. Measurement does not require repeated insertion and/or long-term maintenance of needles or catheters. (2) Safety. Measurement poses no risk or harm to the patient. (3) Mobility. Assessment can be carried out at bedside in an intensive care unit (ICU) environment. (4) Brief test time. Assessments require little time, preferably less than 1 hour and, therefore, do not disrupt ongoing patient intensive care. (5) Objectivity. Test results can be quantified and subjected to mathematical and/or statistical analysis. (6) Reliability. Results are invariant in patients who are neurologically normal or stable, and reliably obtained in all patients. (7) Sensitive and comprehensive index of neurologic status. Method yields information on multiple levels of the central nervous system (CNS) and is sensitive to changes, even subtle ones, in neurologic function. (8) Independence of level of consciousness. Results are not affected by degree of coma. (9) Resistance to drugs. Results are not influenced by commonly used medical therapies in severe brain-injured patients, including chemical paralyzing agents, sedatives, and barbiturates. (10) Cost effectiveness. Modest charge is essential for routine and repeated measurement in intensive care monitoring of a comatose patient.

The auditory brainstem response (ABR), in our experience, meets these criteria and has multiple applications in monitoring neurologic function of comatose patients in the ICU. In this chapter, we first introduce the general concept of monitoring acute, severely brain-injured patients, and present an overview of electrophysiologic procedures applied in comatose patients. Next, we review factors influencing ABR measurements in the ICU, particularly characteristics of the comatose patient and his medical therapy, and possible environmental contaminants. Then, we present original group data and case reports to document the clinical applications of the ABR in monitoring neurologic status of the comatose patient. In the final section, future directions for ABR exploitation in the ICU are suggested.

MONITORING THE PATIENT WITH CEREBRAL FAILURE

Rationale

A patient with central nervous system disease severe enough to result in decreased level of consciousness only occasionally has a process that can be reversed completely with surgery. Often, the process of recovery requires a period of time during which the injured CNS will be more susceptible to further injury. Therefore, it behooves the clinician to develop an environment in which the CNS is protected from additional insult. We can empirically institute a form of therapy based on reasoning or prior experience. However, we must have a way of evaluating how any particular patient is responding to therapy. Monitoring plays a role in the care of any patient but its role is crucial in the care of patients with CNS pathology.

Basic Monitoring

The basic monitor is the physical exam including vital signs. Therefore, whether a patient has a closed head injury or an ear infection, acceptable blood pressure, pulse, and respiratory rate are necessary for the well-being of that patient. For this reason, all patients requiring ICU placement for their intracranial pathology have their blood pressure, pulse, respiratory rate, and temperature monitored frequently, usually every 1 to 2 hours. Another monitor of the patient with cerebral failure is the neurologic exam. Obviously, deviation from the norm of the results of this exam has profound implications for the care and possibly the outcome of these patients. The development of new abnormal responses, such as extensor posturing to noxious stimuli, implies the progression of intracerebral disease and demands immediate action.

Intracranial Pressure (ICP) Monitoring

Beyond monitors that require only a trained observer and some simple equipment, there stretches an ever-enlarging array of highly technical devices of varying degrees of invasiveness, including pulmonary and nutritional monitoring and intracranial pressure monitoring. ICP monitoring is particularly important in the brain-injured, comatose patient.

A frequent injury response of cerebral tissue is swelling, much as with any injured tissue in the body. Swelling is a serious problem for the brain, since it is essentially enclosed by a hard, bony skull. The increase in volume of any intracranial component can adversely affect the rest of the brain by compressing the blood supply. This increase in volume is associated by a rise in ICP, which can be measured continuously by means of an ICP monitor. The most common ICP monitors are ventriculostomies and subarachnoid bolts. These monitors are placed by the neurosurgeon and are connected to a transducer and CRT. Normal ICP is below 15 mm Hg. ICP above 20 to 29 mm Hg has been shown to be correlated to poor outcome in head injuries (Miller, Becker, Ward, Sullivan, Adams, & Rosner, 1977; Saul & Ducker, 1982). The management of elevated ICP has been a major advance in the care of neurosurgical patients.

Several modalities have been used to control elevated ICP. Hyperventilation has been shown to be efficacious in the treatment of some patients with closed head injuries (Gordon, 1971). Hyperventilation decreases cerebral blood flow and, therefore, cerebral blood volume. However, decreasing cerebral blood flow to an injured brain may not always be to every patient's advantage. Another way to reduce the volume inside the cranium is to remove cerebral spinal fluid. This can be done relatively safely if a *ventriculostomy* has been placed for intracranial pressure monitoring. *Steroids* have been quite successful in treating the edema associated with cerebral tumors. Their use in closed head injuries has not been as valuable and, indeed, their efficacy is open to question (Braakman, Schouten, Blaauw-van Dishoeck, & Minderhoud, 1983).

Another therapeutic maneuver that is often successful in reducing intracranial volume and therefore ICP is the use of *diuretics*. Hyperosmolar agents were first used about 60 years ago (Fay, 1923). Today, a hyperosmolar solution of *mannitol* is the most widely administered drug (Marshall, Smith, Rauscher, & Shapiro, 1978). Finally, *barbiturate coma* has been reported to be of significance in the treatment of raised ICP in patients with closed head injuries (Marshall, Smith, & Shapiro, 1979). Barbiturate coma is no small undertaking, as it is essentially an around-the-clock anesthetic. It has been associated with hypothermia and cardiovascular instability, often necessitating invasive cardiovascular monitoring. Since the patient is in a drug-induced coma, the neurologic exam is no longer reliable. Cortical electrical silence is an endpoint of barbiturate coma. This results in a clinical neurologic picture of a patient who does not respond to painful stimuli, who has no posturing, who is not breathing spontaneously, and whose brainstem reflexes are absent except for pupillary response to light in most cases. This seriously limits the clinician's ability to evaluate the effect of therapy on the CNS. The efficacy of barbiturate coma. This results in a clinical neurologic picture of a patient who does not respond injury and factors in outcome see Bruce, Gennarelli, & Langfitt, 1978; Gennarelli, Speilman, Langfitt, et al., 1982; Jennett & Teasdale, 1981).

In summary, pulmonary, cardiovascular, and nutritional system functions, and ICP, are routinely monitored in comatose, brain-injured patients in the ICU. A monitor of neural function is lacking. An adequate cardiac output and excellent cerebral oxygenation are reassuring, but do not directly reflect brain function. Although ICP below 20 mm Hg is considered beneficial, a substantial portion of comatose patients with severe brain injury do not have elevated ICP. Thus, there exists an extremely important need for a clinically feasible monitor of neuronal integrity, particularly, a method that is sensitive to subtle changes in neural function, yet resistant to the influences of treatment modalities, such as barbiturates and chemical paralyzing agents.

ELECTROPHYSIOLOGIC CNS ASSESSMENT

In recent years, a growing number of investigators have reported experiences with electrophysiologic evaluations of neurologic function in comatose patients in the ICU setting. Some have related the pattern of sensory evoked potential outcome with clinical neurologic findings, level of coma, and site of lesion (Britt, Herrick, Mason, & Dorfman, 1980; Greenberg, Becker, Miller, et al., 1977; Greenberg, Stablein, & Becker, 1981b; Hari, Sulkava, & Haltia, 1982; Karnaze, Marshall, McCarthy, Klauber, Bickford, 1982; Klug, 1982; Lütschg, Pfenninger Ludin, & Fassela, 1983; Mjoen, Nordby, & Torvik, 1983; Starr & Hamilton, 1976; Tsubokawa, Nichimoto, Yamamoto, et al., 1980; Uziel & Benezech, 1978; Van Nechel, Deltemre, Strul, & Capon, 1982). The electrophysiologic procedures applied in comatose patients include auditory evoked potentials (Brewer & Resneck, 1982; Hall, Huangfu, & Gennarelli, 1982; Hall, Huangfu, Gennarelli, Dolinskas, Olson, & Berry, 1983; Hall, Morgan, Mackey-Hargadine, Aguilar, & Jahrsdoerfer, 1984; McKay, Hosobuchi, Williston, & Jewett, 1980; Mjoen et al., 1983; Nagao, Sumani, Tsutsui, et al., 1982; Sanders, Smriga, mcCullough, & Duncan, 1981; Seales, Rossiter, & Weinstein, 1979; Tsubokawa et al., 1980; Uziel, Benezech, Loranzo, Monstrey, Duboin, & Roquefeuil, 1982; Walter & Blegvad, 1981), somatosensory evoked potentials (de la Torre, Trimble, Beard, et al., 1978; Greenberg, Newlon, & Becker, 1982; Hume, Cant, & Shaw, 1979), visual evoked potentials (Feinsod & Averback, 1973; Walter & Arfel, 1972; York, Pulliam, Rosenfeld, & Watts, 1981), a battery of multimodality (auditory, somatosensory, and visual) evoked potentials (Greenberg & Becker, 1976; Greenberg et al., 1977; Greenberg, Stablein, & Becker, 1981b; Lindsey,

Carlin, Kennedy, et al., 1981; Lütschg et al., 1983; Narayan, Greenberg, Miller, et al., 1981; Newlon, Greenberg, Hyatt, Enas, & Becker, 1982; Rappaport, Hall, Hopkins, et al., 1977), corneal (blink) reflex assessment (Ongerboer, 1981; Serrats, Parker, & Merino-Canas, 1976; Van Nechel et al., 1982) and electroencephalography, EEG, (Alving, Møller, Sindrup, & Nielsen, 1979; Eng, Dong, Bledsoe, Heavner, Shaw, & Hornbei, 1979; Grossman, 1979; Hari et al., 1982; Westmoreland, Klass, Sharbrough, & Regan, 1975).

The objective of most of these studies was to describe the relationship between electrophysiologic findings and short- and/or long-term neurologic outcome. Indeed, some of the procedures, such as the multimodality evoked potential (MEP) battery, appear to be more powerful prognostic indicators than the neurologic examination (including motor responses, pupillary response, brainstem reflexes, and the Glasgow Coma Scale), computerized tomography (CT), or standard physiologic parameters measured in the ICU, such as ICP. Narayan et al., (1981), for example, found that by evaluating MEPs according to a four-category grading system, it was possible to predict patient outcome at 1 year following severe head injury with 91% accuracy. Furthermore, there were no "false-pessimistic" errors with the MEP battery. That is, none of their 133 patients with predicted poor outcome actually recovered. The prognostic accuracy of the MEP battery compared favorably with the Glasgow Coma Scale (80%), CT (64%), and ICP (75%).

Almost without exception, however, electrophysiologic assessments in acute head-injured patients have been carried out on only one occasion. The few studies of longitudinal electrophysiologic assessments usually began with an initial test in the acute stage following brain injury (the first week), and then follow-up measurements were made months or even a year or more later. The extensive prognostic data reported by Greenberg and colleagues (1977, 1981a, 1982), for example, were collected an average of 3.8 days post-injury. Electrophysiologic measurements have rarely been made within the extremely important 24- to 48-hour post-injury period, and there are no reports of intensive serial monitoring of neurologic status in comatose patients within the first post-injury week.

Among the electrophysiologic procedures, the somatosensory (SSEPs) and auditory evoked potentials (AEPs) have been applied with greatest regularity in comatose patients. These two modalities offer clinical advantages not shared by visual evoked potentials or the standard EEG. The SSEPs and AEPs have peripheral, brainstem, and cortical neuroanatomic components, are relatively easy to interpret (compared to the EEG, for example), and can be reliably recorded in an ICU setting from patients that are deeply comatose (with eyes closed), and often sedated, or under the influence of intoxicants or therapeutic CNS suppressants.

FACTORS INFLUENCING ABR MEASUREMENTS IN THE ICU

The ABR is influenced by myriad factors, including subject characteristics (age, sex, auditory status, body temperature), stimulus parameters (e.g., intensity, frequency, duration, rate), recording parameters (electrode array, neural filtering), and drugs. The effects of these and other factors have recently been summarized (Hall, 1983) and are not described here. However, the five main factors of particular concern with the comatose patient in the ICU environment are the degree of coma, patient characteristics, environmental contaminants, otologic pathology, and therapeutic drugs.

Coma

A commonly used clinical grading system for severity of brain injury is the Glasgow Coma Scale (GCS), shown in Figure 14-1. The GCS, developed by Jennett and colleagues in 1974 (see

FIGURE 14–1.
Glasgow Coma Scale, GCS (Jennett & Teasdale, 1981). A GCS of 8 or less defines severe brain injury and comatose state. See text for detailed description.

Glasgow Coma Scale

Eye Opening	Spontaneous	4	Total Glasgow Coma Scale Points
	To Voice	3	
	To Pain	2	14-15=**5**
	None	1	11-13=**4**
Verbal Response	Oriented	5	8-10=**3**
	Confused	4	5- 7=**2**
	Inappropriate Words	3	3- 4=**1**
	Incomprehensible Words	2	
	None	1	
Motor Response	Obeys Command	6	
	Localizes Pain	5	
	Withdraw (pain)	4	
	Flexion (pain)	3	
	Extension (pain)	2	
	None	1	
Total Trauma Score			**1-16**

Jennett & Teasdale, 1981), is based on the evaluation of eye opening, verbal, and motor responses to sensory stimulation. Patients with the highest possible score (15) are grossly intact neurologically, whereas patients with the lowest score (3) are totally unresponsive to even painful stimulation. The accepted criterion for severe brain injury is a GCS of 8 or less. Patients with severe brain injury are, therefore, comatose, and typically do not open their eyes, do not vocalize (most are intubated for mechanical ventilation), and have only abnormal (posturing) motor responses to painful stimulation. For detailed description of the pathophysiology of coma, the reader is referred to Plum and Posner (1980).

The ABR is not influenced by degree of coma in patients without primary or secondary brainstem injuries. As illustrated in Table 14-1, a completely normal ABR may be recorded in patients with GCSs as low as 3. Indeed, in our series of 200 severely head-injured patients, over 70% initially show a normal ABR. Abnormal ABRs are, of course, commonly recorded in patients with GCS of 3 to 4, probably because this group is more likely to have structural

TABLE 14–1.
Relationship between Glasgow Coma Score (see Figure 14–1) and initial auditory brainstem response (ABR) outcome in 83 comatose, brain-injured patients.

Glasgow Coma Score	No response[b]	Auditory brainstem response[a]			Normal
		Abnormal			
		Missing wave component	Latency prolongation		
9–10					3
7–8					15
5–6		1	2		27
3–4	14	1	3		15

NOTE. ABR data were obtained within 48 hours post-injury.

[a] ABR symmetry was observed in 62 (75%) of the patients. With asymmetrical findings, data from the better side were tabulated.

[b] Wave I only (62% of category) or no response (38% of the category).

brainstem damage, or brainstem dysfunction secondary to massive cerebral swelling. Among the patients with GCSs of 3 are those meeting criteria for brain death. ABR patterns in brain death are discussed in a following section. It is important, however, to bear in mind that a GCS of 3 does *not* imply irreversible brain damage and eminent death or a poor neurologic outcome.

Patient Characteristics

Body temperature. The body temperature must be routinely taken into account in the interpretation of ABR findings in comatose patients. The influence of body temperature on latency of the ABR is well documented (Marsh, Yamane, & Potsic, 1984; Marshall & Donchin, 1981; Stockard, Sharbrough, & Tinker, 1978; Stockard, Stockard, & Sharbrough, 1978), and appears to be greater for later-latency ABR components. Comatose patients, especially those in barbiturate-induced coma, tend to have lower-than-normal body temperatures, and may, for this reason, show increased ABR latencies. Body temperature is usually monitored continuously in ICU patients, and the digitally displayed value should be recorded at the start of the evaluation and periodically checked throughout testing (see ABR data record sheet, Figure 14-2). If body temperature monitors are not available, current data can usually be obtained from ICU patient flow sheets or requested of nursing personnel. Body temperature documentation is extremely important in the interpretation of subtle changes in serially recorded ABR data.

Alcohol. Blood alcohol levels are often excessive upon hospital admission in traumatically head-injured patients. Alcohol abuse is frequently an important factor in motor vehicle accidents and accidental falls. In normothermic patients, alcohol probably does not seriously affect the ABR (Squires, Chu, & Starr, 1978), although chronic alcohol abuse may have an effect (Chu, Squires, & Starr, 1978; Rosenhamer & Silverskiold, 1980). The possible influence of blood alcohol must be considered, however, in the interpretation of auditory middle-latency response (MLR) findings in the acutely injured.

Neuromuscular state. The neuromuscular status varies in the comatose patient. Patients in deep coma, with Glasgow Coma Scores of 8 or less (see Figure 14-1), rarely move spontaneously or to light touch or acoustic stimulation. Some are flaccid. Following severe brain injury, the patient is intubated and placed on mechanical ventilation. Chemical muscle paralyzing agents (such as Metacurine or Pavulon) are frequently administered during this period (see Figure 14-2). For these reasons, muscle artifact is an infrequent problem in ABR measurement in the acute phase after severe brain injury. In less severely injured patients, or those recovering neurologically, ABR recordings can be seriously contaminated by excessive muscle movement. Decorticate or decerebrate posturing, torsion of neck musculature, or a generally agitated, highly active state can all introduce an unacceptable amount of artifact. The best solution to this artifact problem is induced patient relaxation during testing by means of a sedative. Haldol or morphine, for example, is commonly used in the ICU and can usually be administered as needed or immediately prior to evoked response assessment in the neuromuscularly active patient. Sedatives do not, it appears, influence the ABR. They may, however, alter the MLR. This is particularly troublesome as movement artifact often precludes the recording of these later-latency responses. Furthermore, the postauricular muscle (PAM) artifact, in our experience, appears to be more common in muscularly active or tense patients. Muscle paralyzing agents, when medically appropriate, reduce the influence of muscle contamination, including the PAM reflex, without complicating MLR interpretation (Kileny, 1983). If sedatives or chemical paralyzing agents cannot be used, or are not effective, the deleterious influence of muscle artifact on the response can sometimes be reduced by more restricted high-pass neural filtering, for example, changing the

FIGURE 14-2.
Example of auditory brainstem response (ABR) data record sheet used with comatose patients. Note that time of assessment, physiologic patient data, and medical therapies are carefully documented.

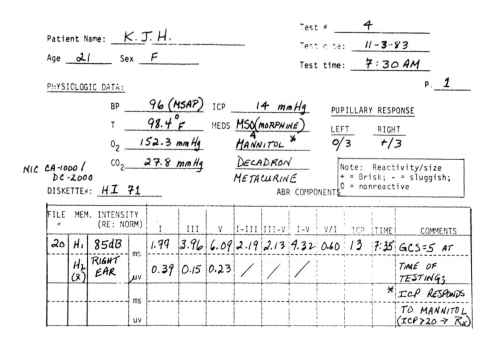

filter setting from 30 to 150, or even 300 to 3000 Hz. It is important to remember, however, that neural filtering will also alter amplitude and latency characteristics of the ABR (Boston & Ainslie, 1980; Laukli & Mair, 1981). Of course, use of artifact rejection features and increasing the number of averages will contribute to signal enhancement and noise reduction.

Environmental Contaminants

The ICU is potentially a hostile environment for evoked response measurement. Nonetheless, we have successfully recorded auditory brainstem, middle-latency, and 40-Hz responses from over 200 comatose patients in a busy ICU (a total of over 500 separate test sessions). In the majority of cases, the test environment was quite acceptable, and comparable to patient rooms or our audiology facility. The key factors for successful ABR measurement in an ICU are quality instrumentation and a flexible test protocol. Airborne *electromagnetic interference* and *60-Hz line noise* are not uncommon in an ICU. There are numerous sources of electrical artifact close to the patient, including fluorescent light, mechanical ventilators, monitoring devices, and thermal blankets. Also, other sources of electrical interference may be located adjacent to, or above or below the ICU, or share power lines with the ICU. We take the following precautions to reduce the deleterious influence of electrical artifact. In addition to using a high-frequency and well-grounded evoked response system (Nicolet CA-1000/DC-2000), we rely on quality, gold cup electrodes (Grass). Before electrode placement with adhering paste and surgical tape, we vigorously prepare the skin with a liquid abrasive (Omni prep). Electrode impedance, including the ground lead, is less than 3000 ohms. A good ground electrode contact is probably the single most important factor in successful evoked response measurement of ICU patients. Earclip electrodes are preferable to mastoid-placed cup electrodes, both in ease and consistency in placement and also for an approximately 30% amplitude-enhancement of the wave I component. Rather than a vertex electrode, we routinely employ a high-forehead positive-voltage electrode. This placement offers two advantages. First, many ICU brain-injured patients have head dressings and/or ICP monitoring devices in the vertex region. Consequently, intra- or interpatient consistency in vertex placement is not possible. Second, electrode contact tends to be better on the smooth, hairless forehead surface. Our normative ABR data were obtained with a high-forehead placement of the vertex-positive electrode, and with earclip electrodes.

In spite of the precautions in electrode type and placement, 60-Hz "hum" and high-frequency "snow" may still be present in evoked response measurement. Therefore, we attempt to locate a power outlet that is not being used for other equipment, perhaps at a nearby empty bed. We also choose stimulus rates that are not evenly divisible into 60 Hz (i.e., 21.1/s for the ABR, 11.1/s for the MLR, and 39.7/s for the 40-Hz response), and average the ABR for at least 2000 repetitions of the stimulus. Routine use of alternating-polarity click stimuli will generally eliminate the stimulus artifact commonly encountered with single polarity stimuli at high intensity levels. Finally, as a last resort, we will set the bandpass neural filter settings to 150 or 300 to 3000 Hz, if 60-Hz artifact is a problem, or 30 to 1500 Hz if high-frequency noise is contaminating measurement. This, in combination with digitally smoothing and adding acquired, replicated, averaged waveforms, generally yields a valid and interpretable ABR. If all of these measures fail to adequately reduce the artifact problems, we recommend returning to the bedside later in the day or, preferably, in the evening for a second attempted measurement.

Otologic Pathology

Peripheral auditory abnormalities are not uncommon following traumatic brain injury (Grove, 1947; Hall et al., 1982; Schuknecht, 1950; Toglia & Katinsky, 1976). Our clinical experience confirms the high incidence of otologic pathology and immittance abnormalities in severe head-injury (Aguilar, Hall, & Mackey-Hargadine, 1983; Hall et al., 1982). For example, two-thirds of a series of 50 severely head-injured patients in our ICU had one or more clinically significant otologic abnormalities. Hemotympanum was the most common (30%) single finding. Yet, a normal ABR was recorded in some patients with distinct otologic pathology, including radiologically confirmed temporal bone fractures (Aguilar et al., 1983). We routinely request otologic consultation for patients with ABR evidence of peripheral auditory dysfunction (e.g., grossly reduced amplitude and prolonged absolute latency of component I), but prior evidence of otologic pathology, even CSF or blood drainage from the ear, does not preclude the successful measurement of clinically valuable ABR data.

In most cases, ABR assessment of our ICU patients is carried out for evaluation of CNS status, rather than peripheral auditory function. Therefore, we typically complete the assessment with high-intensity stimuli (75 to 95 dB re: normal click threshold), and rarely seek ABR threshold. Circumaural earphone cushions are used to reduce the likelihood of collapsing ear canal walls. In patients with excessive head dressings, or neck collars, which partially cover the ear, we use a miniature insert transducer (wide-frequency response hearing and receiver). Normative data for stimulus intensity levels and ABR response parameters with this special earphone must be acquired.

Patients with evidence of middle ear pathology by otologic examination or air-conduction ABR stimuli are assessed by bone-conduction ABR (see chapters 6 and 7), mainly in an attempt to observe wave components I, III, and V, and therefore define brainstem function.

FIGURE 14–3.
Simultaneous four-channel auditory brainstem response (ABR) recordings 12 hours post-injury for a deeply comatose patient with severe closed head injury (GCS = 5). ABR and patient data are documented in Figure 14–2. See text for explanation.

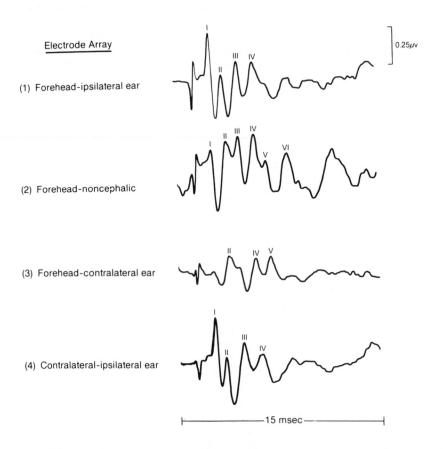

We routinely make simultaneous four-channel ABR recordings in all patients who do not yield well-defined and reliable wave components I, III, and V at standard stimulus intensity levels (75 to 95 dB). Experience with this recording technique from over 200 comatose, head-injured patients has confirmed its clinical value. An example of the ABR waveforms for the four-channel recordings is shown in Figure 14-3. Electrodes are placed on the high forehead (at the hair line), each earlobe, and a noncephalic site (thorax or shoulder). This technique was recently described elsewhere (Hall et al., 1984). The noncephalic and contralateral (to the stimulus) ear arrays tend to enhance resolution of waves IV versus V. We have observed, in selected cases, a reliable wave V with the noncephalic array, yet not with the traditional forehead-ipsilateral array. The horizontal (contralateral-to-ipsilateral earlobe) array augments the early ABR waves (I, II and III) in some patients.

Therapeutic Drugs

The commonly used drugs in comatose ICU patients that act on the nervous system are chemical paralyzers, sedatives, anticonvulsants, and barbiturates. As noted earlier, chemical paralyzing agents do not adversely effect ABR measurement, and actually eliminate bothersome muscle artifact. Likewise, latency of the ABR does not, in our experience, appear to be influenced by sedatives (e.g., Haldol, morphine), or therapeutic doses of anticonvulsants (e.g., Dilantin).

The possible influence of high-dose barbiturates on the ABR has been studied experimentally (Bobbin, May, & Lemoine, 1979; Cohen & Britt, 1981; Sutton, Frewen, Marsh, Jaggi, & Bruce, 1982) but has not been systematically investigated in comatose, brain-injured patients. We have analyzed ABR latency and amplitude for 50 head-injured patients in deep barbiturate coma, and have recorded a well-formed, reliable response in patients with barbiturate blood levels as high as 200 μg/ml. A detailed discussion of the effect of pharmacologic agents on AEPs is found in the preceding chapter (13). A brief case report is presented to illustrate our clinical experiences.

Case study: Barbiturate coma. A 17-year-old male was involved in a motor vehicle accident (MVA) at 2 AM. He was the driver and only person in an automobile and was thrown from the vehicle when it rolled over. There was immediate loss of consciousness. Neurologic examination revealed pinpoint and nonreactive pupils, decerebrate motor response, and an intact corneal reflex. There was no gag reflex and no spontaneous respiration. The patient was treated at the scene with mannitol and Decadron and then transported by helicopter to the Hermann Hospital with a severe closed head injury. Glasgow Coma Score was 6 at the time of admission. Emergency computerized tomography at 4 AM showed multiple scattered hemorrhagic contusions, including a large contusion in the left basal ganglia and smaller contusions in the anterior thalamus, evidence of intraventricular hemorrhage, diffuse cerebral edema with partial effacement of the ventricles and the basal cisterns, and minimal shift of midline structures from left to right. On the second post-injury day, the patient's ICP became elevated (greater than 20 mm Hg). High-dose barbiturate therapy was initiated and was effective in controlling ICP. Repeat CT scans (post-injury Days 3, 12, 17) showed little change. The patient had a moderate neurologic disability at 1 year post-injury.

Serial auditory evoked response assessment was carried out at bedside in the ICU, beginning at 8 AM on the day of the accident (6 hours post-injury). At that time, an otologic examination showed Battle's sign on the right but was otherwise normal. ABR findings for left ear stimulation are illustrated in Figures 14-4 and 14-5. All assessments yielded a symmetrical ABR. The patient was always normothermic (37.9 to 39.5 °C). We repeatedly observed a well-formed ABR with absolute and interwave latency values within normal limits (Figure 14-4), even within the initial 5 days post-injury when CT suggested compression of the basal and perimesencephalic cisterns. ABR latency was not significantly influenced by barbiturates. Before, during, and after barbiturate coma, wave I–V latency values were within ± 0.20 ms and showed no consistent trends. Two major changes in the ABR were noted, however. Amplitude of the wave I component was greatly enhanced in barbiturate coma. Before and after barbiturates, wave I amplitude was less than 0.40 μV, but during barbiturate administration it ranged from 60 to 78 μV, and was grossly abnormal by our clinical standards. Also, there appeared to be suppression of ABR wave components following wave V (perhaps VI and VII) during deep barbiturate coma.

The MLR, in contrast, was profoundly influenced by barbiturates. On the initial assessment, a *Pa* component of prolonged latency and reduced amplitude was reliably observed. By Day 2, there was a distinct bipeaked *Pa* component. However, in barbiturate coma, a *Pa* component was not recorded. The positive-voltage deflection on Days 4 through 11 is most likely a filter-related artifact (see Kileny, 1983), and was not observed with an extended filter setting (5–1500 Hz vs. 30–100 Hz). On Day 12, with a low barbiturate blood level (3 μg/ml), the MLR emerged.

FIGURE 14–4.

Serial auditory brainstem response (ABR) recordings for a severely head-injured patient before, during, and after barbiturate-induced coma. Note stability of latencies and enhancement of wave I amplitude with high barbiturate blood levels.

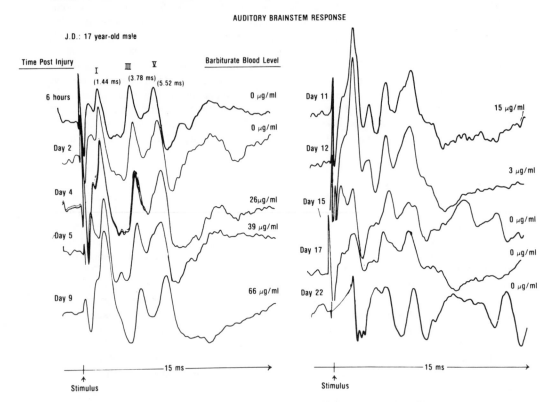

Unexpectedly, there was an abnormally large Pa component on the first day after complete clearance from barbiturates. The patient was chemically paralyzed, reducing the likelihood of a myogenic artifact. Over the next week, a well-formed MLR became apparent.

In our experience, the ABR is extremely resistant to the effects of high-dose barbiturates. Clinically significant changes in the ABR during barbiturate coma, then, may be attributed to neurologic improvement or deterioration. The MLR, in contrast, appears to be suppressed by even low levels of barbiturates (less than 10 $\mu g/ml$), and, therefore, appears to have little value as a monitoring device in barbiturate coma.

MONITORING NEUROLOGIC STATUS WITH THE ABR

Applications of the ABR in comatose patients are varied. In Table 14-2, we show the reasons for ABR assessment/monitoring as indicated by the attending physicians responsible for the care of brain-injured patients in our ICU. Some patients were assessed by the ABR for more than one reason. For example, ABRs were often requested for patients with CT evidence of impending serious neurologic deterioration (e.g., apparent compression of perimesencephalic cisterns and rostral brainstem), particularly when their medical therapy included paralysis or

FIGURE 14–5.
Serial auditory middle-latency response (MLR) recordings for a severely head-injured patient (ABR in Figure 14-4) before, during, and after barbiturate-induced coma. Note suppression of *Pa* component in barbiturate coma.

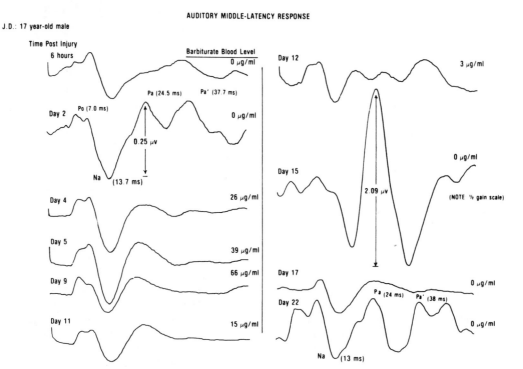

barbiturates. As noted earlier, these drugs render the clinical neurologic examination invalid. Unfortunately, a proportion of patients monitored during neurologic deterioration ultimately underwent ABRs in the determination of brain death. Within these categories, information on CNS function obtained from ABR measurement contributed to medical management of patients. In some cases, patients with GCSs of 3 or 4 at hospital admission, a normal initial ABR within 2 hours post-injury argued for aggressive intensive care and, on occasion, surgical intervention. In fact, as shown in Table 14-1, almost one-half of the patients with GCSs of 3 or 4 had normal ABRs when assessed within 48 hours post-injury. In others, an early finding of gross ABR abnormalities, coupled with supplemental clinical evidence of extensive neurologic dysfunction, lead to the decision to provide supportive care management, or to initiate the assessment of candidacy for organ donation. These applications are illustrated with upcoming case presentations.

Our ICU is in a private urban hospital affiliated with a medical school. These institutions house a regional CNS trauma center. Three helicopters are available to transport patients from the scene of an accident or from an outlying hospital. Average elapsed time from lift-off at the scene to patient admission is 30 min. As a result, we have had experience in monitoring comatose patients with very serious and highly varied brain injuries. Characteristics of a series of 87 patients assessed by ABR in an 8-month period are displayed in Table 14-3. All assessments were carried out at bedside in the surgical ICU by the first author (JWH). Most of the patients

TABLE 14–2.
Reasons for Auditory Brainstem Response (ABR) Assessment and Monitoring in Comatose, Brain-injured Patients (N = 200) as Reported by Referring Physicians.

Reason	% of Patients[a]
Neurologic deterioration	66
Chemical paralysis	50
Barbiturate coma	40
Determination of brain death	34
Glasgow coma score of 3 or 4 (excluding brain death)	20
Hypoxic episodes without increased intracranial pressure	10
Unstable intracranial pressure; risk in transport to computerized tomography	8

[a]A patient may be included in more than one category.

were young adults (mean age 30 years). Approximately two-thirds were male. The majority of the patients (58%) were involved in motor vehicle accidents. At the time of ABR testing, 90% of the group had severe brain injury (GCS of 8 or less). Three-fourths of the patients underwent initial ABR measurement within 48 hours post-injury. The remaining 25% were typically assessed by ABR because of delayed neurologic complications, or lack of neurologic improvement (e.g., static GCS) within the first week. With this introduction to the rationale for ABR assessment in comatose patients, and summary of characteristics of a clinical population in an ICU, we present some cases to illustrate our experiences in monitoring CNS status with the ABR. In select patients, ABR findings are compared with MLR and 40-Hz response outcome, as all patients have received this evoked response test battery.

Medical Management and Neurologic Deterioration

Case report. A 30-year-old male stepped from a moving vehicle and was struck by a second vehicle (12 PM, 9/24). He was intoxicated at the time. The patient was transported to Hermann Hospital within 45 min of the accident via helicopter. Neurologic examination yielded a GCS of 3–4, pupils 2 mm and nonreactive bilaterally, negative oculocephalic reflex (doll's eyes), a flicker-type motor response to pain, and positive gag and corneal reflexes. Emergency CT, illustrated in Figure 14-6a and b, indicated left-sided cerebral contusions and edema, and compression of the perimesencephalic cistern. He was taken to the ICU where initial ABR measurement was made within 2 hours post-injury.

Initial assessment showed a normal ABR bilaterally and a small-amplitude but repeatable MLR. Based on this evidence of brainstem integrity by ABR, a medical decision was made to manage the patient aggressively, despite the low GCS (bear in mind that he was intoxicated at hospital admission). He was immediately taken to the OR for placement of an ICP monitor. Results of subsequent serial ABR findings are illustrated in Figure 14-7. Throughout monitoring, the ABR was symmetrical. Only the ABR waveforms for right ear stimulation are depicted. At 18 hours post-injury (6 PM 9/25), a normal ABR was again observed. The following morning at 10 AM (34 hours post-injury) there was an abnormal prolongation of the wave III–V interval

TABLE 14–3.
Characteristics of 87 brain-injured patients evaluated by auditory brainstem response (ABR) in an 8-month period at Hermann Hospital/University of Texas Medical School, Houston, Texas

Sex	Age	Mode of injury (%)	Severity of injury (GCS by %)[a]		Post-injury time of ABR evaluation	
					Less than	Cumulative %
Male: 61	Mean: 30	Closed head injury: 76				
Female: 26	Mean: 10–79	MVA: 58	3–4:	61	12 hours	23
		MCA: 7	5–6:	18	24 hours	48
		Fall: 9	7–8:	11	48 hours	75
		Assault: 2	9:	10	7 days	91
		Gunshot wound: 13			14 days	98
		CV insult: 11				

[a]GCS = Glasgow Coma Score; MVA = motor vehicle accident; MCA = motor cycle accident; CV = cerebrovascular.

FIGURE 14–6a, b.
Computerized tomography (CT) scan for a 30-year-old male with severe closed head injury obtained within 1 hour post-injury.

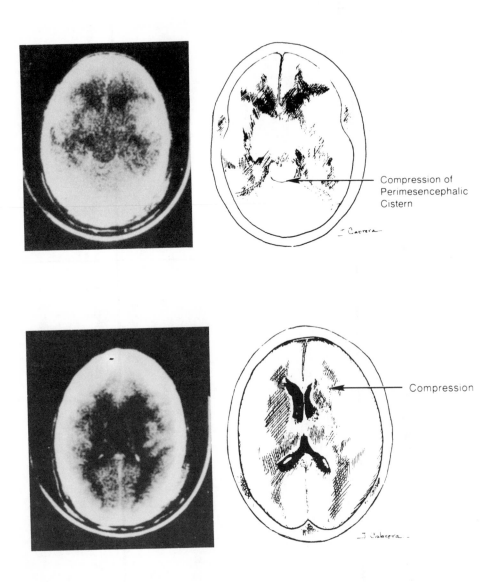

(2.52 ms vs. our 2.32 ms upper limit of normal value). ICP was 41 mm Hg, but pupils at that time were reactive. A total of 50 separate ABR recordings (two averaged runs of 1000 stimuli each per recording) were made during the following 2 hours. By 10:02 AM pupils were fixed and dilated. The wave III–V interval systematically increased and wave V morphology deteriorated

FIGURE 14–7.
Serial auditory brainstem response (ABR) recordings for a 30-year-old male with severe closed head injury, documenting acute neurologic deterioration (see CT in Figure 14–6). Initial assessment was carried out within 2 hours post-injury, and within 30 min of CT.

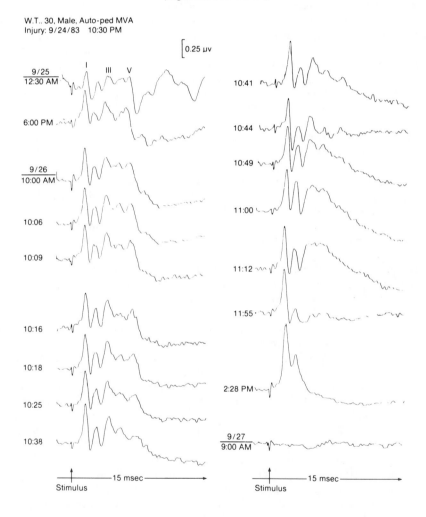

AUDITORY BRAINSTEM RESPONSE
(Right Ear Stimulation)

until, by 10:41 AM no repeatable, distinct wave V was apparent. A similar deterioration of caudal (wave III) auditory brainstem functioning was then observed. The I–III latency value fell outside of the normal region at 11 AM, and the peak became broadly shaped. At noon, only a distinct wave I and II complex was recorded. In fact, during deterioration of the brainstem response, wave I amplitude progressively increased, reaching a maximum of 0.57 μV (vs. 0.26 μV initially). Temperature varied less than 1 °F during this series of recordings. ICP gradually increased from 41 to 60 mm Hg (by noon) while mean systemic arterial pressure decreased (from 100 to 70 mm Hg). Consequently, cerebral perfusion pressure systematically declined from 60 mm Hg to a low of 9 mm Hg (from 11 AM onward). Throughout the afternoon of 9/26 only the waves I and II were present. On the following morning, there was no ABR. Bedside nuclear cerebral angiography at that time showed no evidence of cerebral blood flow. The patient was declared brain dead, was taken off life-support, and expired.

Comment. This case illustrates at least six main points about ABR assessment in comatose patients: (1) Valid ABR measurement is feasible in an ICU setting within hours of severe traumatic brain injury. (2) ABR findings are useful in management of acute brain injury. In this case, a bilaterally normal ABR (and presence of an MLR) was taken as evidence of brainstem integrity, and contributed to a decision to take the patient to surgery, and to manage him aggressively in the ICU. Intoxicants on board at hospital admission may have influenced clinical neurologic findings. In approximately 20% of our patients, medical or surgical therapy has been initiated upon the development of ABR abnormalities, and the effectiveness of therapy confirmed by partial or total reversal of the abnormalities. In other patients (10% of the total), surgical or medical intervention, dictated by CT, has been postponed or deferred entirely on the basis of consistently normal ABRs, particularly in patients with unstable ICP, or some contraindication to surgery, such as sepsis. (3) Initial ABR abnormalities (slight wave III–V prolongation) preceded neurologic (pupillary) changes. Unfortunately, medical therapy (mannitol, barbiturates, hyperventilation) was ineffective and, subsequently, ICP systematically increased while mean arterial pressure decreased, and pupils immediately became fixed and dilated. Neurologic responses thereafter remained nil. The ABR, however, continued to show systematic deterioration. (4) ABR abnormalities can reflect transtentorial herniation associated with increased ICP. There is experimental evidence of a relationship between the ABR and increased ICP (Klug, 1982; McPherson, Blanks, & Foltz, 1984; Nagao, Roccaforte, & Moody, 1979; Raudzens, Schaber, & Erspamar, 1981; Sohmer, Gafni, Goitein, & Feinmesser, 1983). Keith, Jabie, & Heerse (1983), however, reported that elevated ICP (up to 50 cm of H$_2$O) did not affect clinical ABR recordings. Our clinical experience suggests that cerebral perfusion pressure (mean arterial pressure minus ICP) is the critical factor, rather than ICP alone. Increases in ICP with associated increases in arterial pressure (and therefore stable cerebral perfusion pressure) may not produce ABR abnormalities. In close agreement with experimental data (Sohmer et al., 1983), we have found clinically that persistently reduced cerebral perfusion pressure (below approximately 60 mm Hg in this patient) leads to ABR abnormalities, and below 10 mm Hg, the ABR is usually no longer recorded. Presumably, progressive brainstem ischemia is the pathophysiologic basis for this finding (Hassler, 1967). Calculation of accurate cerebral perfusion pressure assumes that monitored ICP and mean arterial pressure values are valid, which may not always be the case clinically. (5) The ABR wave I *and* II components may be observed in patients meeting clinical neurologic criteria for brain death, and with no measurable cerebral blood flow. This observation supports evidence from depth-electrode studies in humans (Møller, Jannetta, Bennett, & Møller, 1981) and recent pathologic ABR findings (e.g., Garg, Markland, & Bustion, 1982) suggesting the wave II component arises from the intracranial portion of the eighth cranial nerve, rather than the cochlear nucleus. Later, with further increases in ICP, and decreases in vertebrobasilar circulation and blood supply to the sensorineural apparatus (Larsen, 1982), only wave I is usually observed, or there is no measurable peripheral component. (6) Inexplicably, with severe brainstem dysfunction, as in deep barbiturate coma, there may be an abnormal augmentation of ABR wave I amplitude. We have observed this phenomenon with other patients during neurologic decompensation, and can only speculate on the possibility that it reflects suppression or elimination of the inhibiting influences of brainstem efferent components of the auditory mechanism (Musiek, Weider, & Mueller, 1983; Warr, 1980).

Assessment of Auditory Function

Case report. A 14-year-old male was involved in a motor vehicle accident and sustained a closed head injury and a fractured pelvis. He was transported to the hospital via helicopter. Upon arrival, GCS was 6. CT showed diffuse edema, but no focal lesion or intracerebral bleed. The patient was taken to the operating room for placement of an ICP monitor (Richmond bolt) and then to the ICU. Hospital course for the first week following admission was uneventful, with ICP adequately controlled medically. However, the GCS had remained essentially unchanged since the injury. There was an eye opening response and localizing motor response to deep pain but, notably, no eye opening or motor response to verbal or loud hand clapping, nor any verbal response (refer again to Figure 14-1). Medical and nursing staff concluded that the patient had an injury-related hearing loss, yet an otologic examination yielded normal findings. An audiologic consult was requested to rule out serious auditory deficit.

Auditory evaluation, carried out in the ICU, consisted of immittance and ABR audiometry. Tympanometry showed negative middle ear pressure bilaterally. Acoustic reflex activity was not observed for ipsilateral or contralateral stimulation at maximum intensity levels. As illustrated in Figure 14-8, a repeatable and well-formed ABR was recorded bilaterally at stimulus intensity levels of 85 down to 35 dB (HL re: click). Lower intensity level stimulation was not used due to time constraints. Brainstem transmission time (wave I–V latency interval) was well within the normal range bilaterally. Likewise, we observed a repeatable MLR at expected latency and amplitude values (see Figure 14-9). Our overall impression was that auditory sensitivity was probably within normal limits, at least in the 1000- to 4000-Hz region, and there was no evidence of auditory brainstem or higher auditory CNS dysfunction, by the auditory evoked responses. In addition to reporting these findings, we recommended that medical/nursing staff and family consistently provide the patient with frequent auditory/verbal stimulation. Two days after testing, the patient showed an eye opening response to speech and began vocalizing spontaneously. Three months post-injury he had good speech and language skills, and only mild cognitive deficits. He intended to return to high school in the fall, and was observed by his mother as "a typical teenager."

Comment. As noted earlier in this chapter, otologic abnormalities and auditory deficits are not uncommon sequelae in traumatic head injury. In a previous paper, we described in detail the relationship between otologic and ABR abnormalities (Aguilar et al., 1983). Unresponsiveness to verbal stimulation is an acute head-injured patient may be a result of auditory deficit and/or neurologic dysfunction, including deep coma. ABR findings can contribute to a better understanding of the patient's auditory and neurologic status, and serial ABR assessment are an effective method for documenting changes in auditory status. In this way, the ABR contributes to rational medical management, and more meaningful family interactions with the patient. For this illustrative case, single-channel, air-conduction ABR assessment was sufficient to rule out significant hearing loss. Occasionally, however, we have had to turn to multichannel and/or bone-conduction ABR recordings to adequately describe peripheral and brainstem auditory functioning (Aguilar et al., 1983; Hall et al., 1984).

The MLR, in our experience, provides a valuable supplement to the ABR in auditory assessment of the comatose, brain-injured patient. Patients showing a repeatedly normal MLR bilaterally on serial assessment during the first week to 10 days of post-injury usually have good

FIGURE 14–8.
Auditory brainstem response (ABR) recordings for a 14-year-old male with severe closed head injury who showed no motor or eye opening response to auditory stimuli (see GCS in Figure 14-1).

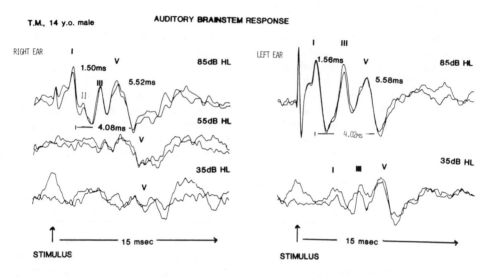

communicative/cognitive outcome. Conversely, our experience suggests that comatose patients with no observable MLR in this time period, excluding those in barbiturate coma, are likely to die or have poor neurologic recovery (at 3 months). Perhaps the association between a normal MLR and favorable communicative outcome is related to generation of this response in a cerebral region vital to language function, such as the primary auditory cortex (Celesia, 1976; Kaga, Hink, Shinoda, & Suzuki, 1980; Lee, Lueders, Dinner, Lesser, Hahn, & Klem, 1984). In any event, assessment of the ABR, in combination with the MLR and immittance measurements, can enhance its clinical value in comatose patients.

Determination of Brain Death

Case report. A 22-year-old male sustained a closed head injury in a motorcycle accident. He was unconscious and hypotensive at the scene. Upon arrival at the hospital via helicopter, GCS was 7. Acute hospital course in the ICU was uneventful. The patient regained consciousness and was transferred to an intermediate care unit. On the eighth post-injury day, however, he developed serious pulmonary complications, and subsequently became hypotensive with an acute deterioration of mental status. CT showed evidence of transtentorial herniation. He was taken to the medical ICU with clinical neurological evidence of brain death. Pupils were fixed and dilated, he was flaccid, and there were no brainstem reflexes. ABRs were then requested.

Results of the initial ABR assessment, and follow-up testing on the next day, are illustrated in Figure 14-10. On the first test day, there was excsssive and apparently asynchronous electrophysiologic activity. A reliable wave I component was recorded but the major brainstem components were grossly abnormal in latency and not clearly repeatable. The ABR recordings were not inconsistent with the pattern associated with excessive electrical or muscular artifact. This patient, however, was entirely flaccid with no muscular response even to deep pain, and there was no evidence of 60-Hz or higher frequency electromagnetic artifact on the oscilloscope during response averaging. Rather, the raw EEG was characterized by a seemingly asynchronous

FIGURE 14-9.
Auditory middle-latency response (MLR) recordings for a 14-year-old male with severe closed head injury (see ABR in Figure 14-8). Communicative/cognitive outcome was good at 3 months post-injury.

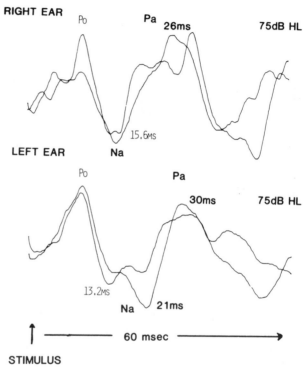

slow wave activity. On the second day, in contrast, testing at bedside in the same ICU environment and with the patient's clinical neurological status unchanged yielded a distinct wave I component with right ear stimulation and no response on the left. The EEG was exceptionally quiet throughout the assessment. We interpreted these latter ABR findings as compatible with electrophysiologic brainstem inactivity. Nuclear cerebral angiography within the hour showed no cerebral blood flow. The patient was declared brain dead.

Comment. A diagnosis of brain death requires evidence of irreversible destruction (or dysfunction) of neurons in the brainstem and cerebrum (Korein, 1980). Cerebral death is not equivalent to brain death. Numerous sets of criteria for definition of brain death have evolved, and are currently used in different locations in the United States and abroad (see Korein, 1980, for review). Most criteria include information from the clinical neurologic examination and several EEG measurements on separate occasions, and ancillary tests when they are available. However, the clinical neurologic examination and EEG are not valid measures of brain integrity in patients who are drug-intoxicated or in barbiturate coma. As noted earlier in this chapter, 40% of our series of head-injured patients were managed with high-dose barbiturates. Also,

FIGURE 14–10.

Auditory brainstem response (ABR) recordings on two successive test days for a 22-year-old male meeting clinical neurologic criteria for brain death.

AW, 22, Male, CHI, neurol brain death

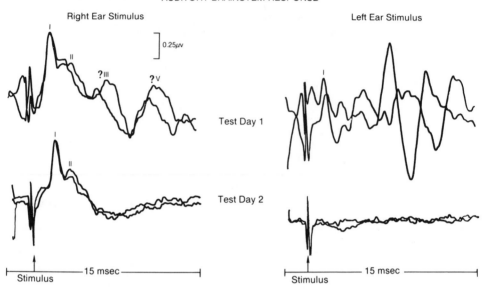

a substantial, but unspecified, proportion are admitted to the hospital with high blood levels of recreational drugs. Furthermore, interpretation of EEG recordings in an ICU environment is often confounded by electrical artifact (Grossman, 1979), and at best provides information only on cerebral functional status.

We have applied the ABR in determination of brain death in over 40 patients to date. Most were victims of traumatic head injury, although approximately one-fourth suffered a severe cerebrovascular insult. In this series of patients, four general patterns of ABR waveforms have been observed (see Figure 14-11). Infrequently, we have recorded a completely normal or mildly abnormal ABR bilaterally in patients meeting valid clinical neurologic criteria for brain death. Waveform 1 in Figure 14-11 is an example of the normal pattern. The patient was a 43-year-old woman involved in an MVA. She had multiple trauma, including severe maxillofacial fractures. At the scene she was hypotensive and required resuscitation. GCS was 3. At the time of initial ABR assessment, pupils were fixed and dilated, there were no brainstem reflexes, and she was flaccid. Follow-up assessments at post-injury Days 2 and 3, however, continued to show a bilaterally normal ABR, and the emergence of a normal MLR and well-formed 40-Hz response bilaterally. The patient was discharged at 5 months after hospital admission with good cognitive/communication function.

Waveform 2 was also measured in a patient meeting clinical neurologic criteria for brain death. This pattern is, in our experience, uncommon and is usually characterized by a reliable wave I component, yet asynchronous, slow wave activity thereafter. Typically, it is recorded in patients who have been hypotensive for an extended period of time and sometimes it follows measurement of a repeatable ABR and precedes the pattern shown in waveform 3. As noted

FIGURE 14-11.

Examples of patterns of the auditory brainstem responses recorded from patients meeting clinical neurologic criteria for brain death. Waveform 3 is compatible with peripheral auditory system integrity and brainstem electrophysiologic inactivity.

AUDITORY BRAINSTEM RESPONSE

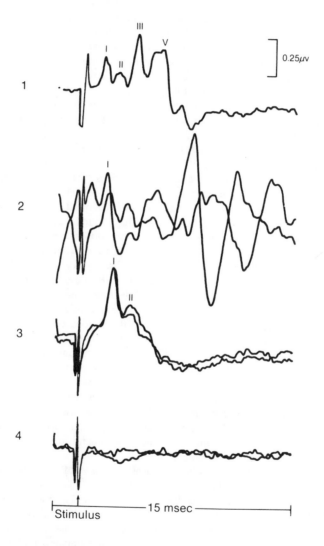

in the discussion of the previous case report, the excessive activity in the recordings appears to be electrophysiologic, rather than muscle or electrical artifact. We can only speculate that the asynchronous activity is a reflection of end-stage neuronal dysfunction secondary to severe brainstem ischemia. Clinically, we do not report this pattern as compatible with brainstem inactivity, but recommend that ABR assessment be repeated within 24 hours.

A reliable recorded wave I, without subsequent brainstem components, is the most clear-cut ABR pattern compatible with brain death (waveform 3 in Figure 14-11). Patients in our series showing this ABR pattern bilaterally have invariably fulfilled clinical neurologic criteria for brain death, and no patient with this finding unilaterally has survived. In the majority of these patients, previous ABR assessment yielded a normal response, or some evidence of auditory brainstem functioning, and then the response progressively deteriorated to the point where only a wave I remained. Presence of a reliable wave I component is extremely valuable clinically as it confirms relative integrity of the peripheral auditory apparatus.

A finding of no ABR, including the absence of wave I on initial assessment (see waveform 4 in Figure 14-11) is equivocal, and does not contribute to the evaluation of brain death. Without the wave I component, serious otologic pathology cannot be ruled out. In the traumatic head-injury patient, the possibility of middle ear or sensorineural dysfunction, with or without temporal bone and/or basilar skull fracture, must always be considered. Therefore, even in patients with no signs of ear disease by otologic examination and no radiographic (CT or X-ray) evidence of skull fracture, we do *not* report this pattern as consistent with brain death.

Fortunately, we have recorded this waveform type bilaterally on initial assessment for only 8 patients out of a series of over 200 with severe head injury. This is in contrast to the experience of Goldie, Chiappa, Young, and Brooks (1981) who reported ABR and somatosensory response findings in brain death. These researchers noted absence of all ABR waves, including wave I, in 77% of 35 presumably brain dead patients, and argued that this outcome, plus excessive measurement artifact in 5 other patients, rendered the ABR relatively ineffective in determination of brain death. We agree with their contention that absence of all ABR components is related to cessation of intracranial circulation and, in fact, have found a perfect correlation between this ultimate ABR outcome and absence of cerebral blood flow as measured by nuclear cerebral angiography. However, in our experience over three-fourths of patients presumably brain dead do, in fact, yield distinct and repeatable wave I. The discrepancy in findings is probably due to differences between studies in the post-injury time of ABR assessment. Goldie et al., according to their subject selection criteria, studied ABR in patients with no clinical neurologic evidence of brainstem or cerebral function "for several hours" before evoked response assessment, lack of spontaneous respiration, *and* a previous finding of electroencephalographic silence on an EEG. Our patients, on the other hand, were assessed at the first appearance of a clinical neurologic pattern consistent with brain death or, more commonly, were monitored by ABR daily or bidaily beginning within 24 hours post-injury, and during neurologic deterioration. In addition, because there is an organ transplantation program at our institution, attempts are often made to maintain the patient's blood pressure and systemic function while suitability for organ donation is evaluated, and the patient's family is counseled. Indeed, the importance of maintaining patient viability for possible organ transplantation has dictated the need for prompt declaration of brain death and contributed to demand for ABR assessment as soon as possible following neurologic decompensation.

The application of ABR findings in brain death is lent validity by the strong association between the ABR and nuclear cerebral perfusion, displayed in Table 14-4. Patients with a normal ABR have invariably had normal cerebral blood flow (CBF) and over 85% of the patients with no response had no CBF. Examination of serial data indicated that patients with no ABR (wave I only in each case), yet some evidence of cerebral blood flow (actually evidence only of sagittal sinus filling), expired within 24 hours of the assessment. In summary, application of the ABR as a measure for determination of brain death is clinically feasible and useful, and is not associated with false-positive errors (no response in a viable patient) when interpreted according to guidelines outlined above. The use of the ABR is particularly valuable clinically when high-dose barbiturate therapy invalidates EEG and the standard neurologic evaluation.

TABLE 14-4.
Correlation of auditory brainstem response and cerebral perfusion outcome in 39 studies of 28 severely brain-injured patients.

	Auditory brainstem response		
Cerebral perfusion	**Normal**	**Abnormal**[a]	**No response**[b]
Normal	8	7	2
Asymmetric	0	2	1
None	0	1	18

[a] Abnormal response = significant unilateral or bilateral prolongation in latency of waves III and/or V, or absence of wave III or V.

[b] No response = no brainstem components, i.e., a wave I (eighth cranial nerve) only or no observable response.

NEW DIRECTIONS FOR CLINICAL APPLICATIONS

There are four potentially promising areas for clinical research on ABR monitoring of neurologic status of the comatose patient. First, the possible influence of medical therapy modes commonly used in the ICU on AEPs needs further description. We have, in this chapter, noted the effect of barbiturates on the ABR versus MLR. Less is known of the influence of hypersmolar drugs, such as mannitol, sedatives (e.g., morphine) or other types of therapy (e.g., hyperventilation) on auditory electrophysiology. This information would aid in confident interpretation of subtle, but perhaps clinically relevant, alterations in the AEPs.

Secondly, correlations among pathophysiologic mechanisms in head injury and AEPs are poorly understood. Among these are cerebral edema, hypoxia, cerebral perfusion pressure, cerebral blood flow, and ischemia (brainstem and cerebral) in general. Presumably, these pathophysiologic processes differentially influence the various AEP neuroanatomic and neurophysiologic substrates because of differences in metabolic requirements, neuron populations, and blood supply (e.g., Makishima, Katz, & Snow, 1976). We have, for example, observed that isolated ABR wave I to III latency abnormalities may develop in patients apparently following repeated hypoxic and/or ischemic episodes, while the rostral brainstem components and even MLR remain normal. Clearly, duration and number of insults, and the timing of AEP assessment in the pathophysiologic process, are also important factors. Investigation of these complex interactions between pathophysiology and the AEP would have readily apparent clinical application and long-term implications for basic neuroscience.

Thirdly, there is an important and well-recognized need for increased knowledge of the neuroanatomy and physiology of the AEPs. This would facilitate their application in localization of brain dysfunction and in providing a functional correlate of CT evidence of structural damage. It would also contribute to a more meaningful and precise electrophysiologic description of neurologic decompensation, as during impending transtentorial herniation. This type of information, in combination with the correlation with pathophysiology noted above, would be particularly valuable in the rational management of acute brain injury. We are now assessing clinical correlations among sites of injury and ABR outcome, to further augment recent depth-electrode findings (Funai & Funasaka, 1983; Hashimoto, 1982; Hashimoto, Ishiyama, Yoshimoto, & Nemoto, 1981).

Finally, application of AEPs in monitoring comatose patients would be strengthened clinically, and be more cost-effective, by automation and computer assistance, rather than the current operator-intensive approach. The demand for ABR monitoring may occur at any time of day or night. And continuous monitoring for 24 hours or more may be required in neurologically unstable patients. To be fully exploited clinically in an ICU, it would be best if ABR recordings could be initiated by the machine at predetermined times, by a simple manual mode (for nursing personnel), or triggered by a predesignated criteria of change in neurologic or physiologic status, such as increased ICP or reduced arterial oxygen values. Naturally, skillful, experienced, and dedicated auditory neurophysiology personnel are a crucial and indispensable factor in the successful clinical application of AEPs in the comatose, brain-injured patient. Accurate and thorough electrophysiologic data from this population are of no use unless they are carefully interpreted in the context of numerous clinical variables, and reported promptly in the form of a patient chart note or, frequently, by telephone contact with managing physicians.

CONCLUSIONS

Our clinical experience with serial ABR measurement in over 200 comatose brain-injured patients may be summarized as follows: (1) Valid ABR recordings within hours of injury are feasible at bedside in an ICU environment. In most cases (85%), standard instrumentation and clinical test protocol ensure adequate recordings. Multichannel measurements and bone-conduction stimulus techniques are valuable clinical adjuncts to this routine protocol. (2) The ABR appears to be independent of depth of coma, including deep barbiturate-induced coma. (3) Changes in ABR latency can be correlated with dynamic pathophysiology in head injury, such as hypoxia, ICP, and cerebral perfusion pressure. (4) ABR abnormalities may precede other clinical evidence of neurologic deterioration, and occur in the presence of normal ICP. (5) Reversible ABR abnormalities in brain injury have been associated with effective medical and/or surgical therapy. (6) As suggested by Starr (1976), the ABR can be effectively applied in the determination of brain death, and offers an objective and cost-effective measure of brainstem integrity that is not influenced by intoxicants and CNS depressants, unlike the clinical neurologic examination. A normal ABR can be recorded in patients meeting clinical neurologic criteria for brain death who may subsequently have good neurologic/cognitive outcome.

Denice P. Brown, PhD, Audiology Supervisor, Hermann Hospital, Susan H. Morgan, M Ed, audiologist, Department of Otolaryngology–Head and Neck Surgery, University of Texas Medical School, and Chaudry Saleem, DVM, research technician, Division of Neurosurgery, University of Texas Medical School, assisted in ABR data acquisition. Otologic examinations were performed by Eugenio A. Aguilar III, MD, Resident, Department of Otolaryngology–Head and Neck Surgery. Julio Cruz, MD, Division of Neurosurgery, is acknowledged for his contribution to the selection of patient material. Juan (Tito) Cabrera, MD, Division of Neurosurgery, prepared the illustrated computerized tomography scans. Some of the clinical findings in this chapter were presented at the 1983 National American Speech–Language and Hearing Association Convention (Cincinnati) and the 1984 Annual Meeting of the American Association of Neurological Surgeons (San Francisco).

REFERENCES

Aguilar, E. A., Hall, J. W. III, & Mackey-Hargadine, J. (1983). *Neuro-otologic evaluation of the acute severely head-injured patient: Correlations among physical findings, auditory evoked responses and computerized tomography.* Paper presented at the Academy of Otolaryngology–Head and Neck Surgery, Anaheim, October.

Alving, J., Møller, M., Sindrup, E., & Nielsen, B. L. (1979). "Alpha pattern coma" following cerebral anoxia. *Electroencephalography and Clinical Neurophysiology, 47,* 95–101.

Bobbin, R. P., May, J. T., & Lemoine, R. L. (1979). Effects of pentobarbital and ketamine on brainstem auditory potentials. Latency and intensity function after intraperitoneal administration. *Archives of Otolaryngology, 105,* 467–470.

Boston, J. R., & Ainslie, P. J. (1980). Effects of analog and digital filtering on brainstem auditory evoked potentials. *Electroencephalography and Clinical Neurophysiology, 48,* 361–364.

Braakman, R., Schouten, H. J. A., Blaauw-van Dishoeck, M., & Minderhoud, J. M. (1983). Megadose steroids in severe head injury. Results of a prospective double-blind clinical trial. *Journal Neurosurgery, 58,* 326–330.

Brewer, C. C., & Resnick, D. M. (1982). *The value of ABR in the assessment of comatose patients.* Paper presented at The Second International Symposium on Evoked Potentials, Cleveland, October 18.

Britt, R. H., Herrick, M. K., Mason, R. T., & Dorfman, L. J. (1980). Traumatic lesion of the pontomedullary junction. *Neurosurgery, 6,* 623–631.

Bruce, D. A., Gennarelli, T. A., & Langfitt, T. W. (1978). Resuscitation from coma due to head injury. *Critical Care Medicine, 6,* 254–269.

Celesia, G. G. (1976). Organization of auditory cortical areas in man. *Brain, 99,* 403–414.

Chu, N. S., Squires, K. C., & Starr, A. (1978). Auditory brain stem potentials in chronic alcohol intoxication and alcohol withdrawal. *Archives of Neurology, 35,* 596–602.

Cohen, M., & Britt, R. (1981). Effects of anesthetics on the brainstem evoked response. *Society of Neuro Science Abstracts, 7,* 282.

de la Torre, J. C., Trimble, J. L., Beard, R. T., et al. (1978). Somatosensory evoked potentials for the prognosis of coma in humans. *Experimental Neurology, 60,* 304–317.

Eng, D. Y., Dong, W. K., Bledsoe, S. W., Heavner, J. E., Shaw, C. M., & Hornbei, D. F. (1979). Electrical and pathological correlates of brain hypoxia during hypotension. *Anesthesiology, 53,* S92.

Fay, T. (1923). The administration of hypertonic salt solution for the relief of intracranial pressure. *JAMA, 80(20),* 1445–1448.

Feinsod, M., & Averbach, E. (1978). Electrophysiological examinations of the visual system in the acute phase after head injury. *European Neurology, 60,* 304–317.

Funai, H., & Funasaka, S. (1983). Experimental study on the effect of inferior colliculus lesions upon auditory brainstem response. *Audiology, 22,* 9–19.

Garg, D. P., Markland, O. N., & Bustion, P. F. (1982). Brainstem auditory evoked responses in hereditary motor-sensory neuropathy: Site of origin of wave II. *Neurology 32,* 1017–1019.

Gennarelli, T. A., Spielman, G. M., Langfitt, T. W., et al. (1982). Influence of the type of intracranial lesions on outcome from severe head injury. *Journal of Neurosurgery, 56,* 26–32.

Goldie, W. D., Chiappa, K. H., Young, R. R., & Brooks, E. B. (1981). Brainstem auditory and short-latency somatosensory evoked responses in brain death. *Neurology, 31,* 248–256.

Gordon, E. (1971). Controlled respiration in the management of patients with traumatic brain injuries. *Acta Anaesthesia Scandinavia, 15,* 193–208.

Greenberg, R. P., & Becker, D. P. (1976). Clinical applications and results of evoked potential data in patients with severe head injury. *Surgical Forum, 26,* 484–486.

Greenberg, R. P., Becker, D. P., Miller, J. D., et al. (1977). Evaluation of brain function in severe head trauma with multimodality evoked potentials. Part II. Localization of brain dysfunction in correlation with post-traumatic neurologic condition. *Journal of Neurosurgery, 47,* 163–177.

Greenberg, R. P., Newlon, P. G., & Becker, D. P. (1982). The somatosensory evoked potential in patients with severe head injury: Outcome prediction in monitoring of brain function. *Annals of the New Academy of Sciences,* 683–688.

Greenberg, R. P., Newlon, P. G., Hyatt, M. S., Narayan, R. D., & Becker, D. P. (1981a). Prognostic implication of early multimodality evoked potentials in severely head-injured patients. A prospective study. *Journal of Neurosurgery, 55,* 227–236.

Greenberg, R. P., Stablein, D. M., & Becker, D. P. (1981b). Noninvasive localization of brain-stem lesions in the cat with multimodality evoked potentials. Correlation with human head-injured data. *Journal of Neurosurgery, 54,* 740–750.

Grossman, R. G. (1979). Electrophysiologic evaluation of the central nervous system after trauma. In G. L. Odom (Ed.), *Central nervous system trauma: Research study report.* NIH, NINCDS, 159–176.

Grove, W. E. (1947). Hearing impairment due to craniocerebral trauma. *Annals of Otology, Rhinology, and Laryngology, 56,* 264–270.

Guerit, J. M., & Mahieu, P. (1981). The use of evoked potentials in the intensive care unit. *Electroencephalography and Clinical Neurophysiology, 52,* 40.

Hall, J. W. III. (1983). Auditory brainstem response audiometry. In J. Jerger (Ed.), *Hearing disorders in adults* (pp. 1–55). San Diego: College-Hill Press.

Hall, J. W. III, Haungfu, M., & Gennarelli, T. A. (1982). Auditory function in acute severe head injury. *Laryngoscope, 92,* 883–890.

Hall, J. W. III, Huangfu, M., Gennarelli, T. A., Dolinskas, C. A., Olson, J., & Berry, G. A. (1983). Auditory evoked responses, impedance measures and diganostic speech audiometry in severe head injury. *Otolaryngology and Head and Neck Surgery, 91,* 50–60.

Hall, J. W. III, Morgan, S. H., Mackey-Hargadine, J., Aguilar, E. A. III, & Jahrsdoerfer, R. A. (1984). Neuro-otologic applications of multi-channel auditory brainstem response recordings. *Laryngoscope, 94,* 883–889.

Hari, R., Sulkava, R., & Haltia, M. (1982). Brainstem auditory responses in alpha-pattern coma. *Annals of Neurology, 11,* 187–189.

Hashimoto, I. (1982). Auditory evoked potentials from the human midbrain: Slow brain stem responses. *Electroencephalography and Clinical Neurophysiology, 53,* 652–657.

Hashimoto, I., Ishiyama, Y., Yoshimoto, T., & Nemoto, S. (1981). Brain-stem auditory-evoked potentials recorded directly from human brain-stem and thalamus. *Brain, 104,* 841–859.

Hassler, O. (1967). Arterial pattern of human brainstem: Normal appearance and deformation in expanding supratentorial conditions. *Neurology, 17,* 368–375.

Hume, A. L., Cant, B. R., & Shaw, M. A. (1979). Central somatosensory conduction time in comatose patients. *Annals of Neurology, 5,* 379–384.

Jennett, B., & Teasdale, G. (1981). *Management of head injuries.* Philadelphia: Davis.

Kaga, K., Hink, R. E., Shinoda, Y., & Suzuki, J. (1980). Evidence for a primary cortical origin of a middle-latency auditory evoked potential in cats. *Electroencephalography and Clinical Neurophysiology, 50,* 254–266.

Karnaze, D. S., Marshall, L. F., McCarthy, C. S., Klauber, M. R., & Bickford, R. G. (1982). Localizing and prognistic value of auditory responses in coma after closed head injury. *Neurology, 32,* 299–302.

Keith, R. W., Jabie, A. F., & Heerse, K. L. (1983). Auditory brainstem response testing in the surgical intensive care unit. *Seminars in Hearing, 4,* 385–389.

Kileny, P. (1983). Auditory evoked middle-latency responses: Current issues. *Seminars in Hearing, 4,* 403–413.

Klug, N. (1982). Brainstem auditory evoked potentials in syndromes of decerebration, the Bulbar syndrome in central death. *Journal of Neurology, 227,* 219–228.

Korein, J. (1980). Brain death. In J. E. Cottrel & H. Turndorf (Eds.), *Anesthesia and neurosurgery* (pp. 282–321). St. Louis: Mosby.

Larsen, H. C. (1982). The effect of intracranial hypertension on cochlear bloodflow. *Acta Otolaryngologica, 93,* 415–419.

Laukli, E., & Mair, I. W. S. (1981). Early auditory-evoked responses: Filter effects. *Audiology, 20,* 300–312.

Lee, Y. S., Lueders, H., Dinner, D. S., Lesser, R. P., Hahn, J., & Klem, G. (1984). Recording of auditory evoked potentials in man using chronic subdural electrodes. *Brain, 107,* 115–131.

Lindsey, K. W., Carlin, J., Kennedy, I., et al. (1981). Evoked potentials in severe head injury: Analysis and relation to outcome. *Journal of Neurology, Neurosurgery, and Psychiatry, 44,* 796–802.

Lütschg, J., Pfenninger, J., Ludin, H. P., & Fassela, F. (1983). Brain-stem auditory evoked potentials and early somatosensory evoked potentials in neurointensively treated comatose children. *American Journal of Diseases in Children, 137,* 421–426.

Makishima, K., Katz, R. B., & Snow, J. B., Jr. (1976). Hearing loss of a central type secondary to anoxic anoxia. *Annals of Otology, Rhinology, and Laryngology, 85,* 826–833.

Marsh, R. R., Yamane, H., & Potsic, W. P. (1984). Auditory brainstem response and temperature: Relationship in the guinea pig. *Electroencephalography and Clinical Neurophysiology, 57,* 289–293.

Marshall, L. F., Smith, R. W., Rauscher, L. A., & Shapiro, H. M. (1978). Mannitol dose requirements in brain-injured patients. *Journal of Neurosurgery, 48,* 169–172.

Marshall, L. F., Smith, R. W., & Shapiro, H. M. (1979). The outcome with aggressive treatment in severe head injuries. Part II: Acute and chronic barbiturate administration in the management of head injury. *Journal of Neurosurgery, 50,* 26–30.

Marshall, N. K., & Donchin, E. (1981). Circadian variation in the latency of brainstem responses and its relation to body temperature. *Science, 212,* 356–358.

McKay, A. R., Hosobuchi, Y., Williston, J. S., & Jewett, D. (1980). Brainstem auditory evoked responses in brainstem compression. *Neurosurgery, 6,* 632–638.

McPherson, D., Blanks, J., & Foltz, E. (1984). Intracranial pressure effects on auditory evoked responses in the rabbit: Preliminary report. *Neurosurgery, 14,* 161–166.

Miller, J. D., Becker, D. P., Ward, J. D. Sullivan, H. G., Adams, W. E., & Rosner, M. J. (1977). Significance of intracranial hypertension in severe head injury. *Journal of Neurosurgery, 47,* 503–516.

Mjoen, S., Nordby, H. K., & Torvik, A. (1983). Auditory evoked brainstem responses (ABR) in coma due to severe head trauma. *Acta Otolaryngologica, 95,* 131–138.

Møller, A. R., Jannetta, P. J., Bennett, M., & Møller, M. B. (1981). Intracranially recorded responses from the human auditory nerve: New insights into the origin of brain stem evoked potentials (BSEP's). *Electroencephalography and Clinical Neurophysiology, 52,* 18–27.

Musiek, F. E., Weider, E. J., & Mueller, R. J. (1983). Reversible audiological results in a patient with an extra-axial brain stem tumor. *Ear and Hearing, 4,* 169–172.

Nagao, S., Roccaforte, P., & Moody, R. A. (1979). Acute intracranial hypertension and auditory brain-stem responses. Part I: Changes in the auditory brain-stem and somatosensory evoked responses in intracranial hypertension in cats. *Journal of Neurosurgery, 51,* 669–676.

Nagao, S., Sumani, N., Tsutsui, T., et al. (1982). Serial observations of brainstem function by auditory brainstem responses in central transtentorial herniation. *Surgical Neurology, 19,* 355–357.

Narayan, R. K., Greenberg, R. P., Miller, J. D., et al. (1981). Improved confidence of outcome prediction in severe head injury. A comparative analysis of the clinical examination, multimodality evoked potentials, CT scanning and intracranial pressure. *Journal of Neurosurgery, 54,* 751–752.

Newlon, P. G., & Greenberg, R. P. (1983). Assessment of brain function with multimodality evoked potentials. In M. Rosenthal, E. R. Griffith, M. R. Miller, & A. Douglas (Eds.), *Rehabilitation of head-injured adults.* Philadelphia: F.A. Davis.

Newlon, P. G., Greenberg, R. P., Hyatt, M. S., Enas, G. G., & Becker, D. P. (1982). The dynamics of neuronal dysfunction and recovery following severe head injury assessed with serial multimodality evoked potentials. *Journal of Neurosurgery, 57,* 168–177.

Ongerboer, B. W. de Visser (1981). Corneal reflex latency in lesions of the lower postcentral region. *Neurology, 31,* 701–707.

Plum, F., & Posner, J. D. (1980). *The diagnosis of stupor and coma* (3rd ed.). Philadelphia: F. A. Davis.

Rappaport, M., Hall, M. K., Hopkins, K., et al. (1977). Evoked brain potentials and disability in brain-injured patients. *Archives of Physical Medicine and Rehabilitation, 58,* 333–338.

Raudzens, P., Schaber, R., & Erspamar, R. (1981). Intracranial pressure effects on brainstem potentials. *Anesthesiology, 51,* S40.

Rosenhamer, H. J., & Silverskiold, B. D. (1980). Slower tremor and related auditory brainstem auditory evoked responses in alcoholics. *Archives of Neurology, 37,* 293–296.

Sanders, R. A., Smriga, D. J., McCullough, D. W., & Duncan, P. G. (1981). Auditory brainstem responses in patients with global cerebral insults. *Journal of Otolaryngology, 10,* 52–58.

Saul, T. G., & Ducker, T. B. (1982). Effect of intracranial pressure monitoring and aggressive treatment on mortality in severe head injury. *Journal of Neurosurgery, 56,* 498–503.

Schuknecht, H. F. (1950). A clinical study of auditory damage following blows to the head. *Annals of Otology, Rhinology, and Laryngology, 59,* 331–357.

Seales, D. M., Rossiter, V. S., & Weinstein, M. E. (1979). Brainstem auditory evoked responses in patients comatose as a result of blunt head trauma. *Journal of Trauma, 19,* 347–353.

Serrats, A. F., Parker, S. A., & Merino-Canas, A. (1976). The blink reflex in coma and after recovery from coma. *Acta Neurochirgica, 34,* 79–97.

Sohmer, H., Gafni, N. I., Goitein, K., & Feinmesser, P. (1983). Auditory nerve–brainstem evoked potentials in cats during manipulation of the cerebral perfusion pressure. *Electroencephalography and Clinical Nuerophysiology, 55,* 198–202.

Sohmer, H., Garni, M., & Chisin, R. (1982). Auditory nerve–brain stem potentials in man and cat under hypoxic and hypercapnic conditions. *Electroencephalography and Clinical Neurophysiology, 53,* 506–512.

Squires, K. C., Chu, M. S., & Starr, A. (1978). Auditory brain stem potentials with alcohol. *Electroencephalography and Clinical Neurophysiology, 45,* 577–584.

Starr, A. (1976). Auditory brain-stem responses in brain-death. *Brain, 99,* 543–554.

Starr, A., & Hamilton, A. E. (1976). Correlation between confirmed sites of neurological lesions and abnormalities of far-field auditory brainstem responses. *Electroencephalography and Clinical Neurophysiology, 41,* 595–608.

Stockard, J. J., Sharbrough, J. W., & Tinker, J. A. (1978). Effects of hypothermia on the human brainstem auditory response. *Annals of Neurology, 3,* 368–370.

Stockard, J. J., Stockard, J. E., & Sharbrough, F. W. (1978). Non-pathologic factors influencing brainstem auditory evoked potentials. Part 1. *Journal of Electrophysiological Technology, 18,* 177–193.

Sutton, L. M., Frewen, T., Marsh, R., Jaggi, J., & Bruce, D. A. (1982). The effect of deep barbiturate coma on multimodality evoked potentials. *Journal of Neurosurgery, 57,* 178–185.

Toglia, J. J., & Katinsky, S. (1976). Neuro-otological aspects of closed head injury. In P. J. Winken & G. W. Bruyn (Eds.), *Handbook of clinical neurology.* Amsterdam: North-Holland.

Tsubokawa, T., Nichimoto, H., Yamamoto, T., et al. (1980). Assessment of brainstem damage by the auditory brainstem response in acute severe head injury. *Journal of Neurology, Neurosurgery, and Psychiatry, 43,* 1005–1011.

Uziel, A., & Benezech, J. (1978). Auditory brainstem response in comatose patients. Relationship with brainstem responses and level of coma. *Electroencephalography and Clinical Neurophysiology, 45,* 515–524.

Uziel, A., Benezech, J., Loranzo, S., Monstrey, Y., Duboin, M. P., & Roquefeuil, B. (1982). Clinical applications of brainstem auditory evoked potentials in comatose patients. In J. Courjon, F. Mauguiere, & M. Revol (Eds.), *Clinical application of evoked potentials in neurology.* New York: Raven Press.

Van Nechel, C., Deltemre, P., Strul, S., & Capon, A. (1982). Value of the simultaneous recording of brainstem auditory evoked potentials, blink reflex, short-latency somatosensory potentials for the assessment of brainstem function in clinical neurology. In J. Courjon, F. Mauguiere, & M. Revol (Eds.), *Clinical applications of evoked potentials in neurology,* New York: Raven Press.

Walter, B., & Blegvad, B. (1981). ABR following head trauma: A study of click-evoked frequency-following responses. *Scandinavian Audiology, Supplement 13,* 125–130.

Walter, S., & Arfel, G. (1972). Responses aux stimulations visuelles dans les etats de coma aiger et de coma chronique. *Electroencephalography and Clinical Neurophysiology, 32,* 27–41

Warr, B. (1980). Efferent components of the auditory system. *Annals of Otology, Rhinology, and Laryngology* (Supplement 74), *89,* 114–120.

Westmoreland, B. F., Klass, D. W., Sharbrough, F. W., & Regan, T. J. (1975). Alpha-coma: Electroencephalographic, clinical pathologic and etiologic correlations. *Archives of Neurology, 32,* 713–718.

Yagi, T., & Baba, S. (1983). Evaluation of the brain-stem function by the auditory brain-stem response and the caloric vestibular reaction in comatose patient. *Archives of Otorhinolaryngology, 238,* 33–43.

York, D. H., Pulliam, M. W., Rosenfeld, J. G., & Watts, C. (1981). Relationship between visual evoked potentials and intracranial pressure. *Journal of neurosurgery, 55,* 909–916.

SECTION IV
PEDIATRIC ASSESSMENT

Chapter 15

Neurologic Applications of the Auditory Brainstem Response to the Pediatric Age Group

Kurt Hecox

INTRODUCTION

Since the introduction of auditory brainstem responses (ABR) more than ten years ago, the number of neurologic and audiologic applications has multiplied. The response is now widely recognized as an important tool in the diagnostic repertoire of many fields (Chiappa, Harrison, Brooks, & Young, 1980; Galambos & Hecox, 1978; Hecox, Cone, & Blaw, 1981; Kaga, Kitazumi, & Kodama, 1979; Sohmer, Feinmesser, Bauberger-Tell, & Edelstein, 1977; Starr & Achor, 1975; Stockard & Rossiter, 1977; Terkildsen, Huis In't Veld, & Osterhammel, 1977). The diagnostic criteria for neurologic applications include the response to changing rate of stimulation, the timing between component peaks (e.g., I to V interval), and the amplitude ratio of wave V to wave I (Jerger & Mauldin, 1978; Starr & Achor, 1975; Stockard & Rossiter, 1977). Audiometric criteria include the slope of the latency-intensity function, thresholds, and absolute latencies (Galambos & Hecox, 1978; Jerger & Mauldin, 1978).

The focus of this chapter is on the neurologic applications of the ABR to the pediatric age group. The separate treatment of neurologic and audiologic disorders in this and other textbooks should not mislead the reader into believing that the auditory system functions can be divided into two clearly defined groups. The integrity of the peripheral auditory system is critical for the normal function and development of the auditory system. The interplay between peripheral and central nervous system components is constant and critical for normal auditory function. Only history, professional boundaries, and convenience have dictated their separation in this and other similar chapters.

With the introduction of a new clinical measure, several criteria should be fulfilled if that measure is to assume an important role in diagnostic evaluation of human disorders. First, the measure must be feasible from a technical standpoint, with respect to both equipment and level of required training. Second, the measure must have sufficiently limited variability to permit the establishment of clinical norms and the recognition of pathologic responses. Third, the new tool should result in minimal risk and discomfort to the patient. Finally, the new measure must target an unserved population for whom alternative tests are inadequate.

The technical feasibility of auditory brainstem responses is established, although standards of performance (technical and interpretative) are not. The extraordinarily limited variability within and between subjects is now well known (Sohmer, Gafni & Chisin, 1978; Starr & Achor, 1975; Suzuki & Suzuki, 1977). The collection of ABRs involves little more than the application of routine EEG electrodes and the placement of standard earphones with no associated risk or discomfort to the patient. The brainstem response fills at least two incompletely met needs— the early detection of hearing impairment in the uncooperative patient and the detection of unsuspected brainstem neurologic abnormalities.

The spectrum of human diseases to which the brainstem response is sensitive is expanding rapidly, and the following paragraphs survey and discuss the application of the auditory brainstem response to pediatric diseases. The chapter is organized according to disease category in terms of diagnostic application, followed by a discussion of the use of the ABR for monitoring purposes.

INFECTIOUS DISEASES

Infectious diseases cause both otologic and neurologic disorders in the pediatric population. The best known relationship is between bacterial meningitis and hearing loss; our experience is that about ten percent of preverbal infants with bacterial meningitis experience hearing loss. Estimates of the incidence of hearing impairment following bacterial meningitis in the infant and young child vary considerably in the behavioral audiometry literature, probably reflecting differences in sampling methods (Smith, Ingram, Smith, Gilles, & Bresnaw, 1973; Sproles, Azerrad, Williamson & Merrill, 1969). For example, in many such studies, patients institutionalized because of severe neurologic deficits are often excluded from follow-up testing. Our experience is that the incidence of serious neurologic deficits more than doubles the likelihood of peripheral auditory disease, although even neurologically normal patients can have severe hearing loss. The estimated incidence of hearing loss secondary to bacterial meningitis, according to the ABR, is also flawed by ascertainment biases, but varies between five and ten percent (Finitzo-Hieber, Simhadri & Hieber, 1981).

We have been able to document impaired peripheral auditory function, excluding middle ear disease, from multiple infectious agents, but there has not been any systematic investigation of the incidence of abnormalities as a function of infecting agent or other clinical signs or symptoms. This information might be helpful in determining more precise criteria for the referral of pediatric patients following bacterial meningitis.

The availability of the brainstem response offers several possible research applications. The pathophysiology of hearing loss in bacterial meningitis is usually attributed to eighth nerve dysfunction secondary to a fibrous reaction with adhesions comprising the auditory nerve (Greenfield, 1966). While the validity of this concept in some patients is not in doubt, the vast majority of patients with hearing loss following bacterial meningitis have exhibited electrophysiologic recruitment, implying inner ear disease. This observation, coupled with the fact that the incidence of hearing impairment in patients exhibiting a "stroke-like" picture is two to three times that seen in similar unaffected populations, suggests that vasculitis of inner ear vessels may be important in the pathophysiology of hearing impairment.

While there is a very real (but small) incidence of central auditory abnormalities of the ABR in patients with bacterial meningitis, these abnormalities often reverse (especially abnormal interwave intervals) and are not necessarily related to the incidence of peripheral auditory impairment. Additionally, the relative incidence of central auditory abnormalities in the same patients should be investigated to determine if indeed there is any relationship between the pathophysiology of the two entities.

As mentioned earlier, many of the central abnormalities seen in this group show reversibility (Hecox et al., 1981). The mechanisms responsible for this reversibility are unknown but may include transiently raised intracranial pressure, toxic effects of antibiotics, vasculitis, or other perfusion factors that may or may not contribute to hypoxia. Of the various central abnormalities, the most commonly encountered are prolonged interwave intervals and rate-dependent abnormalities; both commonly reverse.

A second group of infectious agents that must be considered are the "congenital infections." These include cytomegalovirus, herpesvirus, toxoplasma, and rubella virus. While cytomegalovirus and rubella virus have a well-documented predilection for the auditory system, toxoplasmosis is usually associated with disorders of the visual pathway. Herpesvirus has been described as residing in the eighth nerve ganglion in both animal and human autopsy material, although its relation to hearing disorders is unclear.

The nature of the auditory impairment with cytomegalovirus appears to be peripheral in origin with little evidence of concomitant central disease. Of 18 patients evaluated for congenital rubella, none exhibited central auditory abnormalities. Of 20 patients with cytomegalovirus, two exhibited central auditory disorders. All of the patients with rubella and 12 of the patients with cytomegalovirus demonstrated peripheral auditory disease. The incidence of peripheral auditory impairment should not be estimated on the basis of these figures, however, since there is a clear sampling bias toward patients felt to have auditory dysfunction or patients who have significant neurologic deficits. Nevertheless, it is quite clear that the primary lesion in most congenital infections is an inner ear disorder and not a disorder of the central auditory pathway.

An interesting yet unanswered question concerns the possible progressive nature of the hearing impairment seen in cytomegalovirus or chronic rubella infection. Although this has been a matter of considerable discussion in the past, particularly as it relates to the possibility and role of the carrier-infected state, there are no prospective longitudinal studies of patients infected with cytomegalovirus or rubella virus.

A final group of infection-related disorders comprises the postinfectious diseases of which subacute sclerosing panencephalitis (Greenfield, 1966) is the best known. Central auditory abnormalities are surely seen in this population and would be expected on the basis of the white matter changes seen at autopsy. The occurrence of these abnormalities has, in our experience, been related to the severity of the neurologic picture, and the diagnostic utility of the brainstem auditory response in the early detection and documentation of white matter changes in the population is unevaluated.

TUMORS

Abnormalities of the ABR have been documented in patients with tumors of the cerebellopontine angle, intrinsic brainstem, suprapineal region, and cerebellum and from suprathalamic masses. Tumors need not, therefore, impinge directly upon the brainstem auditory pathways to produce central auditory abnormalities. Mechanical distortion, raised intracranial pressure, and edema are all processes by which tumors may produce their abnormalities from a distance.

Special attention has been given to at least two categories of tumors—the acoustic neuroma and the brainstem glioma. Although estimates of the percentage of patients with known acoustic neuromas displaying abnormalities of the brainstem response vary widely from study to study, at least two recent articles document that greater than 90 percent of patients with definable waveforms have central abnormalities of the ABR (Glasscock, Jackson, Josey, Dickins, & Wiet, 1979; Selters & Brackmann, 1977). These abnormalities are present even when the audiogram is entirely within normal limits. This is a particularly interesting circumstance, since it is an example of how this response may be sensitive to central auditory "dysfunction" that is not necessarily reflected in those processes monitored by a routine behavioral audiogram. A similar circumstance arises in the evaluation of patients with multiple sclerosis, in which patients with no central auditory brainstem evoked potential components may have normal audiograms. This occurrence has been used to emphasize the limitations of the ABR for hearing evaluations. In fact, it only underscores the importance of considering more than one aspect of auditory function when evaluating a patient with auditory system complaints. We have seen only one patient in the pediatric age group with acoustic neuromas, so that the primary utility of this tumor is to serve as a model for the study of other, more common cerebellopontine angle masses in infancy and early childhood.

A more common tumor in the pediatric age group is the brainstem glioma. We have not yet found a case of documented brainstem glioma with normal auditory brainstem responses. In some cases, there was a delay of over one year between the first documentation of central abnormalities on the ABR and the neuroradiologic confirmation of the neuropathology by arteriograms or CT scan. In fact, we are unaware of any published cases of a brainstem glioma at or above the level of entry of the eighth nerve into the brainstem in which the patient has not had associated central abnormalities of the ABR. We conclude, therefore, that the presence of normal auditory brainstem potentials makes unlikely the diagnosis of brainstem glioma.

ASPHYXIA

Hypoxic-ischemic encephalopathy is the most common cause of neurologic problems in the newborn. Until recently, however, hypoxia was thought to be of secondary importance as a cause of hearing loss. The remarkably high incidence of hearing impairment among premature infants evaluated upon discharge from the newborn intensive care unit has resulted in the reinvestigation of the role played by hypoxia, ischemia, acidosis, and so forth, in the production of hearing loss. Hypoxia can also produce brainstem auditory dysfunction. The presence of central auditory pathology on the ABR increases the risk of long-term neurologic deficit, especially when the response abnormality is a decrease of wave V amplitude relative to waves I and III (Finitzo-Hieber, Hecox & Cone, 1979). Outcome for this central abnormality was universally poor, including death, persistent vegetative state, or essentially no developmental progress for all the patients. This relationship does not necessarily apply to the premature infant, nor are other forms of central auditory abnormalities as strongly associated with poor neurologic outcomes. In fact, interwave interval abnormalities and rate-dependent abnormalities are associated with a wide spectrum of outcome. Untested is the possibility that milder degrees of amplitude abnormality are associated with milder degrees of neurologic impairment.

The pathophysiology involved in the production of such markedly abnormal amplitude ratios is not obvious, nor can it be explained on the basis of changing patterns of vascular anatomy. More likely, the extremely high metabolic rates associated with inferior collicular and midbrain auditory centers play an important role in determining the special susceptibility of this region. There has been considerable research effort expended on the separation of several forms of hypoxic encephalopathy in animal models, especially by Windle and colleagues. The assertion that there are two primary forms—the first, cortical in distribution, the second, brainstem in distribution—has received little support from human neuroanatomic literature. Recent reports by Leech and Alford (1977) on the correlates of ABR to neurologic outcomes support this fundamental distinction, however.

A number of very practical questions remain unanswered. The best test time from the standpoint of correlating to neurologic outcome is unknown; so too is whether there is a continuum of amplitude ratio abnormalities associated with a continuum of neurologic impairment. In addition, the determinants of reversibility exhibited by a significant percentage of patients suffering from asphyxia need more careful definition. Nonetheless, the ABR can play a significant role in improving the diagnosis and management of hypoxic encephalopathy in the pediatric patient.

TOXIC-METABOLIC DISORDERS

One of the earliest applications of the ABR was in determining the cause of coma. When the etiology of the coma was drug intoxication, patients were noted to have normal ABRs; when the depressed level of consciousness was secondary to structural disorders (hemorrhage, tumor, or raised intracranial pressure), responses were abnormal (Starr & Achor, 1975). From these studies arose the concept that metabolic disorders do not produce abnormalities of the ABR. As a general rule, this concept has held firm in the adult population, but it is clearly in error for the pediatric age group. The only drug in which ABR abnormalities have been seen at "therapeutic" doses has been lidocaine, according to preliminary reports.

Several of the dysmyelinating metabolic disorders produce central auditory brainstem potential abnormalities (Galambos & Hecox, 1978). Similarly, Wilson's disease is associated with central abnormalities of the ABR (Fujita, Hosoki & Miyazaki, 1981). Unresolved is the importance of alcohol and at least one anesthetic (enflurane) in the production of central abnormalities. Nevertheless, it is important to realize that none of the routinely prescribed sedatives, anticonvulsants, or analgesics, or any of the antibiotics, have been demonstrated to produce central abnormalities of the ABR. Thus, it is not necessary to adjust patient norms on the basis of the patient's medication.

NEURODEGENERATIVE DISORDERS

A number of neurodegenerative disorders have been associated with abnormalities of the ABR. Examples of these disorders include the sphingolipidoses, the leukodystrophies (including metachromatic leukodystrophy and adrenal leukodystrophy), certain of the genetic peripheral neuropathies (e.g., Friedreich's ataxia), Wilson's disease, and multiple sulfatase deficiencies. It is common to most of these disorders that the progression of neurologic impairment is paralleled by the progressive deterioration of the auditory brainstem response. Among the categories of the degenerative disorders that may produce central abnormalities of the ABR, a recurring theme is that the pathologic process must interfere with myelin function. It is pertinent to note at this juncture that the progression of neurologic symptoms often reflects advancing pathology at the supra-brainstem level among patients with these disorders. Thus, it is not reasonable to expect that all forms of neurologic deterioration would be reflected in abnormalities of the ABR. The inclusion of the so-called middle latency evoked potentials and the long latency potentials in a diagnostic battery would more completely sample the entirety of the auditory pathway; their inclusion would be necessary if a more anatomically complete analysis of electrophysiologic and behavioral relationship is to be made. Whether pure grey matter disorders (which leave unaffected myelin maintenance and formation) result in central abnormalities is unanswered, but it is an important issue from the standpoint of differential diagnosis.

An important extension in the use of the ABR would be the creation of an improved nosology for several of the degenerative disorders whose expression is quite diverse. For example, the spinocerebellar disorders can show either normal or abnormal ABRs. Similarly, certain of the peripheral neuropathies have shown central ABR abnormalities while other patients with the same diagnostic label have not shown central abnormalities. Whether this means that the patients were at different stages in the development of their disorder or whether these patients had different underlying diseases is an unresolved issue, but one that can be answered with careful longitudinal studies. Creating an improved nosology is important if the goal is to define a relatively homogeneous subgroup of patients on whom biochemical or other genetic measures can be performed.

TRAUMA

The only available description of ABR changes as a function of closed head injury is for the adult population (Fujita et al., 1981). In the older age group, studies indicate that the ABR is an effective, though imperfect, predictor of neurologic impairment. Several of the published studies include small numbers of children, but the investigators did not treat the pediatric data separately, and the numbers included were insufficient to produce meaningful conclusions. All types of abnormalities of the ABR in pediatric patients with significant head trauma have been observed. Reversals of abnormal amplitude ratios, abnormal interwave intervals, and rate-dependent abnormalities have been seen. In our experience, the relationship between brainstem neurologic signs and abnormalities of the ABR is imperfect at best. The pediatric population, however, has shown a reasonably high sensitivity to rate-dependent stimulus changes. Because of the difficulties of prognostication and the ease with which these evoked potential measures are obtained, it is believed that information will become available concerning the utility of the brainstem potential in the early detection of severe forms of pathology and in providing long-term prognostic information on neurologic outcome.

CHROMOSOMAL DISORDERS AND STRUCTURAL MALFORMATIONS

Many chromosomal abnormalities and malformation syndromes demonstrate central abnormalities of the ABR. The list of such disorders is even longer when peripheral auditory abnormalities are included. Among chromosomal disorders, it is exceedingly common to observe peripheral auditory abnormalities within the Down's syndrome population. Squires and associates have observed an interesting phenomenon in which patients with Down's syndrome show very little change in response to increasing rates of stimulation. The explanation for this finding is unclear, but it is hypothesized to be related to the significant language processing abnormalities exhibited in this population. In more severe malformation syndromes the ABR aberrations are but a small portion of the overall picture of neurologic devastation. In other cases, particularly short- or long-arm deletional abnormalities, the neurologic status of the patient is not sufficiently impaired to prevent the development of general communication skills. It is especially important for this group that auditory abnormalities capable of interfering with the acquisition of language be monitored. Too often the striking morphologic abnormalities apparent in children with these disorders carry with them an assumption of mental subnormality or of an impaired potential for intellectual and communication development. The high incidence of peripheral auditory abnormalities in these populations requires early intervention to optimize speech and language development. There is, unfortunately, little information available on the impact of such interventions in many of the populations for whom such measures might be undertaken.

We have observed progressive changes in the central abnormalities exhibited by several patients with unknown malformation syndromes, despite little evidence of morphologic change or any evidence of deterioration in neurologic skills. Thus, in several cases, the ABR was able to show that a structural malformation syndrome was in fact a progressive degenerative disorder, unsuspected on the basis of routine clinical examination.

To date, there have been no reported studies of the genetic transmission of central abnormalities of the ABR. Similarly, there is little published information on the relationships between observable chromosomal defects and the type of central auditory abnormalities reflected in pathologic ABRs. Studies conducted in our own laboratory have been promising with respect to early detection of progressive genetic disorders, counseling with regard to newborns genetically at risk for hearing loss, and, most recently, the detection of carrier status in selected neurologic disorders. We consider this one of the most promising new areas of application of evoked potentials.

PSYCHIATRIC DISORDERS

The primary diagnostic group to which we would like to address our comments is for those labeled autistic. The inclusion criteria for this disorder vary from laboratory to laboratory. Indeed, there is little or no consensus on a national or international basis concerning the diagnostic criteria for autism. Studying this disorder, especially in a quantitative fashion, is difficult at best. It is well known that many disorders mimic autism, including hearing impairment, mental retardation, and, in some cases, intoxications. Clearly, it would not be surprising to find auditory brainstem response abnormalities in the hearing impaired. Similarly, for the mentally retarded, central abnormalities could be explained on the basis of perinatal events such as hypoxia or ischemia. Therefore, any study addressing the issue of specific changes associated with autism must first address the question of diagnostic criteria in this disorder. Alternative diagnoses that may mimic autism and that have been associated with central abnormalities of the ABR must be explicitly excluded. The only other well-accepted association is between Wilson's disease and ABR abnormalities, particularly at high stimulus rates.

APPLICATIONS TO MONITORING

The initial impact of the ABR in neurology was on diagnostics. More recently, attention has been directed to the use of the ABR in monitoring surgical and nonsurgical therapeutics. The earliest suggestion was that the brainstem response could be used to determine whether steroids were effective in altering the course of multiple sclerosis. Despite early anecdotal evidence to support this contention, controlled studies are absent. The earliest suggestion that the ABR could measure therapeutic efficacy in children was anecdotal evidence from this laboratory that effective dietary therapy is associated with improvement in the ABR in maple syrup urine disease and phenylketonuria. To these can be added pyruvate dehydrogenase deficiency, citrullinemia, and proprionic acidemia. Beyond case reports, there are no published reports of *series* of patients with specific metabolic diseases who have been studied prospectively from the standpoint of correlating evoked potential changes with dietary changes. Salamy and colleagues, however, have demonstrated that kind of relationship in animals.

Another monitoring application is in prognosticating outcome in patients who are undergoing or have undergone asphyxia. In infants (nonpremature) with isolated asphyxia, an amplitude ratio of less than 0.5, when elicited by moderate intensity clicks, is predictive of a very poor outcome. Early reports, and our own experience, also suggest that significant increases in raised intracranial pressure are sometimes reflected in central abnormalities of the ABR that can normalize when the intracranial pressure is normalized.

Anecdotal reports have now been described in which radiation or chemotherapy of brainstem tumors has resulted in improvement of the ABR. This can be especially helpful in the pediatric-aged patient with a known central nervous system tumor who is admitted for the evaluation of vomiting. Tumor growth or recurrence versus intercurrent viral infection is often the differential diagnosis. Worsening of the ABR implies a noninfectious cause for the vomiting.

The most common monitoring application of the ABR in adults is for intraoperative recording. This is not so for the auditory response in the pediatric age group.

SUMMARY

The auditory brainstem response is a widely applied tool for the investigation of neurologic integrity in pediatric populations. The spectrum of disorders to which this response is sensitive is striking, although details regarding percentage of false positives and false negatives are not yet available for many of these disease categories. Clinical tests are often evaluated according to their false negative and false positive rates. The estimation of false negative rates requires external, objective criteria for the targeted disorder with demonstrated sensitivity to the pathology impinging upon auditory pathways—and usually such measures are unavailable or crude. The false positive rate not only depends on the availability of such external measures but also assumes stability of the underlying pathology. In other words, it is very difficult to evaluate false positive rates if the investigator admits the possibility of reversible disorders. The problems are difficult, and to date no adequate solutions have been put forth.

The primary uses of the technique have been in the recognition of unsuspected brainstem neurologic problems and in the detection of unsuspected hearing loss. It is customary to separate these two functions since they depend on different dependent variables, therapeutic interventions, and diagnostic evaluations. One of the assertions of this chapter is that the effective use of this tool cannot be achieved without an understanding of both audiologic and neurologic determinants of response abnormalities. Furthermore, optimization of central auditory development is not possible without consideration of the integrity of the peripheral auditory apparatus.

A major area of future applications is in monitoring of the progression or regression of central pathology. This concept is especially applicable in the case of tumors (therapeutic response to chemotherapy or radiotherapy) and in monitoring the efficacy of dietary therapy in metabolic disorders, the time course and rate of degeneration in neurodegenerative diseases, and the integrity of patients undergoing therapeutic coma.

We optimistically conclude that the auditory brainstem response will continue to play an important role in the areas of diagnostics and monitoring. If, as suspected, this measure proves sensitive when used as a means of monitoring the progress of neurologic improvement or deterioration, we should witness an increase in the popularity and utility of the ABR. As with most clinical measures, the power of the technique depends less on electronic sophistication than on the experience and expertise of those responsible for test interpretation.

This chapter represents a highly personalized description of these responses in our laboratory, and results may not be the same for another laboratory without strict agreement on data collection and interpretation guidelines. Although this chapter is more personal than scholarly, we still conclude that the ABR is and will continue to be a useful tool for the neurologic evaluation of pediatric-aged patients.

REFERENCES

Chiappa, K. H., Harrison, J. L., Brooks, E. B., & Young, R. R. (1980). Brainstem auditory evoked responses in 200 patients with multiple sclerosis. *Annals of Neurology, 7*(2), 135–143.

Finitzo-Hieber, T., Simhadri, R., & Hieber, J. P. (1981). Abnormalities of the auditory brainstem response—post meningitic infants and children. *International Journal of Otorhinolaryngology, 3,* 275–286.

Finitzo-Hieber, T., Hecox, K., & Cone, B. (1979). Brainstem auditory evoked potentials in patients with congenital atresia. *Laryngoscope, 89,* 1151–1158.

Fujita, M., Hosoki, M., & Miyazaki, M. (1981). Brainstem auditory evoked responses in spinocerebellar degeneration and Wilson's disease. *Annals of Neurology, 9,* 42–47.

Galambos, R., & Hecox, K. E. (1978). Clinical applications of the auditory brainstem response. *Otolaryngology Clinics of North America, 11*(3), 709–722.

Glasscock, M. D., Jackson, C. G., Josey, A. F., Dickins, J. R. E., & Wiet, R. J. (1979). Brainstem evoked responses audiometry in a clinical practice. *Laryngoscope, 89,* 1021–1035.

Greenfield, R. (1966). *Neuropathology* (pp. 142–143). Baltimore: Williams & Wilkins Company.

Hecox, K. E., Cone, B., & Blaw, M. E. (1981). Brainstem auditory evoked response in the diagnosis of pediatric neurologic diseases. *Neurology, 31,* 832–839.

Jerger, J., & Mauldin, L. (1978). Prediction of sensorineural hearing level from the brainstem evoked response. *Archives of Otolaryngology, 104,* 456–461.

Kaga, K., Kitazumi, E., & Kodama, K. (1979). Auditory brainstem responses of kernicterus infants. *International Journal of Pediatric Otorhinolaryngology, 1*(3), 255–264.

Leech, R. W., & Alford, E. C. Jr. (1977). Anoxic-ischemic encephalopathy in the human neonatal period. *Archives of Neurology, 32,* 109–113.

Selters, W. A., & Brackmann, D. E. (1977). Acoustic tumor detection with brainstem electric response audiometry. *Archives of Otolaryngology, 103*(4), 181–187.

Smith, D. H., Ingram, D. L., Smith, A. L., Gilles, F., & Bresnaw, M. J. (1973). Diagnosis and treatment-bacterial meningitis (A Symposium). *Pediatrics, 52,* 586–600.

Sohmer, H., Feinmesser, M., Bauberger-Tell, L., & Edelstein, E. (1977). Cochlear brainstem and cortical evoked responses in non-organic hearing loss. *Annals of Otology, Rhinology, and Laryngology, 86,* 227–234.

Sohmer, H., Gafni, M., & Chisin, R. (1978). Auditory nerve and brainstem responses: Comparison in awake and unconscious subjects. *Archives of Neurology, 35,* 228–230.

Sproles, E. T., Azerrad, J., Williamson, C., & Merrill, R. E. (1969). Meningitis due to Hemophilus influenzae: Long-term sequelae. *Journal of Pediatrics, 75,* 782–788.

Starr, A., & Achor, L. J. (1975). Auditory brainstem responses in neurological disease. *Archives of Neurology, 32,* 761–768.

Stockard, J. J., & Rossiter, V. S. (1977). Clinical and pathologic correlates of brainstem auditory response abnormalities. *Neurology, 27*(4), 316–325.

Suzuki, M., & Suzuki, J. I. (1977). Clinical application of the auditory-evoked brainstem response in children. *Aruis Nasus Larynx, 4*(1), 19–26.

Terkildsen, J., Huis In't Veld, F., & Osterhammel, P. (1977). Auditory brainstem responses in the diagnosis of cerebellopontine angle tumors. *Scandinavian Audiology, 6*(1), 43–47.

Chapter 16

Infant Assessment: Developmental and Age-Related Considerations

L. Clarke Cox

In the preceding chapters, the adult auditory brainstem response (ABR) has been detailed primarily as a rather consistent, static response unless acted upon by changes in stimulus or recording parameters or pathology. Responses obtained over time vary by only a small degree. In the infant ABR, however, not only are response morphology and latency different, but in addition the response changes as the infant matures. The infant response is affected by essentially the same factors as the adult response and is compounded by maturation. This creates specific problems that prevent using adult criteria for assessment. Additional variables such as premature birth further compound the problem and dictate separate and specific criteria for ABR testing of the infant.

THE INFANT RESPONSE

Morphology

The infant ABR response differs in virtually all measurement parameters from the adult response. The waveform morphology of a typical infant response (Figure 16-1) consists of three vertex/forehead positive peaks in comparison to the six or seven seen in the adult (Jacobson, Seitz, Mencher, & Parrott, 1981; Salamy & McKean, 1976). These waves correspond to the adult waves of I, III, and V by Jewett–Williston designation (Jewett & Williston, 1971). The absolute and interpeak latencies of these waves are longer than adult waves and the absolute and relative amplitudes are markedly different from those of the adult.

In the preterm infant the response emerges sometime after the 27th to 28th week of gestation. It is not uncommon, however, not to see the response until after 30 weeks (Galambos & Hecox, 1978; Starr, Amalie, Martin, & Sanders, 1977; Stockard & Westmoreland, 1981). The response is elicited only at higher stimulus intensities and is relatively low in amplitude (Stockard & Stockard, 1980). Wave I is usually the most prominent component, while wave V may not be as clearly formed and is smaller in amplitude (Montandon, Cao, Engel, & Grajew, 1979; Stockard & Stockard, 1980; Stockard & Stockard, 1983).

According to Stockard, Stockard, and Coen (1983) wave I makes its appearance between the 27th and 30th weeks of conceptional age (CA). The amplitude doubles during the first 1 to 2 weeks after which it slows to a steady rate of growth. Salamy, Fenn, and Bronshvag (1979) have reported that wave I amplitude reaches a plateau at approximately 3 months of age and decreases through adulthood.

FIGURE 16–1.
Typical infant ABR at 60 dB HL.

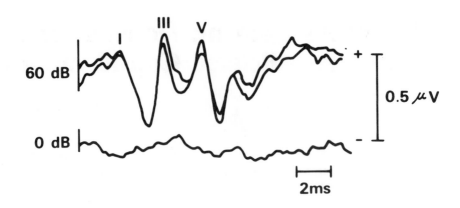

In contrast, wave V develops more slowly but is usually identifiable by 32 weeks CA (Stockard, Stockard, & Coen, 1983). Peak amplitude is not reached until approximately 12 months, and then minimal decreases occur in adulthood (Hecox & Burkhard, 1982).

Wave III has been documented as having similar development as wave I by Salamy et al. (1979), while Hecox and Burkhard (1982) have reported that wave III follows wave V development.

Amplitude

As a general rule, the largest amplitudes are seen in infants and the smallest in neonates, with those of adults falling somewhere in between (Leiberman, Sohmer, & Szabo, 1973). In evaluating absolute amplitude values, the infant wave V is considerably smaller than the adult wave V at comparable levels of intensity. The infant wave I, on the other hand, may be twice the adult amplitude (Salamy & McKean, 1976; Starr et al., 1977; Stockard, Stockard, & Sharbrough, 1978). Speculation regarding the large wave I amplitude includes close electrode approximation to the eighth nerve due to infant head size (Jacobson et al., 1981; Yoshie & Ohashi, 1969).

The variability of response amplitude in the adult has prevented its inclusion in the ABR test battery. In the infant the absolute amplitude variability is even greater due to a number of variables, such as recording procedures, age of the subject, transient changes in peripheral sensitivity (otitis media), and presentation levels (Hecox, Cone, & Blaw, 1981; Stockard & Westmoreland, 1981). At the present time, these variables, given the current levels of information and technology, prevent absolute amplitudes from contributing to infant assessment (Amadeo & Shagass, 1973; Chiappa, Gladstone, & Young, 1979; Rowe, 1978; Stockard, Stockard, Westmoreland, & Corfits, 1979).

In contrast, amplitude ratios have been advocated for adults (Starr & Achor, 1975; Stockard, Stockard, & Sharbrough, 1978) and infants (Hecox & Cone, 1981). The components of logical choice are waves I and V. Since wave I reflects peripheral activity and wave V central activity, comparisons of separate groups of auditory structures are obtained.

The amplitude ratio is smaller in infants (Hecox et al., 1981; Salamy, McKean, Pettett, & Mendelson, 1978) than in adults. The typical adult ratio approximates 3 (Chiappa et al., 1979;

Stockard, Stockard, & Sharbrough, 1978) while that of the infant is about 1 (Hecox et al., 1981). The adult ratio values appear to be reached sometime after the first year of life (Salamy, Mendelson, & Tooley, 1982). Consensus regarding a specific maturational age at which adult ratios are seen does not currently exist. A caveat regarding ratios must be noted here. As with virtually all other ABR measures used in infant assessment, numerous factors (electrode montage and impedance, stimulus level, age of the subject, muscle activity, etc.) can affect the amplitude ratio measurement and as far as possible must be controlled.

Latency

In Table 16-1, typical latencies from various age groups are shown for waves I, III, V, and I–V. The obvious difference between the infant and the adult is the prolonged latency of all components. As noted in the table, with increases in age, the latency of all components decreases. The rate of change occurs in a consistent fashion with wave I reaching adult values by 2–3 months (Jacobson, Morehouse, & Johnson, 1982; Salamy et al., 1982) and wave V sometimes after 1 to 2 years of age (Salamy & McKean, 1976). Wave III follows a timetable similar to wave V. Waves II and IV, which typically are not seen in the newborn, follow maturation schedules which parallel adjacent waves, that is, wave II follows wave I and wave IV follows wave V (Salamy et al., 1982).

Several factors may decrease waveform component latencies: myelination, cochlear maturation, resolution of middle ear abnormalities (fluid, unabsorbed mesenchyme), increased synaptic efficiency, and firing synchrony (Cox, Hack, & Metz, 1981b; Kiang, Watanabe, Thomas, et al., 1965; Salamy & McKean, 1976). Whether individual factors or a combination of factors acting in concert are responsible for these changes is unknown and requires further study.

As in the adult, relative latencies are used to assess brainstem transmission (Salamy & McKean, 1976). The components of choice are again waves I and V. Wave I is used as a point of reference and wave V is used because it is the most stable of the ABR components. In the infant the interpeak latencies (IPL) of waves I and V reflect the integrity of the central auditory system and, when assessed over time, document maturation. IPLs of I–III and III–V have also been used to denote maturation (Jacobson et al., 1982; Salamy et al., 1982).

MEASUREMENT VARIABILITY

The above properties of the ABR response—amplitude, amplitude ratios, latencies, and IPLs—are all affected by many factors, chief among which are age and stimulus intensity. To complete an assessment of an infant, the effects of these various factors must be known and controlled if ABR testing is to be completed. In the following section a number of these factors are discussed.

Age

Age affects both amplitude and latency of the response. By plotting decreases in latency as a function of age, a measure of the maturation of the response and possibly of the auditory system is obtained. The latency–age (L–A) function for wave V has been documented. In the preterm period the reported rate of change has ranged from 0.04 to 0.4 ms decrease per week (Schulman-Galambos & Galambos, 1975; 1979; Starr et al., 1977) with a general consensus of approximately 0.2 ms (Hecox & Burkhard, 1982). For wave I, reports of a 0.45-ms/week decrease up to 32 weeks and a 0.15-ms/week average to term have occurred (Stockard, Stockard, & Coen, 1983). Because the reported data vary, L-A functions are not now clinically useful. A major contributor to the data variability is inexactness in determining the subject's age. Agreement between the ages estimated by the mother's last menstrual cycle and by examination is not good. In spite of numerous studies completed with a variety of procedures, determination of gestational age with less than a 2-week error has not been achieved. Since maturational changes in the infant ABR occur in a 2-week time period (Galambos & Despland, 1980) agreement between studies detailing L-A function is impossible. Speculatively speaking, at some point the L-A function may assist with this problem by serving as a supplementary index of gestational age, barring the presence of pathology.

Maturational changes in the IPL have also been documented (Salamy, McKean & Buda, 1975; Starr et al., 1977; Stockard et al., 1979; Stockard & Westmoreland, 1981). Stockard and Westmoreland (1981) have reported considerable variations among subjects between 32 and 34 weeks CA. The IPL decreased at a rate of 0.45-ms/week while, in contrast, at 40 weeks the change was less than 0.1-ms/week. Both absolute latency and IPLs exhibit decreases in latency from term (approximately 5.0 ms) to a period between 12 and 18 months when adult values (approximately 4.0 ms) are normally reached (Salamy & McKean, 1976; Salamy et al., 1982).

Temperature

Hypothermia has been shown to affect the ABR response. Central temperature reductions to below 35°C produce amplitude reduction and prolonged IPLs (Stockard, Sharbrough, & Tinker, 1978). Unless the core temperature is known, neurologic abnormality may be erroneously inferred. The problem is particularly acute in low-birthweight infants, in whom hypothermia is common (Stockard & Westmoreland, 1981). In this population, normothermia should prevail during ABR testing.

Sex

Adult female IPLs are comparatively less than those of males while wave V latencies are approximately 0.2 ms shorter (Kjaer, 1979; McClelland & McCrea, 1979). In the normal infant and preadolescent child no sex differences have been documented (Jacobson et al., 1982; McClelland & McCrea, 1979; Stockard et al., 1979). Regarding the preterm infant, opinions vary, but differences in latency between male and female subjects have been noted (Cox, Hack, & Metz, 1981a; Pauwels, Vogeleer, Clement, Rousseeuw, & Kaufman, 1982). The differences noted by Cox et al. (1981a) at 33 to 39 weeks CA apparently were transient because retesting of the same subjects at 4 months produced no sex differences. The differences noted are likely due to the higher incidence of neurologic and risk factor involvement seen in the preterm male (Ambramowicz & Barnett, 1970; Fitzhardinge, Pape, Arstikaitis, et al., 1974).

Conductive Hearing Loss

Conductive pathology is only briefly discussed, as a complete treatise is found in chapter 7 of this book. Middle ear disorders reduce stimulus intensity at the cochlea and therefore increase all absolute ABR component latencies (Mendelson, Salamy, Lenoir, & McKean, 1979). Stockard and Stockard (1983) have reported that conductive disorders may decrease IPLs due to greater effects of deficit on wave I. The care of the preterm infant or the infant admitted to the neonatal intensive care unit (NICU) entails a number of factors that predispose to conductive disorder. With intubation for assisted ventilation and tube feeding, decreased swallowing occurs. This,

Table 16–1.
Means and standard deviations of waves I, III, V, and I–V of various age groups at six intensity levels.

db HL		33–34 Wks CA				35–36 Wks CA				37–38 Wks CA				39–40 Wks CA			
		I	III	V	I–V	I	III	V	I–V	I	III	V	I–V	I	III	V	I–V
80	X	2.26	5.01	7.38	5.13	2.13	4.47	7.19	5.06	2.02	4.61	7.01	4.99	1.79	4.26	6.72	4.93
	SD	.81	.74	.72	.67	.69	.71	.48	.56	.53	.47	.48	.48	.59	.62	.40	.59
70	X	2.59	5.22	7.49	4.90	2.33	4.97	7.41	5.08	2.24	4.75	7.17	4.93	1.94	4.57	6.83	4.89
	SD	.84	.79	.56	.75	.68	.55	.61	.64	.67	.41	.47	.54	.51	.44	.48	.46
60	X	3.07	5.38	7.76	4.69	2.73	5.33	7.68	4.95	2.47	5.06	7.28	4.70	2.38	4.71	7.07	4.69
	SD	.69	.84	.87	.91	.71	.63	.41	.52	.89	.43	.55	.71	.58	.62	.49	.51
50	X	3.21	5.79	8.19	4.98	3.18	5.72	8.11	4.93	2.94	5.43	7.65	4.71	2.65	5.01	7.31	4.66
	SD	.88	.64	.56	.73	.51	.84	.56	.77	.64	.73	.72	.68	.72	.59	.53	.60
40	X	3.59	6.17	8.51	4.92	3.57	6.00	8.51	4.94	3.22	5.61	7.95	4.73	3.06	5.36	7.65	4.59
	SD	.97	.63	.77	.78	.89	.71	.60	.73	.78	.66	.69	.71	.87	.74	.55	.66
30	X	4.17	6.46	8.88	4.71	4.06	6.58	8.77	4.72	3.78	6.31	8.39	4.61	3.59	5.79	8.03	4.44
	SD	1.13	1.03	.97	.98	.95	.82	.99	.87	1.04	.78	.88	.90	.81	.84	.72	.69

db HL		2 Months				6 Months				12 Months				Adult			
		I	III	V	I–V	I	III	V	I–V	I	III	V	I–V	I	III	V	I–V
80	X	1.64	4.18	6.39	4.75	1.60	4.10	6.27	4.67	1.62	3.79	5.93	4.31	1.59	3.64	5.57	3.98
	SD	.43	.32	.29	.36	.26	.31	.21	.28	.24	.18	.17	.19	.24	.17	.16	.25
70	X	1.81	4.27	6.51	4.70	1.79	4.26	6.50	4.71	1.81	3.84	6.14	4.33	1.75	2.86	5.67	3.92
	SD	.30	.41	.38	.33	.32	.34	.31	.26	.23	.23	.19	.23	.21	.23	.15	.22
60	X	2.14	4.64	6.69	4.55	1.93	4.46	6.34	4.41	1.91	4.01	6.15	4.24	1.88	4.11	5.81	3.93
	SD	.42	.35	.30	.34	.31	.40	.27	.30	.29	.22	.24	.33	.27	.20	.27	.22
50	X	2.35	4.85	6.91	4.56	2.28	4.75	6.68	4.40	2.18	4.43	6.47	4.29	2.23	4.49	6.12	3.89
	SD	.44	.37	.34	.37	.41	.37	.41	.36	.26	.32	.21	.27	.34	.18	.22	.24
40	X	2.72	5.18	7.23	4.51	2.49	4.93	6.86	4.37	2.43	4.59	6.62	4.19	2.46	4.55	6.29	3.83
	SD	.41	.45	.31	.46	.48	.37	.33	.43	.40	.29	.36	.37	.31	.26	.27	.15
30	X	3.11	5.64	7.58	4.47	2.86	5.08	7.20	4.34	2.90	5.11	7.09	4.19	2.83	5.00	5.79	3.86
	SD	.62	.39	.48	.52	.61	.50	.44	.42	.44	.51	.39	.47	.36	.31	.29	.30

in concert with constant supine positioning, affects ventilation of the middle ear by undermining eustachian tube function (Balkany, Berman, Simmons, & Jafek, 1978; Paradise, 1980).

The incidence of conductive disorder in the NICU has been reported to be as high as 50% (Stockard, Stockard, & Sharbrough, 1980). While other reports give lower percentages (Balkany et al., 1978; Cox et al., 1981b), the figures suggest that conductive disorder commonly occurs in the NICU, particularly in the very low birthweight infant. The major concern with conductive disorder lies with the transient changes in ABR latency. Inappropriate determination of disorder may occur if careful evaluation of the response is not made. Specifically, wave I must be accurately noted for correct identification of peripheral or central disorders.

Stimulus Intensity

Latency. In the adult and infant responses, absolute latency decreases as the stimulus intensity increases (Figure 16-2). Although the changes are nonlinear in the adult, they are consistent. In the infant, however, there is greater variability in the change.

FIGURE 16-2.
Illustration of changes in latency as a function of intensity.

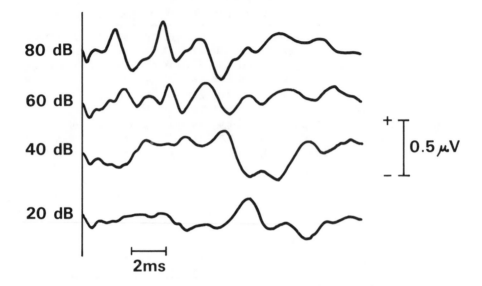

The adult wave I exhibits a "transition zone" between 40 and 50 dB HL (Stockard et al., 1979). This transition zone is characterized by a sudden change in the latency of wave I. Wave V, on the other hand, exhibits a more gradual shift over the intensity range. The infant exhibits similar wave I changes, but has two "transitional zones" at 30–40 and 60–70 dB HL (Stockard & Stockard, 1980; Stockard & Westmoreland, 1981).

With increases in intensity, wave I typically decreases in latency faster than wave V. This difference results in changes in the IPL as a function of intensity. Table 16-1 illustrates the decrease in IPL as the intensity decreases. This action is responsible for the decrease in IPL and the moderate decrease in wave V latency that may be seen in conductive losses. Not all studies have supported the decrease in IPL with decreases in intensity (Jacobson et al., 1982).

Amplitude. The amplitude of the ABR response is affected by intensity in a parallel fashion. Figure 16-3 illustrates that as intensity decreases, amplitude does also. The amplitude of wave I exhibits a "transitional" response similar to the latency response. A doubling in amplitude has been reported at between 60 and 70 dB HL in both infants and adults (Stockard, Stockard, & Coen, 1983). The amplitude ratio in the infant is also affected by stimulus intensity in an inverse fashion—as intensity increases the amplitude ratio decreases (Jacobson et al., 1982). This effect occurs primarily due to differential reduction in amplitude. Stockard et al. (1978b) reported a one-third reduction in wave V amplitude as intensity was reduced by 50 dB while wave I exhibited a 10-fold reduction in amplitude.

Slope. The slope of the infant wave V latency–intensity (L-I) function has been the subject of considerable attention and disagreement. In adults the L-I function has been used in differentiating cochlear and conductive pathology (Galambos & Hecox, 1978; Picton & Smith, 1978). The L-I slope in adults has been reported to be between 0.28 (Pratt & Sohmer, 1976) and 0.40 ms/10 dB (Galambos & Hecox, 1978) while Stockard, Stockard, and Coen (1983) have reported a case of 0.14 ms/10 dB. In the infant the slope has been documented as being approximately 0.007 ms/dB slower than in adults by Hecox and Burkhard (1982), indicating

FIGURE 16–3.
Effects of intensity on absolute amplitude of the infant wave V.

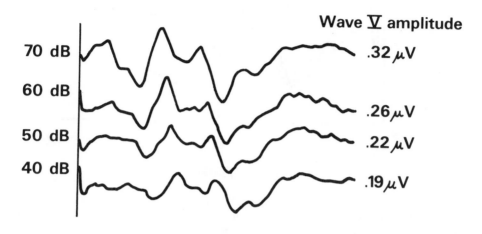

a 0.28 ms/10 dB function. Other studies (Hecox & Galambos, 1974; Stockard, Stockard, & Coen, 1983) have reported just the opposite: 0.28 ms/10 dB for adults and 0.36 ms/10 dB for newborns. Stockard, Stockard, & Coen (1983) have reported the slope in preterm infants to be steeper than in term newborns, while Lee and Cox (1982) found preterm L-I functions identical to those of 1- to 2-month-old infants. Because the amount of shift is not stable over a given intensity range (40 dB), L-I functions obtained over smaller ranges doe not correlate. Until the intensity range of the L-I function has been equated across studies, L-I agreement will not be reached.

Stimulus Polarity

The polarity of the stimulus typically used has been either condensation (C), rarefaction (R), or alternating. Single-polarity stimuli produce different initial movements of the basilar and tympanic membranes related to onset of firing of the auditory nerve. Initial firing of the nerve coincides with R stimuli (Kiang et al., 1965). Waveform morphology differences between single- and alternating-polarity clicks have been recognized and generally accepted (Picton, Stapells, & Campbell, 1981; Stockard et al., 1979). Polarity effects on latency have not been afforded similar agreement (Weber, Seitz, & McCutcheon, 1981). Stockard et al. (1979) have reported that the R/C difference is particularly evident in infants. Figure 16-4 illustrates the differences between R and C waveforms. The reported latency difference of wave I between R and C is 0.12 ms (Stockard et al., 1979; Stockard, Stockard, & Coen, 1983). Because polarity primarily affects wave I, the IPLs also exhibit polarity effects. Although consistent documentation has been published of wave V insensitivity to polarity effects (Ornitz, Mo, Olson, & Waller, 1980) and shorter wave I latency to R clicks (Coats & Martin, 1977; Stockard et al., 1980), disagreement exists regarding the degree of effect (Jacobson et al., 1982).

In advocating the use of single-polarity clicks, Stockard et al. (1980) have suggested that, because wave I is attenuated to a greater degree than wave V with alternating clicks, the amplitude ratio will be affected. They also report that alternating clicks distort the newborn response. Jacobson et al. (1982) advocate alternating-polarity clicks because of the variability of single-polarity stimuli. For example, in the Stockard et al. (1979) study, approximately 17% of normals

FIGURE 16–4.
Differences in R and C waveforms.

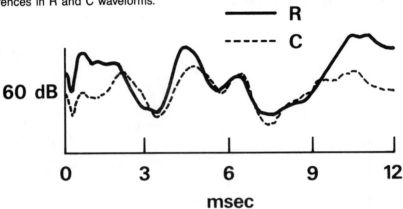

had shorter wave I latencies to C clicks while 22% exhibited no differences. Furthermore, in some normals, wave V may be absent or the amplitude ratio reduced with R stimuli and present with C or alternating stimuli (Stockard, Stockard, & Coen, 1983). One advantage of using alternating stimuli lies in the reduction of stimulus artifact, particularly with tone burst stimuli. Figure 16-5 illustrates the effects of using alternating stimuli to reduce artifact.

The question as to which polarity is optimal for infant testing remains unsettled. The differences between the reported data are not great; therefore single- or alternating-polarity stimuli can be used with confidence. If a wave I response is not clear with alternating stimuli, single-polarity measurement data should be obtained. Conversely, if a response is absent or stimulus artifact is excessive with single-polarity stimuli, alternating-stimuli data should be obtained. Additional techniques of enhancing wave I are found in chapter 6.

Stimulus Frequency

Clicks. The most common stimulus used to elicit the ABR has been the broad band click generated by exciting a transducer with a rectangular voltage plus (100 μs rise–fall). To obtain a satisfactory response, synchronous activity of individual neural units of the acoustic nerve and brainstem must occur (Picton et al., 1981). Although very short duration clicks are ideal for eliciting synchronous neural activity, frequency specificity is sacrificed.

Click stimuli have been acceptable in spite of the lack of frequency-specific information. The problems that arise are localized to endeavors to estimate hearing sensitivity for discrete frequencies based on the click ABR. In the hearing-impaired infant, habilitation/rehabilitation has traditionally relied on frequency-specific information. Click ABRs can overestimate hearing sensitivity with precipitous hearing losses above 2000–3000 Hz and low-frequency hearing loss below 1000 Hz. Since the latter case occurs infrequently and the former is also not common in infants, the problem is relatively minor in infant assessment.

Frequency Specificity. Stimuli such as tone burst, tone pip, or filtered click produce adequate synchronization but their brief duration results in the spread of the frequency spectrum (Eggermont & Don, 1980). In the normal ear, intensity affects frequency specificity by increasing cochlear participation (basal shift) as the intensity increases. Only at very low levels is there a consistent relationship between stimulus frequency and region of basilar membrane displacement (Eggermont & Don, 1980). In cochlear pathology, these relationships may differ, however.

FIGURE 16–5.
Illustration of stimulus artifact reduction with alternating-polarity tone burst.

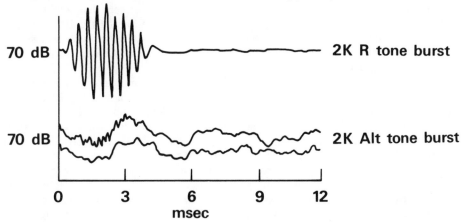

Brief tone stimuli produce poorer thresholds than clicks and are longer in latency (Suzuki, Harai, & Horiuchi, 1977). Wave V latency increases with decreases in frequency (Kodera, Yamana, Yamana, & Suzuki, 1977), for example, 10.6 ms at 1000 Hz and 8.44 ms at 4000 Hz (Stockard, Stockard, & Coen, 1983). Data describing tonal stimuli in the infant population are scant and studies of the effects of age are lacking. Tonal responses can be obtained consistently at 1000 Hz and possibly at 500 Hz in the infant (Yamada, Hidemichi, Kodera, & Yamane, 1983), but further research is needed.

Stimulus Temporality

Stimulus duration has limited effects on ABR latency and amplitude since it is an onset response (Brinkman & Scherg, 1979). Few reports address rise–fall effects on the infant ABR. Hecox and Burkhard (1982) have reported on/off effects that are peculiar to neonates but only on a preliminary basis.

In adults and infants, increasing the rise time increases response latency while amplitude remains unaffected (Brinkman & Scherg, 1979; Suzuki & Horiuchi, 1981). Neonates exhibit a rise time/latency effect that differs from the adults; increases in rise time produce smaller increases in latency. Cochlear and/or middle ear immaturity have been suggested as factors (Hecox & Burkhard, 1982).

Stimulus Rate

Changes in stimulus rate affect the latency and/or amplitude of virtually all ABR components (Figure 16-6). The more immature the auditory system, the greater the effects (Stockard et al., 1979). While wave V amplitude is least affected by rate, increases in the latency of wave V do occur with increases in presentation rate (Despland & Galambos, 1980; Fujikawa & Weber, 1977; Stockard et al., 1979).

Wave I shows a slower or reduced latency shift with rate changes in comparison to wave V. This results in the IPLs increasing with faster rates. Wave I amplitude also decreases with increased stimulus rates, resulting in an increase in the V/I amplitude ratio (Stockard, Stockard, & Coen, 1983).

The slope of the latency–rate (L–R) function is between 60 and 79 μs/decade for adults and from 140 to 163 μs/decade for term infants (Hecox & Burkhard, 1982; Lasky, 1983). For preterm infants the slope has been reported to be considerably steeper than adults or term newborns—227 μs/decade (Lasky, 1983). Within restricted intensities (30–70 dB), the L–R is linear and consequently expected functions can be predicted based on the subject's age. This provides the potential to assess central nervous system maturation and abnormality in infants using the L–R function.

The click rate for infant assessment is chosen by the amount of accuracy and information desired. If wave V is the only component of interest, as is sometimes the case in ABR screening procedures, faster click rates of 30–40/s can be used. Although test time is reduced, definition of earlier waves generally will be inconsistent because they are degraded at the faster rate. Above 30/s wave I is reduced in amplitude, threshold may increase, and peak definition is degraded. In testing infants, particularly neonates and preterms, slower click rates are usually necessary for consistent peak definition. For neurologic applications 10/s is a popular rate (Stockard & Westmoreland, 1981). For term and stable preterm infants, 21/s has been shown to be a good compromise between peak definition and test time (Lee & Cox, 1982). With poor waveform definition at faster rates, the logical approach is to reduce the presentation rate. Figure 16-7 illustrates the effects of a rate change of only 10/s.

Stimulus Presentation Mode

Because binaural stimulation produces as much as a 60% increase in amplitude while latency is unaffected (Møller & Blegvad, 1976; Starr & Achor, 1975; Van Olphen, Rodenburg, & Verwey, 1978), it has been suggested by Pauwels et al. (1982) that binaural testing be used with infants to increase the percentage of "interpretable" records. There is no doubt (with binaural stimulation) that response amplitude will increase and waveform definition may be easier. The trade-off in information lost would lead us to seriously question this practice, however. With binaural stimulation, unilateral peripheral hearing loss and possibly central auditory disorders could be missed. The strength and uniqueness of ABR testing are diluted without information about each ear. Binaural stimulation is not recommended as the standard mode of presentation, particularly with screening procedures. As an adjunct procedure, binaural derived ABRs may contribute to the assessment.

While discussing binaural presentation, a brief mention of binaural interaction should be made. Binaural interaction is determined by subtracting the summed monaural responses from binaural responses. The obtained difference is the binaural interaction (Dobie & Berlin, 1979; Van Olphen et al., 1978). In the adult, binaural interaction is not without controversy and consequently has not enjoyed clinical acceptance. Binaural interaction has been observed in the infant (Ainslie & Boston, 1980) but little else has been reported. With the interest in ABR-measured neuromaturation, the potential of binaural interaction should be further explored.

Electrode Configuration

The position of the electrodes interacts with and affects waveform morphology and latency (McPherson, Hirosugi, & Starr, 1984; Stockard et al., 1980; Stockard, Stockard, & Coen, 1983). Wave I amplitude is larger in a horizontal montage—earlobe to earlobe, or mastoid to mastoid—than in the standard vertical montage—vertex to mastoid/earlobe (Terkildsen & Osterhammel, 1981). When wave I is difficult to detect in the standard montage, a change to a horizontal montage may be helpful (McPherson et al., 1984). On the other hand, maximum wave V amplitude is seen with the vertical montage—vertex (Cz) or forehead (Fz) to mastoid/earlobe

FIGURE 16–6.
Effects of stimulus repetition rate changes.

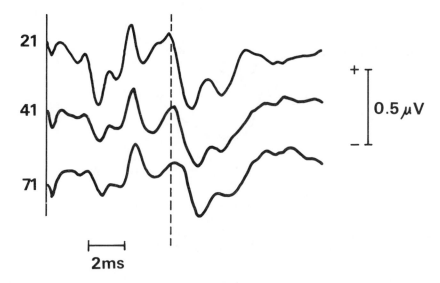

(Martin & Moore, 1977). In the adult, wave V amplitude is almost never larger with a horizontal montage. In infants, however, as many as 40% have a greater wave V amplitude with a horizontal montage (Hecox & Burkhard, 1982).

There is some difference of opinion in the literature regarding position of the positive electrode. Some authors are proponents of vertex placement (Barden & Peltzman, 1980; Despland & Galambos, 1980; Galambos & Hecox, 1978; Hecox & Cone, 1981; Kileny, Connelly, & Robertson, 1980; Morgan & Salle, 1980; Salamy, 1981, Salamy et al., 1982) while others recommend forehead placement (Cox, Hack, & Metz, 1982; Harris, Mollerstrom, Reimer, & Grennert, 1981; Jacobson et al., 1982; Kaga & Tamaka, 1980; Kodera et al., 1977; Marshall, Reichert, Kerley, & Davis, 1980; Mjoen, 1981; Pauwels et al., 1982; Roberts, Davis, Phon, et al., 1982).

Changes in amplitude and latency with different negative electrode sites have been well documented (Stockard et al., 1980; Stockard, Stockard, & Coen, 1983; Stockard & Westmoreland, 1981). Similar waveform changes between the vertex and forehead have not been seen. McPherson et al. (1984) noted no significant differences between vertex and an anterior electrode site (nasion). For convenience, some authors have suggested using forehead sites to eliminate fontanel problems (Jacobson et al., 1982). If the positive electrode site is not used interchangeably, either vertex or forehead electrode placement is acceptable.

Electrode Impedance

The general rule for ABR electrode impedance is that values above 5000 ohms are unacceptable. Frequently this maximal level is exceeded. This is particularly true in the neonate because of tenderness of the skin. The level of 5000 ohms is not sacred; in fact it is an arbitrary level. Eccard and Weber (1983) have reported satisfactory ABR results with impedances above 5000 ohms.

The impedance balance, however, is a critical factor. Unbalanced impedance between electrodes is considerably more detrimental to "pure" ABR recordings than is high impedance.

FIGURE 16–7.
Changes in waveform morphology seen with a 10 per second change in repetition rate.

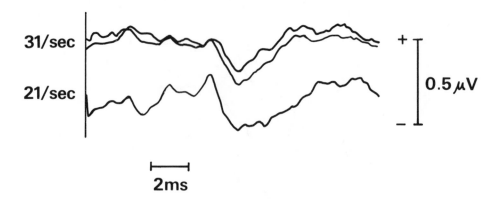

If possible, impedance should be less than 10,000 ohms and equal at each electrode site or else the chance of increased noise levels at the preamplifier will exist.

Number of Samples

The infant response amplitude is generally lower than that of the adult and the morphology is immature. In addition, most infant ABR testing (specifically neonatal) is not accomplished in a sound-treated environment. The net effect is that the number of samples averaged must be increased to obtain definable peaks. In a quiet infant 2000 samples may be adequate. If there is muscle activity, high electrode impedance, electrical noise, and so forth, 4000 or 8000 samples may be needed. The test time will increase in the latter cases, but whenever possible accuracy takes precedence over time.

Frequency Filter Settings

Absolute and relative amplitude and absolute latency are affected by frequency filtering. Amplitudes decrease, absolute latencies increase, and thresholds increase when the low-frequency filter setting exceeds 100 Hz or if the high-filter setting falls below 3000 Hz (Stockard et al., 1978b). Lower filter settings (5 Hz) may minimize phase shifts and waveform distortion caused by analog high-pass filters (McPherson et al., 1984). In a nursery or NICU, however, a higher cut-off is desirable (150 Hz) to reduce line noise (60 Hz). Filter settings of 150–3000 Hz appear to be most popular with infant testing.

Ambient Acoustic Noise

Background masking is a problem in infant testing because, as mentioned previously, frequently the ABR data are gathered in the nursery. Regardless of the type of earphone used, the typical ambient noise levels found in nurseries create ipsilateral masking. Wave I, which is associated with the acoustic nerve, is unaffected by noise (Kiang et al., 1965). Wave V is affected by noise (prolonged latencies) and may result in both relative and absolute latency shifts (Stockard & Westmoreland, 1981). This differential effect may contribute to the variety of values seen in published normative data. Since ambient noise levels vary among settings, the masking effects also vary. To maintain reliability of established norms, testing should be carried out in similar levels of ambient noise (or, preferably, in quiet).

Ambient Electrical Noise

In addition to acoustic noise, a multitude of other problems can arise due to ambient electrical interference. In the nursery and especially the NICU, the environment can be very hostile when attempting ABR. Various monitors (heart rate, respiration, etc.), IVs, and other equipment produce electrical interference, which can contaminate or obscure the ABR response. The introduction of 60-Hz notch filters, isolation transformers, earphone shielding, electrode braiding, repositioning the subject or test equipment or both, and similar tactics have been used to reduce electromagnetic interference. On occasion it may even be necessary (with medical approval) to shut the monitor equipment off during testing.

To control for these problems it is paramount that silent runs and trial replication occur. It is risky to suggest that silent runs or trial replications are not required, as some have done (Zubick, Fried, Epstein, et al., 1982). Figure 16-8 illustrates this problem.

Contralateral Masking

The effects of contralateral masking on the infant ABR are not entirely known. At high intensities, however, a contralateral ABR can be seen with a "dead" ear (Chiappa et al., 1979). This suggests that at stimulus levels above 60–70 dB HL, contralateral masking may be needed to prevent the non-test ear from producing or contributing to the obtained response. Routine masking of stimulus intensities below 60–70 dB is not warranted.

THE ESTABLISHMENT OF NORMATIVE DATA

Establishing the normality or abnormality of ABR responses is based on comparison to what is considered typical for the subject being tested. Full-term neonates and older infants need norms that reflect their age. As mentioned previously, precise determination of age at birth is difficult so the norms must reflect approximate rather than exact ages. Each clinic or laboratory must obtain exclusive normative data. Because of the number of factors that influence the ABR (equipment, ambient noise, stimulus frequency, intensity, rise–fall, etc.), norms obtained from one test location cannot be used at another. Data obtained at other locations may be helpful for comparison.

The preterm infant presents a very difficult group from which to obtain norms. A major problem arises from the fact that an infant born prematurely is not normal (Cox et al., 1981a). Furthermore, a considerable number of risk factors (hyperbilirubinemia, hypoxia, respiratory distress, acidosis, aminoglycoside therapy, etc.) that occur in the preterm population may affect the ABR (Cox, Hack, & Metz, 1984). In principle, norms can be established. One possible approach is to obtain mean data from preterm infants who are healthy and free from as many risk factors as possible (Cox et al., 1981a). One should not expect the data to be absolutely predictive. Longitudinal data (Cox, Hack, & Metz, 1982; Stockard, Stockard, Kleinberg, & Westmoreland, 1983) have shown that ABR abnormalities noted in the NICU do not have a perfect correlation with subsequent hearing loss. Furthermore, infants at risk without auditory

FIGURE 16-8.
Example of electrical interference. The lower trace appears to be a response when in fact
no stimulus was delivered to the subject.

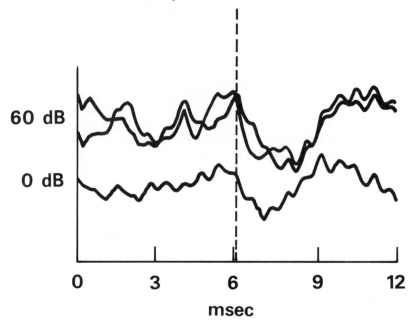

deficits or neurologic difficulties still have a sufficiently different ABR response as to distinguish
them from term infants who are not at risk (Salamy, Mendelson, Tooley, & Chaplin, 1980).

The mean data obtained from preterm infants will also be approximate due to problems
related to age determination, which is itself much more problematical that in the full-term infant.
Mean data (norms) for preterms can be obtained from published reports and utilized with some
degree of confidence. Experiments over the years at many different laboratories support this
approach (Cox et al., 1982; Despland & Galambos, 1980; Kaga & Tamaka, 1980; Pauwels et
al., 1982; Schulman-Galambos & Galambos, 1975; Weber, 1982). Also, obtained theoretical
distributions of the various ABR components in infants have all been Gaussian (Cox et al.,
1981a; Salamy, 1981; Stockard, Stockard, & Coen, 1983). This distribution adds to the confidence
of the above procedure.

The factors that have been discussed have generally been recognized as affecting the infant
ABR. Those mentioned by no means complete the list. There are perhaps other factors whose
effects are not fully understood or are yet to be identified. As the effects of these factors become
known, the ABR test paradigm will change.

One of these factors that is yet to be fully understood is cochlear maturation and its impact
on the infant ABR. Developmentally the inner ear is recognized as being complete by the 20th
week of gestation (Elliot & Elliot, 1964). Yet at birth, responsivity across frequency is not uniform.
At birth the infant appears more responsive to low-frequency stimuli. As the infant matures,
it has been suggested that the cochlea does also and becomes more responsive to high-frequency
stimuli (Cox et al., 1981b; Hecox, 1975; Hecox & Burkhard, 1982; Morgon & Salle, 1980; Starr
et al., 1977; Stockard et al., 1980). Rubel and Ryals (1982), however, have suggested that it is
the basal, not the apical, end that is responding to low-frequency stimuli in the infant. Phase
studies, on the other hand, suggest that the apical regions mature earlier than the basal regions
(Stockard et al., 1980).

Behavioral (Franklin & Bremer, 1982) and electrophysiologic (Wolf & Goldstein, 1980) studies have demonstrated a better response consistency to low-frequency stimuli than to high-frequency stimuli. Animal studies have shown that although, morphologically, cochlear development occurs from base to apex (Pujol & Marty, 1970; Sanders, Coles, & Gates, 1973), at birth the cochlear response is oriented toward lower frequencies (Aitkin & Moore, 1975; Konishi, 1973).

The recent work of Hooks and Weber (1984) with human subjects would appear to parallel the animal studies. With bone-conduction stimuli, these authors found the ABR response latencies shorter than air-conduction latencies. These results are directly opposite to those of adult bone-conduction ABR latencies. The major concentration of energy in the air-conduction click is approximately 4000 Hz (Cox & Metz, 1980). In the bone-conduction click, the major portion of the energy lies below 2500 Hz (Mauldin & Jerger, 1979). The shorter latency of the bone ABRs may have been due to the lower frequency of the stimulus. This would support the notion of apical maturation occurring first in the infant or the basal end representing more low-frequency components and with maturation shifting in frequency to apical regions. The full implications of these data have not been realized. Further research is needed, particularly with respect to control of the filtering (is the response maximized or created by the filter settings?), before practical application can occur.

STANDARDIZATION

Currently there are no published standards for adult or infant ABR parameters such as stimulus frequency, rise/fall, intensity reference, or stimulus phase. With time, standards very likely will be adopted and published. Until then, data using carefully controlled designs must be obtained. For those involved in clinical ABR testing of infants the process of standardization will be facilitated if careful documentation is made of the results using currently available procedures. Utilizing esoteric procedures will not expedite the development of standards. There is currently an adequate body of literature from which test procedures can be extracted.

CONCLUSIONS

The literature describing the infant ABR is replete with studies that extol its virtues, studies that question its utility, studies that recommend universal use, and studies that recommend cautious, conservative application. Regardless of the various opinions expressed regarding the ABR, the fact that the procedure has not fallen into disfavor as have other auditory evoked potentials speaks to the status of the procedure. The majority of all published literature is favorable and indicates that the ABR is the test of choice for newborn and infant assessment. Cautious interpretation and application of the ABR is logical. Yet at the same time, the literature supports optimism as the potential of the procedure begins to be realized.

The contributions of the ABR to early identification of hearing impairment are such that it appears firmly entrenched in the NICU and nursery. The ABR has established the incidence of hearing loss for NICU graduates and is the most powerful tool currently available for assessment of infant auditory function. Estimation of hearing sensitivity and determination of pathology are now routine ABR procedures. The potential of neurologic and developmental evaluation appears promising. With the continuation of aggressive research its full potential can be realized.

REFERENCES

Ainslie, P. J., & Boston, J. R. (1980). Comparison of brainstem auditory evoked potentials for monaural and binaural stimuli. *Electroencephalography and Clinical Neurophysiology*, *49*(3), 147–150.

Aitkin, L. M., & Moore, D. R. (1975). Inferior colliculus II. Development of tuning characteristics and tonotopic organization in central nucleus of the neonate cat. *Journal of Neurophysiology*, *38*, 1208–1216.

Amadeo, M., & Shagass, C. (1973). Brief latency click-evoked potentials during waking and sleep in man. *Psychophysiology*, *10*, 244–260.

Ambramowicz, M., & Barnett, H. L. (1970). Sex ratio of infant mortality. *American Journal of Diseases of Children*, *119*, 314–315.

Balkany, T., Berman, S., Simmons, M., & Jafek, B. (1978). Middle ear effusions in neonates. *Laryngoscope*, *88*, 398–405.

Barden, T. P., & Peltzman, P. (1980). Newborn brain stem auditory evoked responses and perinatal clinical events. *American Journal of Obstetrics and Gynecology*, *136*, 912–919.

Brinkman, R. D., & Scherg, M. (1979). Human auditory on and off potentials of the brainstem. *Scandinavian Audiology*, *8*, 27–32.

Chiappa, K. N., Gladstone, K. J., & Young, R. R. (1979). Brain stem auditory evoked responses: Studies of waveform variations in 50 normal human subjects. *Archives of Neurology*, *36*, 81–87.

Coats, A. C., & Martin, J. L. (1977). Human auditory nerve action potentials and brainstem evoked responses. *Archives of Otolaryngology*, *103*, 605–622.

Cox, L. C., Hack, M., & Metz, D. A. (1981a). Brainstem-evoked response audiometry: Normative data from the preterm infant. *Audiology*, *20*, 53–64.

Cox, L. C., Hack, M., & Metz, D. A. (1981b). Brainstem evoked response audiometry in the premature infant population. *International Journal of Pediatric Otorhinolaryngology*, *3*, 213–224.

Cox, L. C., Hack, M., & Metz, D. A. (1982). Longitudinal ABR in the NICU infant. *International Journal of Pediatric Otorhinolaryngology*, *4*, 225–231.

Cox, L. C., Hack, M., & Metz, D. A. (1984). Auditory brainstem response abnormalities in the very low birthweight infant: Incidence and risk factors. *Ear and Hearing*, (5), 47–51.

Cox, L.C., & Metz, D.A. (1980). ABER in the prescription of hearing aids. *Hearing Instruments*, *31*, 12–15, 55.

Despland, P., & Galambos, R. (1980). The auditory brainstem response (ABR) as a useful diagnostic tool in the intensive care nursery. *Pediatric Research*, *14*(2), 154–158.

Dobie, R. A., & Berlin, C. I. (1979). Binaural interaction in the brainstem evoked responses. *Archives of Otolaryngology*, *105*, 391–398.

Eccard, K. D., & Weber, B. A. (1983). Influence of electrode impedance on auditory brain stem response recordings in the intensive care nursery. *Ear and Hearing*, *4*(2), 104–105.

Eggermont, J. J., & Don, M. (1980). Analysis of click-evoked brainstem potentials in humans using high-pass noise masking. *Journal of the Acoustical Society of America*, *68*(6), 1671–1675.

Elliot, G.B., & Elliot, K.A. (1964). Some pathological, radiological and clinical implications of the precocious development of the human ear. *Laryngoscope*, *74*, 1160–1171.

Fitzhardinge, P. M., Pape, K., Arstikaitis, M., et al. (1974). Mechanical ventilation of infants less than 1501 gram birthweight: Health, growth and neurologic sequelae. *Journal of Pediatrics*, *88*, 531–541.

Franklin, B., & Bremer, D. (1982). *Newborn responses to acoustic stimuli*. Paper presented at the annual meeting of the American Speech-Language-Hearing Association, Toronto, November.

Fujikawa, S. M., & Weber, B. A. (1977). Effects of increased stimulus rate on brainstem electric response (BER) audiometry as a function of age. *Journal of the American Auditory Society*, *3*(3), 147–150.

Galambos, R. G., & Despland, P. A. (1980). The auditory brainstem response (ABR) evaluates risk factors for hearing loss in the newborn. *Pediatric Research*, *14*(3), 159–163.

Galambos, R. G., & Hecox, K. (1978). Clinical applications of the auditory brainstem response. *Otolaryngology Clinics of North America*, *11*, 709–722.

Harris, S., Mollerstrom, B., Reimer, A., & Grennert, L. G. (1981). Auditory brainstem response and gestational age in the newborn. *Scandinavian Audiology*, *13*, 147–148.

Hecox, K. (1975). Electrophysiological correlates of human auditory development. In L. B. Cohen & P. Salaptex (Eds.), *Infant perception: From sensation to cognition* (Vol. III). New York: Academic Press.

Hecox, K., & Burkhard, R. (1982). Developmental dependencies of the human brainstem auditory evoked response. *Annals of the New York Academy of Sciences*, *388*, 538–556.

Hecox, K., & Cone, B. K. (1981). Prognostic importance of brainstem auditory evoked response after asphyxia. *Neurology*, *31*, 1429–1439.

Hecox, K. E., Cone, B., & Blaw, M. E. (1981). Brainstem auditory evoked responses in the diagnosis of pediatric neurologic diseases. *Neurology*, *31*, 832–840.

Hecox, K., & Galambos, R. (1974). Brainstem auditory evoked responses in human infants and adults. *Archives of Otolaryngology*, *99*, 30–33.

Hooks, R. G., & Weber, B. A. (1984). Auditory brainstem response of premature infants to bone conducted stimuli: A feasibility study. *Ear and Hearing*, *5*, 42–46.

Jacobson, J. T., Morehouse, C. R., & Johnson, M. J. (1982). Strategies for infant auditory brain stem response assessment. *Ear and Hearing*, *3*(5), 263–270.

Jacobson, J. T., Seitz, M. R., Mencher, G. T., & Parrott. (1981). Auditory brainstem response: A contribution to infant assessment and management. In G. Mencher & S. Gerber (Eds.), *Early management of hearing loss*. New York: Grune & Stratton.

Jewett, D.L., & Williston, J.S. (1971). Auditory evoked potentials for far fields averaged from the scalp of humans. *Brain, 94*, 681–696.

Kaga, K., & Tamaka, Y. (1980). Auditory brainstem response and behavioral audiometry. *Archives of Otolaryngology*, *106*, 564–566.

Kiang, N., Watanabe, T., Thomas, E., et al. (1965). Discharge patterns of single fibers in the cat's auditory nerve. *Research Monographs* (35). Cambridge: MIT Press.

Kileny, P., Connelly, C., & Robertson, L. (1980). Auditory brainstem responses in perinatal asphyxia. *International Journal of Pediatric Otorhinolaryngology*, *2*, 147–159.

Kjaer, M. (1979). Differences of latencies and amplitudes of brainstem evoked potentials in subgroups of a normal material. *Acta Neurologica Scandinavica*, *57*, 72–79.

Kodera, K., Yamana, H., Yamana, O., & Suzuki, J. (1977). Brainstem response audiometry at speech frequencies. *Audiology*, *16*, 469–479.

Konishi, M. (1973). Development of auditory neuronal responses in avian embryos. *Proceedings of the National Academy of Sciences*, *70*, 1795–1798.

Lasky, R. E. (1983). *Rate effects on auditory brainstem evoked responses: Adult, term and preterm newborns*. Paper presented at the meeting of the Society of Research in Child Development, Detroit, April.

Lee, S. H., & Cox, L. C. (1982). Latency–intensity functions of the auditory brainstem evoked response in premature infants. *Florida Language Speech and Hearing Association Journal*, *3*, 15–19.

Leiberman, A., Sohmer, H., & Szabo, G. (1973). Cochlear audiometry (electrocochleography) during the neonatal period. *Developmental Medicine and Child Neurology*, *15*, 8–13.

Marshall, R. E., Reichert, T. M., Kerley, S. M., & Davis, H. (1980). Auditory functions in newborn intensive unit patients revealed by auditory brainstem potentials. *Journal of Pediatrics*, *96*, 731-735.

Martin, M. E., & Moore, E. J. (1977). Scalp distribution of early (0-10 msec) auditory evoked responses. *Archives of Otolaryngology*, *103*(6), 326-328.

Mauldin, L., & Jerger, J. (1979). Auditory brainstem evoked responses to bone conducted signals. *Archives of Otolaryngology*, *105*, 656-661.

McClelland, R., & McCrea, R. (1979). Intersubject variability of the auditory-evoked brainstem potentials. *Audiology*, *18*, 462-471.

McPherson, D. L., Hirosugi, Y., & Starr, A. (1984). Scalp distribution of auditory brainstem response (ABR) in neonates and adults. Manuscript submitted for publication.

Mendelson, T., Salamy, A., Lenoir, M., & McKean, C. (1979). Brain stem evoked potential findings in children with otitis media. *Archives of Otolaryngology*, *105*, 17-20.

Mjoen, S. (1981). ABR in pediatric audiology. *Scandinavian Audiology*, *13 (Supplement)*, 141-146.

Møller, K., & Blegvad, B. (1976). Brainstem responses in patients with sensori-neural hearing loss. *Scandinavian Audiology*, *5*, 115-127.

Montandon, P., Cao, M., Engel, R., & Grajew, T. (1979). Auditory nerve and brainstem responses in the newborn and in preschool children. *Acta Otolaryngologica*, *87*, 279-286.

Morgan, A., & Salle, B. (1980). A study of brain stem evoked responses in prematures. *Acta Otolaryngologica*, *89*, 370-375.

Ornitz, E., Mo, A., Olson, S., Waller, D. (1980). Influence of click sound pressure direction on brain stem responses in children. *Audiology*, *19*, 245-254.

Paradise, J. (1980). Otitis media in infants and children. *Pediatrics*, *65*, 917-943.

Pauwels, H. P., Vogeleer, M., Clement, P. A. R., Rousseeuw, P. J., & Kaufman, L. (1982). Brainstem electric response audiometry in newborns. *International Journal of Pediatric Otorhinolaryngology*, *4*, 317-323.

Picton, T. W., & Smith, A. D. (1978). The practice of evoked potential audiometry. *Otolaryngology Clinics of North America*, *11*, 263-282.

Picton, T. W., Stapells, D. R., & Campbell, K. B. (1981). Auditory evoked potentials from the human cochlea and brainstem. *Journal of Otolaryngology*, *10*, (Supplement 9), 1-41.

Pratt, H., & Sohmer, H. (1976). Intensity and rate functions of cochlear and brainstem evoked responses to click stimuli in man. *Archives of Oto-Rhino-Larynogology*, *212*, 85-93.

Pujol, R., & Marty, R. (1970). Postnatal maturation in the cochlea of the cat. *Journal of Comparative Neurology*, *139*, 115-126.

Roberts, J. L., Davis, H., Phon, G. L., et al. (1982). Auditory brainstem responses in preterm neonates: Maturation and follow-up. *Journal of Pediatrics*, *101*, 257-263.

Rowe, M. J. (1978). Normal variability of the brainstem auditory evoked response in young and old adult subjects. *Electroencephalography and Clinical Neurophysiology*, *44*, 454-470.

Rubel, E. W., & Ryals, B. M. (1982). Development of the place principle: Acoustic trauma. *Science*, *4584*, 512-514.

Salamy, A. (1981). The theoretical distribution of evoked brainstem activity in preterm, high-risk, and healthy infants. *Child Development*, *52*, 752-754.

Salamy, A., Fenn, C. B., & Bronshvag, M. (1979). Ontogenesis of human brainstem evoked potential amplitude. *Developmental Psychobiology*, *12*(5), 519-526.

Salamy, A., & McKean, C. M. (1976). Postnatal development of the human brainstem potentials during the first year of life. *Electroencephalography and Clinical Neurophysiology*, *40*, 418-426.

Salamy, A., McKean, C. M., & Buda, F. B. (1975). Maturational changes in auditory transmission as reflected in human brainstem potentials. *Brain Research*, *96*, 361-366.

Salamy, A., McKean, C. M., Pettett, C., & Mendelson, T. (1978). Auditory brainstem recovery processes from birth to adulthood. *Psychophysiology*, *15*(3), 214–220.

Salamy, A., Mendelson, T., & Tooley, W. H. (1982). Developmental profiles for the brainstem auditory evoked potential. *Early Human Development*, *6*, 331–339.

Salamy, A., Mendelson, T., Tooley, W. H., & Chaplin, E. R. (1980). Contrasts in brainstem function between normal and high-risk infants in early postnatal life. *Early Human Development*, *4*(2), 179–185.

Sanders, J. C., Coles, R. B., & Gates, G. R. (1973). The development of auditory evoked responses in the cochlea and cochlear nuclei of the chick. *Brain Research*, *63*, 59–74.

Schulman-Galambos, C., & Galambos, R. (1975). Brain stem auditory-evoked responses in premature infants. *Journal of Speech and Hearing Research*, *18*, 456–465.

Schulman-Galambos, C., & Galambos, R. (1979). Brainstem response audiometry in newborn hearing screening. *Archives of Otolaryngology*, *105*, 86–90.

Starr, A., & Achor, L. J. (1975). Auditory brainstem responses in neurological disease. *Archives of Neurology*, *32*, 761–768.

Starr, A., Amalie, R. N., Martin, W. H., & Sanders, S. (1977). Development of auditory function in newborn infants revealed by auditory brainstem potentials. *Pediatrics*, *60*, 831–839.

Stockard, J. E., & Stockard, J. J. (1980). Brainstem auditory evoked potentials in normal and otoneurologically impaired newborns and infants. In C. E. Henry (Ed.), *Current clinical neurophysiology update on EEG and evoked potentials*. New York: Elsevier North.

Stockard, J. E., & Stockard, J. J. (1983). Recording and analyzing. In E. J. Moore (Ed.), *Bases of auditory brain-stem evoked responses*. New York: Grune & Stratton.

Stockard, J. E., Stockard, J. J., & Coen, R. W. (1983). Auditory brain stem response variability in infants. *Ear and Hearing*, *4*(1), 11–23.

Stockard, J. E., Stockard, J. J., Kleinberg, F., & Westmoreland, B. F. (1983). Prognostic value of brainstem auditory evoked potentials in neonates. *Archives of Neurology*, *40*, 360–365.

Stockard, J. E., Stockard, J. J., Westmoreland, B. F., & Corfits, J. L. (1979). Brainstem auditory-evoked response. Normal variations as a function of stimulus and subject characteristics. *Archives of Neurology*, *36*, 823–831.

Stockard, J. E., & Westmoreland, B. F. (1981). Technical considerations in the recording and interpretation of the brainstem auditory evoked potential for neonatal neurologic diagnosis. *American Journal of EEG Technology*, *21*, 31–54.

Stockard, J. J., Sharbrough, F. W., & Tinker, J. H. (1978). Effects of hypothermia on the human brainstem auditory-evoked response. *Annals of Neurology*, *3*, 368–370.

Stockard, J. J., Stockard, J. E., & Sharbrough, F. W. (1978). Non-pathologic factors influencing brainstem auditory evoked potentials. *American Journal of EEG Technology*, *18*, 177–209.

Stockard, J. J., Stockard, J. E., & Sharbrough, F. W. (1980). Brainstem auditory evoked potentials in neurology: Methodology interpretation, clinical application. In M. J. Aminoff (Ed.), *Electrodiagnosis in clinical neurology*. New York: Churchill Livingstone.

Suzuki, T., Harai, Y., & Horiuchi, K. (1977). Auditory brainstem responses to pure tone stimuli. *Scandinavian Audiology*, *6*(1), 51–56.

Suzuki, T., & Horiuchi, K. (1981). Rise time of pure-tone stimuli in brainstem response audiometry. *Audiology*, *20*, 101–112.

Terkildsen, K., & Osterhammel, P. (1981). The influence of reference electrode position on recordings of the auditory brain stem responses. Ear and Hearing, *2*, 9–14.

Van Olphen, A. F., Rodenburg, M., & Verwey, C. (1978). Distribution of brainstem responses to acoustic stimuli over the human scalp. *Audiology*, *17*, 511–518.

Weber, B. A. (1982). Comparison of auditory brain stem response latency norms for premature infants. *Ear and Hearing*, *3*(5), 257–262.

Weber, B. A., Seitz, M. R., & McCutcheon, M. J. (1981). Quantifying click stimuli in auditory brainstem response audiometry. *Ear and Hearing*, *2*, 15–19.

Wolf, K. E., & Goldstein, R. (1980). Middle component AERs from neonates. *Journal of Speech and Hearing Research*, *23*, 185–201.

Yamada, O., Hidemichi, A., Kodera, K., & Yamane, H. (1983). Frequency-selective auditory brainstem response in newborns and infants. *Archives of Otolaryngology*, *109*, 79–85.

Yoshie, N., & Ohashi, T. (1969). Clinical use of cochlear nerve action potential responses in man for different diagnosis of hearing loss. *Acta Otolaryngologica (Supplement)*, *252*, 71–87.

Zubick, H. H., Fried, M. P., Epstein, M. F., et al. (1982). Normal neonatal brainstem auditory evoked potentials. *Annals of Otology, Rhinology and Laryngology*, *91*, 485–488.

Chapter 17

Identification of Congenital Hearing Loss With The Auditory Brainstem Response

Thomas J. Fria

BACKGROUND

Congenital hearing loss constitutes a significant threat to a child's ability to develop and function in today's society. Without adequate auditory input, the infant cannot receive and therefore process those fragments of speech and language which can form the conceptual foundation for growth in communication. Furthermore, linguistic development in childhood can suffer potentially insurmountable lags if such sensory deficiencies are not detected and managed at the earliest opportunity. To be maximally successful, it can be argued that efforts such as amplification, infant stimulation, parental guidance and counselling, and plans for educational placement should be launched during the first year of the affected child's life (Downs, 1974).

Collectively, these considerations serve as reasonable grounds for screening newborns for congenital hearing loss. Initially, such attempts were aimed at all newborns (Downs & Sterritt, 1967; Feinmesser & Tell, 1976) whereby literally thousands were screened by visually observing sound-induced reflexive behaviors. These efforts were soon shown to yield unreasonably high numbers of false alarms, and far too many babies had to be retested to detect an impaired child (Feinmesser, Tell, & Levi, 1982).

The High-Risk Newborn

In 1973, the Joint Committee on Infant Hearing of the American Academy of Pediatrics reported that due to the high frequency of false alarms, mass screening of the normal newborn population could not be "universally recommended." Instead, the Committee recommended identifying infants "at risk" for congenital hearing loss by using five high-risk categories and following the identified infants until a definitive diagnosis could be determined. By definition, high-risk newborns harbor a significantly greater likelihood of congenital hearing loss than members of the general newborn population. Included are newborns who present with one or more conditions of a prenatal or perinatal nature that are associated with insults to the auditory system.

Downs and Silver (1972) referred to these factors as the ABCD'S of congenital hearing loss with each letter designating a different factor—(A) standing for affected family members or the presence of childhood hearing loss in family members, (B) for excessive bilirubin during the perinatal period, (C) for congenital infections such as rubella, cytomegalovirus, toxoplasmosis, or herpes, (D) for defects of the ears, nose, and throat, and (S) for the small baby, that is, less than 1500 grams at birth.

Gerkin (1984) recently reported a revision of the ABCD'S designation which includes the updated suggestions made by the Joint Committee in 1982 (American Academy of Pediatrics, 1982). In the same mnemonic format, these factors include (A) neonatal asphyxia, (B) bacterial meningitis, especially *Hemophilus influenzae,* (C) congenital infection such as syphilis, toxoplasmosis, rubella, cytomegalovirus, and herpes, (D) defects of the head or neck such as craniofacial abnormalities associated with various genetic and metabolic syndromes, cleft palate, and malformations of the pinna, (E) elevated bilirubin to an extent that requires an exchange transfusion, (F) a family history of childhood hearing loss, and (G) a gram birthweight of less than 1500.

Newborns who present with one or more of these factors are considered to be "at risk" for severe, congenital hearing loss. In other words, the risk of such impairment is perhaps 1 in 20 or 1 in 50 instead of the 1 chance in approximately 2000 usually expected for the general newborn population. Pragmatically, the majority of high-risk newborns can be found in the newborn intensive care nursery, the graduates of which comprise the target population for screening purposes. Many authors extend the screen to the normal care nurseries but only for newborns who present with one or more high-risk factors.

During the later part of the 1970s, two international conferences on newborn screening were convened; one in Nova Scotia (Mencher, 1976) and the other in Saskatoon (Gerber & Mencher, 1978). The conferees resolved that the auditory brainstem response (ABR) was a viable screening test for the high-risk newborn population. In its 1982 statement, The Joint Committee on Infant Hearing subsequently endorsed the "audiologic testing" of high-risk newborns because of the 2.5 to 5.0% associated incidence of moderate to profound hearing loss, and suggested that the initial screening of these newborns should include the observation of behavioral *or* electrophysiologic responses to sound.

With the early reports of Hecox and Galambos (1974), Schulman-Galambos and Galambos (1975), and Salamy and associates (Salamy & McKean, 1976; Salamy, Mckean, & Buda, 1975), which demonstrated the apparent ease with which the auditory brainstem response could be recorded in young infants, came the understandable motivation for subsequent attempts to use this electrophysiologic response in newborn screening. Since that time, arguments for and against screening with the ABR have appeared. Some have emphasized that it inherently involves the use of expensive equipment, preferably skilled personnel, and the test itself can be time-consuming and yield results for which a straightforward interpretation is lacking (Jacobson, Seitz, Mencher, & Parrott, 1981). Moreover, evidence has appeared (Cox, Hack, & Metz, 1982; Roberts, Davis, Phon, Reichert, Sturtevant, & Marshall, 1982) that challenges the reliability of ABR findings obtained in the nursery.

Alternatively, Galambos (1978) suggested that nearly every newborn with hearing impairment could be identified by administering an ABR screening test to babies who (1) are graduates of the newborn intensive care unit (NICU), (2) appear on a high-risk register, (3) fail behavioral screening, and (4) are considered suspect for whatever reason. Attempts have also been made to initiate widespread use of ABR screening in hospitals throughout the country, using volunteers to administer the tests and providing less expensive equipment to participating facilities. However, no data exist that confirm or deny the feasibility of this approach.

Previous Experience with ABR Screening

Efforts to screen high-risk newborns with the ABR have continued in the company of these disparate viewpoints. As we shall see later, screening programs which employ the ABR can be expensive and for that reason alone their feasibility may be limited to centers where large numbers

TABLE 17–1.
Previous Studies Using the ABR as a Screening Tool in High-Risk Newborns

Study		N	Pass	Fail	%	Cutoff
Schulman-Galambos & Galambos,	1979	75	71	4	5.33	30 dB
Jacobson, Seitz, Mencher, & Parrott,	1981	96	84	12	12.50	30 dB
Galambos, Hicks, & Wilson,	1982	890	749	141	15.84	30 dB
Mjoen, Langslet, Tangsrud, & Sundby,	1982	60	50	10	16.67	40 dB
Roberts, Davis, Phon, et al.,	1982	75	31	44	58.67	40 dB
Alberti, Hyde, Corbin, et al.,	1983	234	204	30	12.82	40 dB
Durieux-Smith, Edwards, Hyde, et al.,	1983	1564	1270	294	18.80	30 dB
Stein, Ozdamar, Kraus, & Paton,	1983	100	89	11	11.00	40 dB
Dennis, Sheldon, Toubas, & McCaffee,	1984	200	177	23	11.50	30 dB
Shannon, Felix, Krumholz, et al.,	1984	168	147	21	12.50	25 dB
Fria, Kurmin, Ashoff & Sinclair-Griffith,	1984	500	434	66	13.20	30 dB
Jacobson & Morehouse,	1984	176	141	35	19.88	30 dB

of high-risk infants are born. Aside from the expense involved, critics have claimed that far too many babies fail the ABR screening, and the number of false failures seriously jeopardizes the utility of the response as a screening tool.

Table 17-1 presents a list of studies which have directly addressed the problem. Also shown for each project are the number of newborns tested, the number who passed, the number and percentage who failed, and the pass/fail cutoff employed. Only those studies dealing with the identification of congenital hearing loss in newborns are listed. Attempts to identify newborns with neurological impairments by using the absolute and interwave latency characteristics of the response (e.g., Despland & Galambos, 1979) are dealt with in another section of this text.

The projects shown in Table 17-1 typically used a pass/fail cutoff involving the presence or absence of wave V of the ABR in one or both ears at a given stimulus intensity. The cutoff intensity was 30 or 40 dB nHL in all but one study (Shannon, Felix, Krumholz, Goldstein, & Harris, 1984), which used 25 dB nHL. In other words, newborns who did not yield the criterion response in one or both ears at this level were considered failures. The number of newborns tested ranged from 75 to 500 in individual projects. Galambos, Hicks, and Wilson (1982) reported on a composite group of 890 newborns composed of infants from two separate screenings, and Durieux-Smith, Edwards, Hyde, Jacobson, Kileny, Picton, and Sanders (1983) reported on a total of 1,564 newborns representing five separate screening programs.

With the exception of two projects, between 11 and 19% of the newborns failed the ABR screening. Only 5.3% failed in the Schulman-Galambos and Galambos (1979) study, and Roberts and colleagues (1982) uncovered a failure rate of 58%. Closer examination of the data represented in Table 17-1 reveals a notable trend that might explain the former of these two exceptions. In the majority of reports, the failures comprised two subgroups; those failing only at the lower cutoff (30 or 40 dB nHL) but passing at a higher stimulus intensity (e.g., 60 or 70 dB nHL), and those newborns who failed to respond at both the lower and higher stimulus levels. Fria, Kurmin, Ashoff, and Sinclair-Griffith (1982) found that of the 13.2% who failed, 6.6%, respectively, fell into these two categories. The same trend has been reported by others (Dennis, Sheldon, Toubas, & McCaffee, 1984; Mjoen, Langslet, Tangsrud, & Sundby, 1982; Stein, Ozdamar, Kraus, & Paton, 1983). Without exception, the four failures observed by Schulman-Galambos and Galambos (1979) yielded no ABR below 70 dB nHL, and it is reasonable to assume that

TABLE 17–2.

The Number of Screening Failures Receiving Retests and the Number and Percentage of Over-Referrals and the Total Percentage Who Were Eventually Found to be Impaired in Previous Studies Using the ABR to Screen

Study		Cutoff	N Followed	N Over ref	$\%$ Over ref	$\%$ Impaired
Schulman-Galambos & Galambos,	1979	30 dB	4	0	.00	2.1
Jacobson, Seitz, Mencher, & Parrott,	1981	30 dB	4	1	.25	3.6
Galambos, Hicks, & Wilson,	1982	30 dB	60	16	.27	4.8
Mjoen, Langslet, Tangsrud, & Sundby,	1982	30 dB	10	1	.10	—
Roberts, Davis, Phon, et al.,	1982	40 dB	23	22	.96	2.3
Alberti, Hyde, Corbin, et al.,	1983	40 dB	16	6	.38	1.5
Stein, Ozdamar, Kraus, & Paton,	1983	60 dB	8	4	.50	2
Dennis, Sheldon, Toubas, & McCaffee,	1984	30 dB	15	5	.33	5
Shannon, Felix, Krumholz, et al.,	1984	25 dB	19	18	.95	2.2
Fria, Kurmin, Ashoff, & Sinclair-Griffith,	1984	30 dB	31	10	.32	4.2
Jacobson & Morehouse,	1984	30 dB	33	9	.27	4.0

the 5.3% failure rate may represent the second of the two failure subgroups. Therefore the probability was high initially that these infants were severely impaired; they would have failed even if the cutoff had been 60 dB nHL instead of 30 dB nHL.

Roberts and associates (1982) screened a group of 75 babies in the NICU, and, astoundingly, 44 infants (58.7%) failed the screen at 40 dB nHL in one or both ears. These failures consisted of 29 infants (38.7%) with no response at 40 dB nHL and 15 infants (20.0%) failing only at 70 dB nHL. Neither of these failure rates are consistent with any of the other studies shown in Table 17-1. The explanation for this discrepancy is very difficult to discern but some possibilities will be offered later.

The majority of studies conducted thus far, then, would indicate that between 10 and 20% of high-risk newborns will fail an ABR screen when the criterion for failure is an absence of wave V in one or both ears for a click stimulus at 30 to 40 dB nHL. Of these, one can expect that approximately half will fail only at this lower cutoff level, and the remaining half will fail at an even higher cutoff such as 60 or 70 dB nHL.

The issue of over-referrals is addressed in Table 17-2. Shown is the number of newborns who initially failed the screen and who passed a retest following discharge from the nursery. Note that this rate of over-referral ranged from 0 to 96% suggesting that in selected instances fully 9 out of 10 initial failures passed on retest subsequent to discharge. At first glance, these are alarming data because they presumably cast doubt on the reliability of ABR results obtained in the nursery. However, to a certain degree, this discrepancy can be accounted for on the basis of percent follow-up and at what point in time were retest ABRs scheduled. In only two projects did the rate exceed 50%; it was approximately 30% in six of the 11 projects and 10% or less in 2 of the reports.

In the context of the disproportionate number of failures uncovered by Roberts and colleagues (1982), it is not surprising that so many of the newborns who failed their screen were over-referrals. However, only 10 of the original 44 who failed were actually retested; 21 were lost to follow-up and parents of 13 were contacted by phone. Of the 10 who were retested, 6 had originally failed at 40 dB nHL only, and the remaining 4 failed at 70 dB nHL. All six of the 40-dB failures and three of the four 70-dB failures (75%) were over-referrals.

Shannon and associates (1984) also observed a 95% over-referral rate. Twenty-one infants originally failed their screen; two of these were lost to follow-up, and 18 of the remaining 19 newborns were normal at subsequent retest. It is not clear from their report exactly how many of the original 21 failed at 25 versus 65 dB nHL, but the authors state that the majority of the normal retests were those babies who had either unilateral or mild impairments at the original screen. Presumably, then, a large proportion of the original 21 who failed did so only at 25 dB nHL. The one severely impaired infant who was confirmed at follow-up gave no response at 80 dB nHL on the original screen.

Fria and colleagues (1982) found that 21 of 23 newborns (91%) who initially failed at 60 dB nHL were later confirmed to be severely hearing impaired, thereby yielding an over-referral rate of only 9%. In the same study, however, only 3 of the 14 followed who had failed at 30 dB nHL but passed at 60 dB nHL still had a mild impairment on a subsequent retest; 11 (78.6%) were over-referrals. Very similar findings were reported by Dennis and associates (1984) and Jacobson and Morehouse (1984). Consequently, the proportion of over-referrals would appear to be related to the two failure categories previously discussed. The over-referral rate can be expected to be considerably higher in the first group than in the second. Transient middle ear involvement resulting in a mild conductive hearing loss which resolves by the time of the follow-up evaluation may be the most reasonable explanation for this over-referral trend (Stein et al., 1983).

Despite the wide range of over-referrals, it is interesting to note the comparative agreement among studies with regard to the prevalence of congenital hearing loss. This ranged from 1.5 to 5.0% in individual projects. Five of the 12 reports uncovered a prevalence of approximately 2.0% (Alberti, Hyde, Corbin, Riko, & Abramovich, 1983; Schulman-Galambos & Galambos, 1979; Shannon et al., 1984; Roberts et al., 1982; Stein et al., 1983), five observed approximately 4.0% (Fria et al., 1982; Jacobson et al., 1981; Jacobson & Morehouse, 1984; and three of the five projects represented by Durieux-Smith et al., 1983), and the remaining two projects found a prevalence of approximately 5.0% (Dennis et al., 1984; Galambos et al., 1980). Notably, the over-referral rate tended to be higher for the projects where the prevalence was closer to 2.0%.

Were these false failures due to faulty technique, inexperienced testers, bad equipment, a noisy test environment, an immature auditory system in the newborn which may not respond "normally" when screened? Or is the ABR just a poor screening test because the results in the newborn are inherently unreliable? The present author contends that much of the confusion can be clarified by what we already know about screening and screening tests.

THE PRINCIPLES OF SCREENING

Informative discussions of the principles of screening and the characteristics of tests are not commonly found in the audiologic literature. Much of the material that follows was adapted from the paper by Thorner and Remein (1982) and a chapter that appeared in a text by Northern and Downs (1974).

The main objective of screening is to rule out disease or impairment in a population that consists of both impaired and unimpaired individuals. This can be done in a number of ways. For example, generating a list or register of newborns who present with one of the high-risk factors for congenital hearing loss is a form of screening because babies who appear on the list are followed until a diagnosis can be made. To avoid losing babies to follow-up, however, some sort of test can be administered when the newborns are still available for screening, that is, in the nursery.

To determine whether a given test, such as the ABR, is appropriate for screening purposes, one must clearly distinguish between screening and diagnosis. One way to distinguish the two is to think of diagnosis as the process of confirming a specific impairment in an individual.

Screening, on the other hand, subdivides a population into two groups of individuals: (1) those who probably are unimpaired, and (2) those who probably are impaired. As a result of screening, the second group is referred for diagnosis. Consequently, a good screening test is one that assures with very high probability that those individuals who pass are not impaired. Remember, these individuals will not be referred for diagnosis! A good diagnostic test, however, is one that assures with very high probability that those who fail truly have the impairment or disease in question.

Perhaps the most apparent example of the confusion of the ABR as a screening tool versus diagnostic test is the critique of ABR testing in the NICU by D. Downs (1982). Downs questions the validity, reliability, norms, utility, safety, and relevance to intervention of the ABR in newborns. However, his efforts are clearly indicative of (1) a lack of understanding of the distinction between screening and diagnosis, and (2) a superficial grasp of the principles of screening and test characteristics. The majority of Downs' remarks address the ABR as a diagnostic tool, and in that context his statements are well taken and do underscore the need for caution when testing newborns. However, using the test to rule out congenital hearing loss in newborns is an entirely different issue.

A test can be used for both screening and diagnostic purposes. The suitability of a test for either purpose will depend on its operating characteristics, which in turn are determined by the way the results are interpreted. These characteristics can be quantified, and the test can be rendered more suitable for screening, by manipulating the interpretation of the findings.

The Operating Characteristics of a Test

There are two main operating characteristics of a test. The first is called *sensitivity* and denotes the probability that truly impaired individuals will fail the test. The second is called *specificity* and designates the probability that truly unimpaired individuals will pass the test. When a test operates at 90% sensitivity, 9 out of 10 truly impaired individuals will fail the test. When the same test operates with 90% specificity, then 9 out of 10 truly unimpaired individuals will pass the test.

Figure 17-1 shows a four-box matrix, sometimes called a decision matrix, which can clarify these operating characteristics. Each box in the matrix corresponds to a test result, whereas (A) designates the number of impaired individuals who fail the test (i.e., true positives), (B) the number of unimpaired individuals who fail the test (i.e., false positives), (C) the number of impaired individuals who pass (i.e., false negatives), and (D) the number of unimpaired individuals who pass the test (i.e., true negatives). The percent sensitivity of the test is determined by dividing the number of impaired individuals who fail by the total number of impaired individuals: $A/A+C \times 100$. Percent specificity is determined by taking the ratio of the number of unimpaired individuals who pass to the total number of unimpaired individuals: $D/B+D \times 100$.

Consequently, the percent sensitivity is also the true-positive rate, and the reciprocal is called the *false-negative rate*. The percent specificity is the true-negative rate, and the reciprocal is called the *false-positive rate*. A test with 95% sensitivity has a false-negative rate of 5%. In other words, there is a 5% probability that truly impaired individuals will pass a test having 95% sensitivity. If the same test happens to have a specificity of 80%, it will have a false-positive rate of 20% meaning that there is a 20% chance that truly unimpaired individuals will fail the test.

The Cutoff Score

It is important to understand the implications of choosing the test score which will serve as the "cutoff" between pass and fail. On the basis of this choice, a given test will operate

FIGURE 17–1.
A decision matrix demonstrating the computation of a test's operating characteristics. Sensitivity is the ratio of true positives (A) to the total number of impaired newborns (A + C). Specificity is the ratio of true negatives (D) to the total number of unimpaired newborns (B + D). False positives are represented by B, and false negatives are represented by C.

STATUS OF NEWBORN

	IMPAIRED	UNIMPAIRED
ABR FAIL	A	B
ABR PASS	C	D

Sensitivity = (A/A+C) × 100
Specificity = (D/B+D) × 100

with a certain sensitivity and specificity. Moreover, a change in the cutoff score will have a predictable influence on these operating characteristics.

Figure 17-2 shows the distribution of ABR thresholds for unimpaired and impaired newborns who coexist in a hypothetical target population. A cutoff score of 40 dB nHL is represented by the vertical line B. Those who score to the right of this cutoff will fail the test, and those who score at 40 dB nHL or less will pass. Clearly, using this cutoff will fail nearly all of the impaired newborns, and the false-negative rate will be very low. With this cutoff, then, the test is operating with high sensitivity. However, a significant proportion of the unimpaired newborns will also fail with this cutoff score, and the false-positive error rate will be correspondingly high because of the reduced specificity.

Adjusting the test cutoff point toward the impaired newborns to line *C* (60 dB nHL) will markedly increase specificity and decrease sensitivity. This is because none of the unimpaired babies will now fail the test, but a larger proportion of impaired newborns will pass with this

FIGURE 17–2.
Hypothetical distributions of ABR thresholds for unimpaired (top) and impaired (bottom) newborns. Screening cutoff points representing 30 dB nHL (A), 40 dB nHL (B), and 60 dB nHL (C) are shown as vertical lines. See text for explanation.

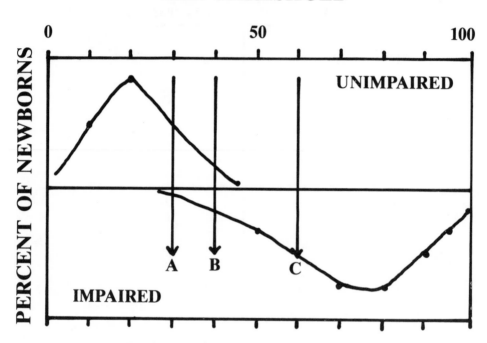

cutoff. It is important to note that this change will result unavoidably in a much lower false-positive rate and a higher false-negative rate.

Moving the cutoff point toward the unimpaired newborns will have just the opposite effect. Sensitivity will increase because the probability increases that an impaired baby will fail the test. As a direct result, fewer unimpaired babies will pass and specificity decreases. Accordingly, this adjustment of the cutoff will increase the false-positive rate and decrease false-negative rate.

Since the main objective in screening is to maximize the confidence in negative results, an ABR cutoff score close to the unimpaired newborns should be selected if we want to eliminate even mild hearing loss. By now it should be apparent that this alteration will have predictable consequences. By increasing the confidence in the negative result we are decreasing the confidence in the positive result. In other words, the false-positive error rate will inherently be increased.

Therefore the increase in false-positive rate associated with an increase in the sensitivity of a test is difficult to avoid. If we wish to rule out only moderate to severe loss, then the overlap between the two populations in Figure 17-2 will be reduced. In other words, it may be possible to increase specificity without a marked reduction in test sensitivity. This will reduce the false-positive error rate, but the identification of newborns having mild congenital hearing loss is sacrificed.

The Influence of the Prevalence of Impairment

It is important to remember that these test characteristics are based on probabilities, and as a result they may be only indirectly related to clinical outcome. That is, there is a tendency to view these probabilities in clinical terms, and this can lead to pertinent misconceptions. The most pertinent misconception is that sensitivity and specificity will change when the test is administered to different populations. Quite possibly, this notion stems from the practice of equating the false-positive rate with the so-called "over-referral" rate. When a test is understood to have 90% specificity it follows that it also has a 10% false-positive rate. However, this does not mean that 10% of those who fail the test will be unimpaired or over-referrals.

The over-referral rate carries a markedly different connotation in terms of clinical outcome. It is the reciprocal of the *predictive value of a positive test result* and is equal to the ratio of the number of unimpaired individuals who fail the test to the total number of individuals who fail. The most important fact to remember is that the over-referral rate is markedly influenced by the prevalence of the impairment in the population being tested, but the false-positive rate is not, assuming the same cutoff point is employed. Therefore, the over-referral rate can change markedly when the false-positive rate of a test does not change at all. The reason is that the sensitivity and specificity of a test do not change when the prevalence of impairment changes. Consequently, the false-positive and false-negative rates do not change.

As an example of these principles, another decision matrix is shown in Figure 17-3. This time a hypothetical population of 1,000 newborns is depicted, of which 25% are truly impaired. In other words, the prevalence of impairment is 25%. If we assume for discussion purposes that the ABR operates with 95% percent sensitivity and 90% specificity, then 238 of the 250 truly impaired newborns will fail and 675 of the 750 truly unimpaired newborns will pass. Consequently, the screen will wrongly classify 12 of the impaired newborns and 75 of the unimpaired newborns. Take a closer look at these findings. The decision matrix also shows that a total of 313 newborns failed the ABR screen, and 238 (76%) were truly impaired; the remaining 75 were unimpaired. That is, the predictive value of a positive ABR screen was 76%, and the *over-referral rate* was 24%. In the same manner, a total of 687 newborns passed the screen, and of these, 675 (98%) were truly unimpaired; the remaining 12 were impaired. Therefore, the predictive value of a negative result for this population was 98%, and the *under-referral* rate was only 2%.

What happens if the same ABR screen is administered to a population of 1,000 newborns in which the frequency of occurrence of congenital hearing loss is much lower? Table 17-3 gives the answer for prevalences of impairment ranging from 1.5 to 5% including the range of reported values. The top section of the table illustrates the consequences of using a 30-dB nHL cutoff, which *hypothetically* corresponds to 98% sensitivity and 90% specificity. The middle and bottom sections, respectively, represent the estimates based on moving the cutoff point toward the impaired newborns to 45 and 60 dB nHL. The assumption is made that the intent is to rule out moderate to severe impairment; therefore, moving the cutoff toward the impaired newborns increases specificity without a marked reduction in sensitivity.

If the top section of the table is entered at 2.5% prevalence, we see that approximately 12% of newborns will fail the test. Based on the presumed sensitivity and specificity, 25 of the failures are true positives and 98 are false positives. Consequently, the over-referral rate would be 80%! Sound familiar? We can do one of two things from here. We can either use a higher cutoff or test a population having a different prevalence. If we use the same cutoff

FIGURE 17–3.
A decision matrix showing the ABR screening results for a hypothetical population of 1,000 newborns of which 25 percent are impaired. The over-referral rate would equal the ratio of false positives (75) to the total number of ABR failures (315). The under-referral rate would be the ratio of false negatives (12) to the total number of ABR passes (687). The reciprocals of these two ratios are the predictive value of a positive and negative test result, respectively.

STATUS OF NEWBORN

	IMPAIRED	UNIMPAIRED	
ABR FAIL	**238**	**75**	313
ABR PASS	**12**	**675**	687
	250	**750**	

and test a population where the prevalence is only 1.5% then 11.3% will fail; this percentage comprises 15 true positives and 99 false positives. This translates to an over-referral rate of 87%! If the same cutoff is used with a 5% prevalence group, then the over-referral will fall to 66%. It is apparent, then, that the number of over-referrals does not necessarily indicate that the test is inaccurate. Very high over-referral rates can be expected when the prevalence of impairment is very low, even though the test is performing very well. Moreover, when the same cutoff point is used to screen populations having a 1.5% versus a 5.0% prevalence, over-referrals will markedly increase, but the proportion of failures will change very little.

If instead we change the cutoff to 45 dB nHL and test the same 2.5% population, we can see from the middle section of Table 17-2 that only 7.3% will fail and the over-referral rate will fall to 67%. The bottom frame of the table shows that moving to a cutoff of 60 dB nHL with a 2.5% prevalence will result in 4.4% failures and 45% over-referrals.

It is consequently important in clinical terms to be mindful of the relationship between the operating characteristics of a test, the selection of the pass/fail cutoff point, and the

TABLE 17–3.
A Breakdown of ABR Screening Results for a Hypothetical Population of 1,000 High-Risk Newborns.

98% Sensitivity, 90% Specificity — 30 dB Cutoff

Prevalence	Abn	Nml	tp	fn	fp	tn	OR	PPV	UR	NPV	EFF	% fail
1.5	15	985	15	0	99	887	.87	.13	.00	1.00	.981	.113
2	20	980	20	0	98	882	.83	.17	.00	1.00	.902	.118
2.5	25	975	25	1	98	878	.80	.20	.00	.999	.902	.122
3	30	970	29	1	97	873	.77	.23	.00	.999	.902	.126
3.5	35	965	34	1	97	869	.74	.26	.00	.999	.903	.131
4	40	960	39	1	96	864	.71	.29	.00	.999	.903	.135
4.5	45	955	44	1	96	860	.68	.32	.00	.999	.904	.140
5	50	950	49	1	95	855	.66	.34	.00	.999	.904	.144

97% Sensitivity, 95% Specificity — 45 dB Cutoff

Prevalence	Abn	Nml	tp	fn	fp	tn	OR	PPV	UR	NPV	EFF	% fail
1.5	15	985	15	0	49	936	.77	.23	.00	1.00	.950	.064
2	20	980	19	1	49	931	.72	.28	.00	.999	.950	.068
2.5	25	975	24	1	49	926	.67	.33	.00	.999	.951	.073
3	30	970	29	1	49	922	.63	.38	.00	.999	.951	.078
3.5	35	965	34	1	48	917	.59	.41	.00	.999	.951	.082
4	40	960	39	1	48	912	.55	.45	.00	.999	.951	.087
4.5	45	955	44	1	48	907	.52	.48	.00	.999	.951	.091
5	50	950	49	2	48	903	.49	.51	.00	.998	.951	.096

96% Sensitivity, 98% Specificity — 60 dB Cutoff

Prevalence	Abn	Nml	tp	fn	fp	tn	OR	PPV	UR	NPV	EFF	% fail
1.5	15	985	14	1	20	965	.58	.42	.00	.999	.980	.034
2	20	980	19	1	20	960	.51	.49	.00	.999	.980	.039
2.5	25	975	24	1	20	956	.45	.55	.00	.999	.980	.044
3	30	970	29	1	19	951	.40	.60	.00	.999	.979	.048
3.5	35	965	34	1	19	946	.36	.64	.00	.999	.979	.053
4	40	960	38	2	19	941	.33	.67	.00	.998	.979	.058
4.5	45	955	43	2	19	936	.31	.69	.00	.998	.979	.062
5	50	950	48	2	19	931	.28	.72	.00	.998	.979	.067

KEY:
Abn	abnormal
Nml	normal
tp	true positives
fn	false negatives
tn	true negatives
OR	over-referral rate
PPV	positive predictive value
UR	under-referral rate
NPV	negative predictive value
EFF	overall efficiency
% fail	overall percentage who fail

prevalence of the impairment in the population being screened. These factors have a substantial influence on the predictive value of positive and negative screening results. Moreover, it is this author's contention that these principles can explain the varying screening results of different investigators which were discussed earlier.

Based on the estimates in Table 17-2 and the collective findings shown in Table 17-1, a comment can be made about the operating characteristics of the ABR. Invariably, investigators report a very low under-referral rate, meaning that very few if any impaired newborns pass the ABR screen. We now know that this indicates very high test sensitivity. It is not unreasonable to assume, then, that the ABR operates at approximately 98% sensitivity when a cutoff score close to that of the unimpaired newborns is employed (i.e., 30 or 40 dB nHL). Specificity is more difficult to estimate, but there are a few clues. Presumably the incidence of moderate to severe impairment in the NICU graduates is nearly 5%, and with this prevalence most investigators report that between 10 and 20% failed the screen and about half of these were over-referrals. This would correspond to a specificity of between 90 and 95%!

These estimates directly relate to the concern over the proportion of over-referrals on ABR screening. Clearly, the number of over-referrals can be substantial even though the test is operating at maximum efficiency. Over-referrals depend on the cutoff point employed and the prevalence of impairment in the population tested. If the cutoff point is very low, such as the 25 dB nHL cutoff employed by Shannon and colleagues (1984), then the over-referral rate will soar, especially if newborns outside the NICU are screened, thereby lowering the prevalence of impairment even more.

The very high over-referral rate shown by Roberts and associates (1982) was unique among the others' projects. Typically, an excessively high failure rate in combination with a high over-referral rate indicates poor test specificity. In other words, too many unimpaired newborns failed the screen. A reasonable solution to this problem is to adjust the cutoff ABR score toward the abnormal group, but these investigators already used 40 dB nHL, a level used by many others who did not observe an excessive failure rate. One can only speculate about the findings of Roberts and colleagues; however, the data clearly are not representative of the majority of attempts to screen with the ABR.

MECHANICS OF A SCREENING PROGRAM

Following the preliminary decision to initiate a screening program aimed at a target population of newborns, each facility must, of course, make its own decision about which test to employ in that endeavor. It is worth noting, however, that in terms of general concepts, programs which use the ABR are no different from those which utilize behavioral responses or some other means for screening newborns. The nature and implementation of the ingredients of the program often determine its success or failure, no matter which test is employed. The ABR is merely a tool that constitutes one of the ingredients of a potentially successful program. Therefore, using the ABR in screening entails much more than buying the latest machine and then commencing with a barrage of screening tests. Table 17-4 presents a series of activities which are the prerequisites of an effective program, and the following discussion outlines the mechanics of such a venture.

Determination of Costs

Although the thought of cost in a screening program may seem callous, it is a paramount consideration in the minds of the administrative personnel. You must eventually deal with these officials with regard to your screening intentions, and it is therefore wise to have a firm grasp of just what the program will cost and how that cost will be covered.

There are three main cost aspects: equipment, personnel, and indirect expenses. These costs must be considered in the context of the number of babies you intend to screen over a given

TABLE 17–4.
Prerequisite Activities for a Screening Program which Utilizes the ABR in High-Risk Newborns

1. Establish cost factors
2. Establish screening and follow-up protocols
3. Contact key hospital personnel
4. Collect ABR normative data
5. Inservice conferences for hospital personnel
6. Modify screening protocol
7. Contact primary care physicians
8. Modify follow-up protocol
9. Determine logistical aspects
10. Begin screening

period of time, usually 1 year. If we assume that an ABR system typically costs $20,000 and we would like to earn this money back in the first 5 years of operation, then $4,000 in direct equipment expense is estimated in each of the first 5 years. In addition, the equipment must then be depreciated, typically over a period of 5 years. In other words, one-fifth of the cost of the equipment ($4,000) must be assigned to each of the first 5 years of operation so that a new device can be purchased when the present one wears out! Therefore, the total cost of equipment in this hypothetical situation is $8,000 per year.

The cost of personnel must then be estimated. Let us say that we plan to have a person spend 20 hours a week (approximately "half time") conducting the tests and coordinating the program. If this person is paid $12,300 (including 23% fringe benefits) then this figure must be added to the total cost per year. This brings the total to $20,300, including equipment and personnel.

Indirect costs also enter into the picture. These expenses are attributed to the costs of running the hospital, costs such as salaries of people who do not see patients (administration, housekeeping, maintenance, etc.) and miscellaneous expenses such as utilities. Usually these expenses are estimated at 25% of the direct costs (equipment and personnel). Consequently, we have to add 25% of $20,300, or approximately $5,000, to our total. Finally, we have to add one more indirect cost, which is sometimes called a "bad debt" allowance. This is the cost of not collecting all the money owed to the hospital and is usually estimated as an additional 25%.

Therefore, the total annual screening program costs will be approximately $30,300. The cost per test, then, would equal this amount divided by the number of anticipated ABR screening tests in 1 year. For example, if 500 tests are anticipated then the cost per test would be approximately $60. If, however, only 100 tests are planned, the cost per test will increase dramatically. Consequently, the cost per infant may realistically preclude using the ABR at your facility unless a fairly large number of babies require screening, or the program can be subsidized in other ways.

Preliminary Contacts

In addition to administrative officials, it is also important to contact the medical personnel who have a vested interest in your planned screening. Included in this group are neonatologists, pediatricians, and nursing supervisors. These people must be aware of what you intend to do and how you plan to do it. Neonatologists and pediatricians may need to be informed about congenital hearing loss, high-risk factors, alternative screening procedures, and your specific plans. The nursing supervisor is interested in the same information, but is equally interested in what role nurses will play in the program. You may have to hold conferences for these purposes.

Needless to say, there is little purpose in screening at all if the plans for follow-up are unclear. The involved medical personnel will be keenly interested in this aspect of your program. These preliminary contacts can serve to inform them of your provisions for diagnosis for those babies who fail the screen, exactly where, when, and how often all of the high-risk newborns will be followed.

Collection of Normative Data

When these aspects have been addressed and preliminary approval has been given to proceed, the first activity should be the generation of your own control sample of ABR data on newborns. These data can be collected in the term nursery while the in-service conferences are being held, and other preliminary contacts are being made. These sessions may require the approval of your facility's human rights committee. This step is vitally important, and the work involved should not pose a source of anxiety. You simply must determine the validity and reliability of your own equipment and procedures in the context of your own facility and personnel. Your main objective is to determine the minimum stimulus intensity at which virtually all of the term newborns yield an ABR. This is the only way of assuring a cutoff point that will afford maximum specificity. Some critics suggest that data from term babies cannot serve as legitimate norms for newborns in the NICU (Downs, 1982), but you are not interested in interwave latency data as much as determining minimum response stimulus levels for screening purposes.

It is not satisfactory to use the norms of other facilities even if such norms appear to be based on established physiologic principles. This incorrectly assumes that adequate standards exist pertaining to the suitability of ABR equipment, personnel, and procedures, thereby permitting the comparison of ABR results between centers. Such practices seriously endanger the operating characteristics of the ABR for screening purposes.

By taking the time to collect these norms, you can also determine those factors which undermine the reliability of your test. The results for a given newborn should not vary markedly from one test to another, assuming the status of the newborn has not changed in the interim. Obvious gremlins such as the influence of electrical artifact or electrical ground problems can surface during these activities, and it is far better to detect such problems and take corrective action at this stage than when screening has begun. A test must be reliable to have any utility, and far too often this relatively direct method for assuring reliability is overlooked.

You may need to modify the screening protocol following the collection of the control sample data. This may relate to the type of stimulus, stimulus level, or presentation rate. You may also find need for other changes such as the type of electrodes used, earphone arrangements, and so forth. These modifications are very easy to implement and serve to increase confidence in your results.

Primary Care Physicians and Parents

You must also discuss the intended screening with the primary care physicians in your community. This accomplishes two important things. It gives these physicians a chance to point out practical and philosophical objections to your intended protocols, thereby avoiding unpleasant confrontations in the future. Moreover, it provides the opportunity to initiate confidence in the results of the ABR screen. This is crucial to successful implementation of the program inasfar as optimizing the number of failures who will eventually be seen for diagnosis. You may want to meet personally with these individuals. Primary care physicians will also have an opinion about what parents should be told and how referrals for diagnosis should be made. Plan to modify your intended follow-up protocol following these sessions.

The nature and extent of interactions with parents are vital to any screening endeavor, and those programs using the ABR are no exception. Information pamphlets that describe the screening program and the meaning of ABR results are especially helpful and can easily be distributed following approval by hospital officials. Pamphlets can also be used to instruct parents on what reactions their baby should exhibit during the early months of life.

You must decide what to actually "tell" parents when the ABR test has been completed. The reader is referred to an excellent treatment of this very important area by Stein and Jabaley (1981). Above all, it must be remembered that failure on the ABR screen is *not* diagnostic of a hearing loss! The discussion given in previous sections of this chapter should make this perfectly clear by now. Consequently, the parents of babies who fail the screen should *never* be told that the infant has a "hearing loss." They should be told that there are a number of reasons why the baby may not have responded, and the result only means that it is necessary to conduct further tests when the baby is older. Carelessness is unforgivable in this area. Absolutely nothing should interfere with the very delicate phenomenon of mother-infant bonding at this time. Over-referrals are bothersome from a statistical standpoint, but they can be devastating to a mother whose child has been acutely ill since birth, if her baby's screening failure has not been portrayed with honesty. Consequently, you may want to assure that all the nursery staff, including attending physicians, understand exactly what the results mean. They will be talking to mothers about the test, and you do not want another source of possible misconceptions. In our own experience, we have found that reprinted cards with a clear explanation of the meaning of the ABR results can be distributed to incoming residents and fellows to counteract this potential misunderstanding.

Logistical Considerations

The logistics of screening with the ABR can pose a significant challenge to a fledgling program. Equipment aspects include a place to store the ABR system when not in use, sterilization of the equipment during use, and a complete safety check of the device by the appropriate hospital personnel. These are thorny details, but their importance merits preliminary attention.

You must also decide when the test will be done. Usually the afternoon is the best time. Rounds are often held in the morning and other nursery activity can interfere with your attempts, or vice versa. Also, the newborns are fed in the late morning and early afternoon and sleep thereafter, presenting an ideal opportunity for optimum ABR testing.

From a nursing standpoint, you must determine who will be your primary contact. It is invaluable to have a nurse advocate when problems and questions arise. The implementation of revisions is greatly facilitated if someone in nursing knows who you are and believes in your cause. You must also designate who in the clerical area of the NICU will assist with the identification of newborns who require the test. And you must determine how the results will be charted.

Finally, there are a few financial details to attend to. It is important to determine how a charge will be generated for the ABR test, and who in the accounting office will facilitate processing. It is unfortunate when 3 months of tests have been conducted and you discover that a bill was not posted for any of this work.

Pitfalls to Avoid

It should be apparent from the above discussion that a substantial amount of work precedes the first ABR screening test. One of the first pitfalls to avoid is to circumvent any of these steps. They are truly time consuming and challenging, but the rewards will be substantial for time well spent.

There are additional pitfalls to avoid. The ABR screening should not be conducted when the newborn is acutely ill. Newborns who are acutely ill are often the smallest and youngest and are simply too immature to yield consistent results. In addition, they are usually attached to monitoring equipment that can be a source of excessive electrical artifact. Obviously, these factors endanger the reliability of the test. It is far better to conduct the test when the infant is in the graduated care section of the NICU, is breathing room air, and is at least 35 weeks postconception (gestational age + chronological age). In other words, wait until the baby is ready to be discharged from the nursery.

Do not use a cutoff point that is too close to the normal newborn. This will result in excessive over-referrals because of (1) undetected, transient middle ear involvement, or (2) varying ambient noise levels, or both. If a baby fails at 30 or 40 dB nHL but passes at 60 or 70 dB nHL, he or she should be considered in the "observe" category. Infants with such results cannot be classified in the same category as those who fail at the higher levels; these are true "failures" and must be followed more aggressively.

It is wise to avoid the overuse of interwave latencies in the NICU, especially if you have the misguided hope of using them diagnostically. Due to a combination of maturation and a host of pathologic influences, interwave latencies are far too variable at this stage. As discussed in other sections of this text, the operating characteristics of ABR interwave latency indices in the NICU are just beginning to be defined, and these data must consequently be used with caution. This is clearly an area in which further research is vital, but care must be taken not to confuse diagnosis and screening.

SUMMARY AND CONCLUSIONS

In summary, the ABR can serve as a valuable tool in programs aimed at screening high-risk newborns for congenital hearing loss. However, the test is merely part of the program and will function in a manner proportional to the effort applied to the entire program. Criticisms of the ABR as a screening tool would appear to be based on an understandable, but unfortunate, confusion between screening and diagnosis. To date, the ABR is the best tool available to *exclude* congenital hearing loss in both ears of the suspect newborn. Because the test performs so well, over-referrals are unavoidable. This means that we must not expect too much from the test. Failure must not be interpreted as de facto evidence of hearing loss, and there is nothing whatsoever wrong with this position. Failure indicates the need for *subsequent* diagnosis, as it should in an appropriate screening program.

It is hoped that this chapter will stimulate a healthy concern for the use of the auditory brainstem response in the assessment of pediatric populations and a scientific concern for its rightful merits and limitations in this context.

REFERENCES

Alberti, P. W., Hyde, M. L., Corbin, H., Riko, K., & Abramovich, M. B. (1983). An evaluation of BERA for hearing screening in high-risk neonates. *Laryngoscope, 93,* 1115–1121.

American Academy of Pediatrics (1982). Joint Committee on Infant Hearing, Position Statement 1982. *Pediatrics, 70,* 496–497.

Cox, L. C., Hack, M., & Metz, D. (1982). Longitudinal ABR in the NICU infant. *International Journal of Pediatric Otorhinolaryngology, 4,* 225–231.

Dennis, J. M., Sheldon, R., Toubas, P., & McCaffee, M. A. (1984). Identification of hearing loss in the neonatal intensive care unit population. *American Journal of Otology, 5,* 201–205.

Despland, P., & Galambos, R. (1980). The auditory brainstem response (ABR) is a useful diagnostic tool in the intensive care nursery. *Pediatric Research, 14,* 154–158.

Downs, D. W. (1982). Auditory brainstem response testing in the neonatal intensive care unit: A cautious response. *American Speech-Language-Hearing Association, 24(12),* 1009–1016.

Downs, M. P. (1974). Early identification of hearing loss: Where are we? Where do we go from here? In G. T. Mencher (Ed.), *Early identification of hearing loss.* Basel, New York: Karger.

Downs, M.P., & Silver, H.K. (1972). The A.B.C.D's to H.E.A.R.: Early identification in nursery, office and clinic of the infant who is deaf. *Clinical Pediatrics, 11,* 563–566.

Downs, M. P., & Sterritt, G. M. (1967). A guide to newborn and infant hearing screening programs. *Archives of Otolaryngology, 85,* 37–44.

Durieux-Smith, A., Edwards, C., Hyde, M., Jacobson, J. T., Kileny, P., Picton, T., & Sanders, R. (1983). *Canadian experience in neonatal hearing screening.* Paper presented at the VIIIth Biennial Symposium of the International Electric Response Audiometry Study Group, Ottawa, Canada, July.

Feinmesser, M., & Tell, L. (1976). Neonatal screening for detection of deafness. *Archives of Otolaryngology, 102,* 297–299.

Feinmesser, M., Tell, L., & Levi, H. (1982) Follow-up of 40,000 infants screened for hearing defect. *Audiology, 21,* 197–203.

Fria, T. J., Kurmin, K., Ashoff, V., & Sinclair-Griffith, L. (1982). *Newborn screening with the auditory brain stem response (ABR).* Miniseminar presented at the Convention of the American Speech-Language-Hearing Association, Toronto, November.

Galambos, R. (1978). Use of the auditory brainstem response (ABR) in infant hearing testing. In S. E. Gerber & G. T. Mencher (Eds.), *Early diagnosis of hearing loss.* New York: Grune & Stratton.

Galambos, R., Hicks, G., & Wilson, M. J. (1982). Hearing loss in graduates of a tertiary intensive care nursery. *Ear and Hearing, 3,* 87–90.

Gerber, S. E., & Mencher, G. T. (1978). *Early diagnosis of hearing loss.* New York: Grune & Stratton.

Gerkin, K. P. (1984). The high risk register for deafness. *American Speech-Language-Hearing Association, 26(3),* 17–24.

Hecox, K., & Galambos, R. (1974). Brainstem auditory evoked responses in human infants and adults. *Archives of Otolaryngology, 99,* 30–33.

Jacobson, J. T., & Morehouse, C. R. (1984). A comparison of auditory brainstem response and behavioral screening in high risk and normal newborn infants. *Ear and Hearing, 5* (4), 247–253.

Jacobson, J. T., Seitz, M. R., Mencher, G. T., & Parrott, V. (1981). Auditory brainstem response: A contribution to infant assessment and management. In G. T. Mencher & S. E. Gerber (Eds.), *Early management of hearing loss.* New York: Grune & Stratton.

Mencher, G. T. (1976). *Early identification of hearing loss.* Basel, New York: Karger.

Mjoen, S., Langslet, A., Tangsrud, S. E., & Sundby, A. (1982). Auditory brainstem responses (ABR) in high-risk neonates. *Acta Paediatrica Scandinavica, 71,* 711–715.

Northern, J. L., & Downs, M. P. (1974). *Hearing in children.* Baltimore: Williams & Wilkins.

Roberts, J. L., Davis, H., Phon, G. L., Reichert, T. J., Sturtevant, E. M., & Marshall, R. E. (1982). Auditory brainstem responses in preterm neonates: Maturation and follow-up. *Journal of Pediatrics, 101,* 257–263.

Salamy, A., & McKean, C. M. (1976). Postnatal development of human brainstem potentials during the first year of life. *EEG & Clinical Neurophysiology, 40,* 418–426.

Salamy, A., McKean, C. M., & Buda, F. B. (1975). Maturational changes in auditory transmission as reflected in human brain stem potentials. *Brain Research, 96,* 361–366.

Schulman-Galambos, C., & Galambos, R. (1975). Brainstem auditory-evoked responses in premature infants. *Journal of Speech & Hearing Research, 18,* 456–465.

Schulman-Galambos, C., & Galambos, R. (1979). Brain stem evoked response audiometry in newborn hearing screening. *Archives of Otolaryngology, 105,* 86–90.

Shannon, D. A., Felix, J. K., Krumholz, A., Goldstein, P. J., & Harris, K. C. (1984). Hearing screening of high-risk newborns with brainstem auditory evoked potentials: A follow-up study. *Pediatrics, 73,* 22–26.

Stein, L. K., & Jabaley, T. J. (1981). Early identification and parent counseling. In L. K. Stein, E. D. Mindel, & T. J. Jabaley (Eds.), *Deafness and mental health.* New York: Grune & Stratton.

Stein, L., Ozdamar, O., Kraus, N., & Paton, J. (1983). Follow-up of infants screened by auditory brainstem response in the neonatal intensive care unit. *Journal of Pediatrics, 103,* 447–453.

Thorner, R. M., & Remein, Q. R. (1982). Principles and procedures in the evaluation of screening for disease. In J. B. Chaiklin, I. M. Ventry, & R. F. Dixon (Eds.), *Hearing measurement: A book of readings (2nd ed.).* Reading, MA: Addison–Wesley.

SECTION V
SPECIAL APPLICATIONS

Chapter 18

Auditory Brainstem Response Measures with Multiply Handicapped Children and Adults

Laszlo Stein
Nina Kraus

INTRODUCTION

The major audiometric application of auditory brainstem response (ABR) is with the difficult-to-test patient: the infant at risk for hearing impairment or the child or adult too impaired physically or mentally to cooperate for behavioral testing. Although the clinical value of ABR with both the infant and multiply handicapped child or adult was recognized early (Hecox & Galambos, 1974; Schulman-Galambos & Galambos, 1975), the potential of ABR with the multiply handicapped, despite the pressing need for electrophysiologic measures of cochlear and brain function in this population, is only now beginning to be fully realized.

Because ABR is at the same time a test of audiologic and neurologic function, investigation of the electrophysiologic signs of both the hearing impairment and the brain dysfunction, presumed to be common in many subpopulations of the neurologically, mentally, or behaviorally impaired, can yield findings of clinical as well as neuroanatomic and neurophysiologic importance. Clinically, ABR offers the means to identify hearing loss in populations often poorly served owing to the limitations of existing diagnostic procedures. Not only can individual patients be identified and treated, but also the true incidence of hearing loss among the physically or mentally retarded—a question never completely answered by studies that had to rely on behavioral tests—can be determined. In addition, ABR, possibly in conjunction with the middle and late auditory evoked potentials, may provide information on the neuroanatomic locus or neurophysiologic nature of the pervasive brain dysfunction suggested by the sensory, cognitive, and motor deficits found among the developmentally disabled or multiply handicapped. Finally, ABR may reveal forms of auditory processing deficits unique to subpopulations of the retarded, those with psychopathology, or children with language-learning disorders.

BACKGROUND

The introduction of averaging computers in the late 1950s provided clinicians for the first time with the potential to assess auditory function by electrophysiologic and presumably more objective means than by behavioral and largely subjective methods. Rapin and her colleagues (Rapin & Graziani, 1967; Rapin, Graziani, & Lyttle, 1969; Rapin, Ruben, & Lyttle, 1970) were among the first to use the late auditory evoked potentials (AEPs) occurring 50 to 250 ms following stimulus onset (Picton, Hillyard, Krauz, & Galambos, 1974) to investigate auditory behavior in several groups of infants and young children with severe neurologic impairment. Although these investigators were able to conclude that hearing thresholds obtained with the late AEP or cortical evoked potential in severely retarded infants and children were often lower than behavioral thresholds, they and others soon found that the presence of abnormal brain wave patterns (electroencephalograms or EEGs) either masked or precluded generation of the late AEP, thus making threshold detection unreliable. In some brain damaged children likely to have sustained damage to both the cochlea and cerebral structures, it was impossible to determine whether late AEPs obtained at elevated thresholds were the result of pathology to the auditory periphery or to the central nervous system. The effects of sleep, sedation, attention, and general state of arousal on the late AEPs posed additional problems (Picton & Hillyard, 1974; Picton et al., 1974; Williams, Tepas, & Morlock, 1962). Subsequently, Cohen and Rapin (1978) investigated the clinical usefulness of the late AEP in combination with the early response (ABR) as an approach to electrophysiologic audiometry with multiply handicapped children. The combined use of ABR, the middle latency response (MLR), and the late AEP will be discussed in greater detail in a subsequent section.

Early attempts at assessing auditory function in difficult-to-test patients also included electrocochleography (ECochG). For detailed descriptions of the ECochG technique, the interested reader is referred to other publications (Eggermont, Odenthal, Schmidt, & Spoor, 1974; Naunton and Zerlin, 1978; Zerlin and Naunton, 1978).

The works of Lyons, Berlin, Lousteau, Ellis, and Yarbrough (1974) and Cullen, Berlin, Gondra and Adams (1976) exemplifies the use of ECochG to assess cochlear function in children and retardates in whom reliable behavioral audiograms were difficult or impossible to obtain. Although ECochG was judged a useful and important contribution in assessing peripheral hearing loss or normal cochlear function in children otherwise unresponsive to auditory stimulation, it was recognized that ECochG did not measure hearing in the sense of behavioral audiometry. Cullen and associates (1976) cited two cases illustrating that the presence of an eighth nerve action potential elicited by click stimuli may not rule out deaf-like behavior due to a central disorder, nor did the absence of an ECochG response rule out the possibility of unusual forms of residual high frequency hearing, limitations that also apply to ABR. The major limitation of ECochG, however, was and continues to be the need to place the child under general anesthesia in order to perform either a transtympanic or tympanic membrane measure. Despite the estimate by Crowley, Davis, and Beagley (1975) that anesthetic complications occur in less than one percent of patients tested by ECochG, its use with children even in major hospital centers was limited to a select few. The introduction of ABR in the early 1970s with its inherent advantages of being able to assess cochlear and brainstem function through surface electrodes under sleep or sedation, thus obviating the need for a surgical procedure or general anesthesia, soon made it the method of choice for the majority of clinicians.

SPECIAL POPULATIONS

Down's Syndrome. Characteristic genetic, physical, and behavioral signs clearly identify Down's syndrome from other and often less well defined forms of retardation. Because diagnosis is less problematic, Down's syndrome has been extensively investigated. It is an especially interesting subpopulation for study of the auditory system because of evidence suggesting a higher incidence of hearing loss (Brooks, Wooley, & Kanjilal, 1972) and reports of anatomic abnormalities in cochlear and neural structures—shortened cochlear spirals and disorders of the vestibular system (Igarashi, Takahashi, Alford, & Johnson, 1977); reduced weight of the cerebellum and brainstem, suggesting lack of development of these structures (Crome, Cowie, & Slater, 1966); and instances of generalized cellular agenesis and abnormal or incomplete myelination (Banik, Davison, Palo, & Savolainen, 1975; Benda, 1969).

Squires, Aine, Buchwald, Norman, and Galbraith (1980) compared the ABRs of 16 Down's syndrome retarded male adults and 15 male adults with retardation of unknown etiology, with 15 nonretarded control subjects as a function of stimulus intensity and repetition rate. Absent ABRs suggested profound hearing loss in one or both ears of four Down's syndrome subjects and in two subjects with retardation of unknown etiology, lending further support to the generally reported higher incidence of hearing loss among retarded populations.

Of greatest interest, however, were findings suggesting functional abnormalities in the auditory brainstem pathway of the Down's syndrome group and, to a lesser extent, in the unknown etiology group. Although a number of subjects in the unknown etiology group showed abnormal neural conduction times (prolonged wave I–V interval), the Down's syndrome group demonstrated shorter interwave intervals (IWI) and an overall decrease in central conduction time as reflected by a shortened wave I–V interval. The abnormal transmission time was not produced by systematic reduction in all IWIs, but by a selective shortening of the I–II and III–IV intervals (Squires, Buchwald, Liley, & Strecker, 1982). The Down's syndrome group also differed from the unknown etiology and control groups by showing significantly less change in wave V latency with increased rate of stimulation (over a 20–50/s range). Thus, the Down's syndrome group was characterized by abnormally short central transmission time and a differential resistance to fast click rates.

Consistent with these findings by Squires and colleagues (1980) are those reported by Folsom, Widen, and Wilson (1983) of shorter absolute wave V latencies in a group of infants with Down's syndrome. ABR results with 38 Down's syndrome infants across three age groups (3 weeks, 6 weeks, and 12 months) were compared with age-matched controls. At 12 months of age, the group with Down's syndrome showed shorter wave V latencies and steeper wave V intensity-latency functions at 40 and 60 dH nHL than the controls. As in the study by Squires and co-workers (1980), caution must be exercised as to whether these data imply abnormalities of peripheral, central, or peripheral and central origin, especially in the absence of audiometric data.

Further evidence of differences in the ABR patterns of individuals with Down's syndrome was found by Galbraith, Aine, Squires, and Buchwald (1983) in a study extending their earlier work (Squires et al., 1980). Among 35 male retarded subjects (14 with Down's syndrome and 21 with retardation of unknown etiology), Down's syndrome individuals were found to have significantly smaller amplitude waves II and III, shorter latencies for waves III and V, and shorter interwave conduction times (I–III and I–V) compared with the unknown etiology retarded group. The normal group showed good definition of waves I and II (90 and 86 percent, respectively), the retarded of unknown etiology group showed poor definition (43 and 52 percent, respectively), and the Down's syndrome group showed extremely good definition of wave I (100 percent) and poor definition of wave II (50 percent). The result of the main focus of the study, the assessment of binaural interaction, was that retarded individuals with Down's syndrome and those with retardation of unknown etiology did not differ from nonretarded individuals in their response to binaural stimulation. Although the assumption that binaural interaction, considered by some as an operational measure of neural efficiency reflected by the convergence of binaural inputs into the brainstem neuronal pool, would differ in degree among retarded individuals was not substantiated, the authors did propose that the significantly smaller overall amplitude of ABR waves in the Down's syndrome subjects suggests that the brainstem pool generating the ABR may be abnormally small or variable.

ABR studies to date generally report significantly shorter latencies, smaller amplitudes, and reduction in certain interwave intervals in Down's syndrome individuals. Interestingly, these abnormal ABR patterns are the inverse of those found for the late AEPs in this population. Latencies for P100, N100, and P200 have been found to be significantly longer (Yellin, Lodwig,

& Jerison, 1980) and amplitudes for the late components P60–N100, N100–P170, P170–N250 have been found to be larger (Dustman & Callner, 1979) in Down's syndrome subjects than in nonretarded subjects. A similar trend of large amplitude evoked potentials in Down's syndrome subjects is also reported for the visual and somatosensory modalities (Dustman & Callner, 1979). Whereas obvious amplitude reductions occur with maturation and aging among nonretarded subjects, such age-related amplitude changes in visual, auditory, and somatosensory evoked responses are generally absent among Down's syndrome subjects (Callner, Dustman, Madsen, Schenkenberg, & Beck, 1978).

Down's syndrome adults also fail to show the fast habituation of cortical potentials evoked by repetitive auditory stimuli characteristic of nonretarded persons (Schafer & Peeke, 1982). Together with the observation that wave V latency showed a significant lack of sensitivity to increases in rate of stimulation, it appears that brainstem as well as cortical neurons are deficient in their response to repetitive stimuli in Down's syndrome patients. Such findings have prompted several investigators to suggest that an abnormality in the ability to adapt and inhibit neural responses to redundant sensory information may underlie behavioral mental retardation.

Infantile Autism. Over the past 20 years, the direction of research seeking to explain the etiologic factors of infantile autism has shifted from psychoanalytic (environmental) to neurobiologic (genetic, neurochemical, and electrophysiologic) studies. There has emerged general agreement that the cognitive and language handicaps and the unusual responsivity to human contact that typify infantile autism are the result of brain dysfunction. Uncertain, however, are the anatomic or neurophysiologic mechanisms underlying the pathophysiology of the syndrome. Currently, neurobiologic theories range from forebrain (failure to develop hemispheric specialization, dysfunction of the frontolimbic system or of specific nuclear groups of the thalamus, and so forth) to brainstem (auditory, vestibular, cardioregulatory dysfunction, and so forth) models. Although it is difficult to ascribe a functional role to brainstem structures in cognition and language, there is growing belief that brainstem dysfunction may result in altered auditory input severe enough to account for the failure of autistic children to develop specific skills in these areas. This belief stems principally from an expanding body of electrophysiologic data.

One of the earliest studies to record ABR in infants and children with various types of psychopathology, including autism, was that of Sohmer and Student (1977). Three groups of children (13 with autism, 16 diagnosed as having minimal brain dysfunction, and 10 having psychomotor retardation) were tested. Specific findings with the autistic group included absent ABRs in four of the children, suggesting the possibility of profound cochlear hearing loss in addition to autistic traits. The remaining nine autistic children all had ABRs at normal threshold values, but the latency of each response wave was significantly longer than normal. Similar findings of longer brainstem transmission time were obtained for the minimal brain damage and retarded groups in comparison with the control group. The authors interpreted these findings as evidence supporting the hypothesis that the abnormal behavior seen in these children was due to an organic brain lesion.

In a study that matched six autistic children by age and sex with six normal children and carefully controlled for possible hearing impairment, Rosenblum, Arick, Krug, Stubbs, Young, and Pelson (1980); significantly longer ABR latencies and central conduction times were also found for the autistic group. In addition to prolonged wave latencies, the autistic children showed significantly more variability than did the normal control group. Rosenblum and colleagues (1980) believed that their findings confirmed those of Sohmer and Student (1977) and extended the evidence for brainstem dysfunction in autistic children (suppression of vestibular nystagmus) described by Ornitz, Brown, Mason, & Putnam (1974).

Tanguay and Edwards (1982), despite their acknowledged earlier skepticism about the brainstem model, accepted the possibility that some autistic children may have abnormalities in auditory reception due to abnormal brainstem processing of auditory input. Their acceptance was based on the study by Rosenblum and co-workers (1980), the work of Skoff, Mirsky, and Turner (1980), who also found prolongation of neural conduction times in autistic children, and their own study. Utilizing 16 autistic and 16 matched control subjects, Tanguay and Edwards found two types of ABR abnormalities in the autistic group: (1) a delay in wave I latency primarily in response to right ear stimulation; and (2) increased interwave latencies for waves I–III, III–V, or I–V. Although Tanguay and Edwards acknowledged the possibility that these brainstem findings may not underlie the child's autistic handicaps but simply be another manifestation of pervasive pathology affecting many parts of the brain, they advanced an interpretation that brainstem dysfunction leading to distortion in auditory input to the forebrain may have been present during a critical phase of early postnatal development. Citing animal research that has demonstrated the importance of environmental stimulation in the developing organism (Hirsch & Spinelli, 1970; Hubel & Wiesel, 1970; Werman & Clopton, 1977), they speculate that the resultant disruption in normal neural connections during such a critical period of development could be a major pathophysiologic factor in infant autism.

Deaf-Blind. In a 1981 publication, Stein, Ozdamar, and Schnabel reported ABR findings with 79 severely developmentally delayed infants and children suspected of being both blind and deaf. All demonstrated signs of cerebral dysfunction, and all 56 children in the two year and older age groupings were judged to fall into the trainable or upper trainable classification (Stein, Palmer, & Weinberg, 1982).

Of the 79 children, 34 (43.0 percent) demonstrated click thresholds in the 0–30 dB HL range, 16 (19.5 percent) in the 40–70 dB HL range, 3 (4.6 percent) in the 80–90 dB HL range, and 26 (32.9 percent) no response to 90 dB HL stimuli. Twenty-six of the 34 children yielding ABR click thresholds at normal to borderline-normal levels (0–30 dB HL) ranged in age from three to 12 years. On the basis of extensive behavioral audiometric testing and teacher reports, all 26 children were judged to be severely hearing impaired or deaf. The ABRs of all 34 infants and children with click thresholds in the 0–30 dB HL range were judged to be audiologically and neurologically normal.

According to the following criteria, (1) no ABR at maximum stimulus intensities, (2) wave I only, or (3) prolonged wave V but no detectable wave I, 26 children with absent ABR and five with elevated ABR thresholds were classified as audiologically or neurologically abnormal, or both. It was reasoned that although absent ABR or elevated wave V thresholds are generally believed to reflect hearing loss, it is not always possible to determine whether concomitant brainstem involvement may have compromised the ABR, thereby leading to an overestimation of the severity of the hearing loss. Prolonged I–V wave intervals occurred in only three subjects, a relatively small number, given the severity of the neurologic and developmental handicaps in the study population.

The principal conclusion of the study by Stein and colleagues was that a high percentage of multiply handicapped children who appear to be deaf and are so labeled in fact may not be hearing impaired, at least as that term is commonly defined. Sohoel, Mair, Everland, and Laukli (1979) and Harris, Broms, and Mollerstrom (1981) also reported findings with similar implications. In 12 of 22 children earlier regarded as having some degree of hearing loss, Sohoel and co-workers reported ABR thresholds consistent with normal hearing sensitivity. Harris and associates found that in 5 of 13 children with suspected or diagnosed hearing loss, ABR findings indicated normal peripheral auditory function, and training with hearing aids was therefore discontinued.

Infantile Spasms. The clinical picture of infantile spasms includes motor abnormalities, abnormal EEG, and mental retardation. Infants with infantile spasms are frequently suspected of having an associated hearing impairment because they tend to be behaviorally unresponsive to sound. Kaga, Marsh, and Fukuyama (1982) compared ABR and behavioral audiometric findings in 30 infants. They found that although thresholds were severely elevated by behavioral audiometry in 86 percent of the subjects, ABR thresholds were elevated in only 27 percent.

The investigators concluded that the threshold elevation seen in behavioral audiometry is seldom caused by peripheral lesions. They also reported ABR evidence for brainstem dysfunction in 30% of the patients with infantile spasms.

Hydrocephalus. Hydrocephalus, in which enlargement of the ventricular system occurs as a result of an imbalance between production and absorption of cerebrospinal fluid (CSF), is associated with several multihandicapping conditions. ABR was measured in 40 patients (80 ears) with confirmed hydrocephalus by Kraus, Ozdamar, Heydemann, Stein, and Reed (1984). Fully 88 percent of the patients showed some form of ABR abnormality. Responses indicative of brainstem dysfunction consisted of prolonged I–V interwave latency (38 percent), reduced V/I amplitude ratio (33 percent), and abnormal morphology of waves III (27 percent) and V (53 percent). ABR threshold abnormalities were observed in 70 percent of these patients: 45 percent had responses in excess of 20 dB HL, and ABRs were absent in the remaining 25 percent. The results were compared with ABRs obtained in 60 postmeningitic patients and 100 multiply handicapped institutionalized children tested under similar conditions, in whom the incidence of intrinsic brainstem abnormalities was one third and two thirds that of the hydrocephalic group, respectively. The authors concluded that ABR can be used to document clinically unsuspected brainstem pathology that may accompany hydrocephalus, and that dysfunction of the auditory brainstem is likely to complicate the assessment of hearing sensitivity in hydrocephalic patients.

ABR has also been proved to be clinically useful in the diagnosis, localization, and monitoring of intracranial pathology in a number of other multiply handicapping conditions. These include myelin disorders, such as maple syrup urine disease, phenylketonuria, Leigh disease, and the leukodystrophies (Hecox, Cone, & Blaw, 1981; Kaga, Tokoro, Tanaka, & Ushijima, 1980b; Ochs, Markand, & DeMyer, 1979).

ABR, MLR, AND LATE AEP

Apparent from the preceding reviews of the use of ABR as both an audiologic and neurologic test with various subpopulations of the mentally and physically handicapped are its advantages as well as its limitations.

As an audiologic test, ABR is a measure of the synchronous neural activity of the eighth nerve and the auditory brainstem. In general, when there is no indication of brainstem neuropathology, ABR and audiologic findings are usually in close agreement. Yet, as we (Stein et al., 1981) and others (Galambos & Hecox, 1977; Harris et al., 1981; Sohoel et al., 1979) have reported, there are exceptions—instances in which an apparently clinically hearing impaired or deaf individual yields audiologically normal ABRs. The converse is also true—instances of waves I and II only or absent ABRs in individuals who behaviorally respond to tones at normal or near-normal levels (Davis & Hirsh, 1979; Lenhardt, 1981; Worthington & Peters, 1980). Kraus, Ozdamar, Stein, & Reed (1984a) have shown that 15 percent of patients with absent ABRs or waves I and II only and no other clinical evidence of brainstem dysfunction demonstrate behavioral hearing sensitivity ranging from normal hearing to moderate impairment. This estimate represents 1.3 to 1.8 percent of the total 543 children tested by ABR for hearing by the authors during a three year period. Both Kraus and associates (1984) and Blegvad, Svane-Knudsen, and Børre (1984) provide behavioral evidence suggesting that such aberrant ABRs may underlie auditory processing deficits and speech retardation.

As a neurologic test of brainstem function, ABR can provide useful information only if the patient has a functioning cochlea and auditory nerve. Hearing loss, especially high frequency loss, can compromise click-elicited ABR components (Coats & Martin, 1977) and invalidate estimates of central conduction time for neurologic purposes. Several of the earlier cited reports on Down's syndrome subjects included a caution about the possible effects of undetected hearing loss on central conduction time.

It is clear that ABR has largely supplanted the middle latency response (auditory evoked potentials occurring 8 to 50 ms after onset of acoustic stimuli) and the late auditory or cortical potential (50 to 250 ms poststimulus) as a clinical test of hearing sensitivity. It is also apparent that ABR does not provide information concerning the electrophysiologic state of the higher levels of the auditory pathway and, by inference, the ability of the subject to understand acoustic information.

As indicated earlier, Cohen and Rapin (1978) and their colleagues were among the first to advocate the combined use of early and late auditory evoked potentials with multiply handicapped children. They believed that ABR and late AEP were complementary methods, especially in children with complex communication disorders, in which late AEPs might provide supplemental information about the functioning of the cortical portion of the auditory system. Their experience suggested that ABR and late AEP thresholds generally agree. Exceptions occurred in children with abnormal EEGs whose ABRs indicated normal auditory sensitivity but whose late AEPs were abnormal, indicating possible dysfunction at the cortical level. In children with severe brain damage in whom both ABR and late AEPs were absent, it was unclear whether the site of pathology was in the cochlea, brainstem, or higher auditory centers.

Although described more than 25 years ago (Geisler, Frishkopt, & Rosenblith, 1958), relatively little is known about the MLR in comparison to the ABR and the late AEP. Recently, however, interest in the MLR has been renewed, not necessarily as a threshold test, but as a means for assessing the electrophysiologic status of the auditory system central to the brainstem. Suzuki, Yasuhito, and Horiuchi (1981) and Ozdamar and Kraus (1983) described a method permitting simultaneous recording of ABR and MLR, thus facilitating comparisons between the two responses. The recording technique utilizes wide bandpass filters (3-2000 Hz, 6 dB/octave). Sleep and mild sedatives do not appear to affect the MLR (Harker, Hosick, Voots,& Mendel, 1977; Ozdamar & Kraus, 1983). Although the MLRs are thought to be generated central to the brainstem, an understanding of the specific generator sites is necessary before they can be maximally utilized clinically. At present, consensus is lacking regarding the origin of MLRs in humans (Celesia, 1976; Cohen, 1982; Goff, Matsumiya, Allison, & Goff, 1977; Kraus, Ozdamer, Hier, & Stein, 1982; Ozdamer, Kraus, & Curry, 1982; Picton et al., 1974; Vaughn & Ritter, 1970; Wood & Wolpaw, 1982) or animals (Arezzo, Pickoff, & Vaughn, 1975; Buchwald, Hinman, Norman, Huang, & Brown, 1981; Hinman & Buchwald, 1983; Kaga, Hink, Shinoda, & Suzuki, 1980a; Teas & Kiang, 1964). Proposed generator sites include primary auditory cortex, association cortex, and thalamus (primary auditory and reticulothalamic pathways). Although the exact generators of the MLR are unknown, clinical data obtained by Kraus and associates (1982) from patients with anatomically defined cortical lesions suggest that Pa (the vertex-positive component of the MLR occurring at approximately 30 ms poststimulus) is affected by temporal lobe lesions involving auditory cortex and thalamic projections.

Although MLRs have been recorded successfully in infants and children (Frye-Osier, Goldstein, Hirsch & Webster, 1982; McRandle, Smith, & Goldstein, 1974; Mendelson & Salamy, 1981; Wolf & Goldstein 1980), it is becoming increasingly recognized that MLRs in children may differ substantially from those of adults (Davis, 1976; Engel, 1971; Kraus, Reed, Smith, Stein, & Cartee, 1984b; Skinner & Glattke, 1977; Suzuki, Hirabayashi, & Kobayashi, 1983). MLR components Na and Pa (at approximately 17 and 30 ms, respectively) are reliably obtained in adults (Mendel & Hosick, 1975; Picton et al., 1974; Ozdamar & Kraus, 1983); however, MLRs are often inconsistently obtained in children. Whether this variability is due to the different energy concentrations of the EEG in children versus adults (Graziani, Katz, Cracco, Cracco, & Weitzman, 1974) or to maturation of the generator sources of the MLRs remains to be determined. The manner in which MLRs obtained from normal subjects compare to the responses from retarded individuals must also be investigated before the potential of the MLR as a diagnostic tool can be fully realized.

Clinical application of combined recording of ABR, MLR, and late AEPs with multiply handicapped patients has been recently extended by several investigators. Kileny and Berry (1983) report ABR, MLR, and late AEPs obtained on 15 children aged six weeks to 15 years with evidence of neurologic involvement in the form of hypotonia, spasticity, or convulsive disorder primarily due to anoxia. ABR was consistent with normal hearing in all subjects, with two exceptions suggestive of mild hearing loss. Prolonged interwave latencies were observed in six cases. MLR was absent in two and abnormal in three of the 11 patients tested. The late AEP was either absent or abnormal in all 15 patients. The authors concluded that MLR and late AEPs are better suited to determining function rather than threshold or the specific site of lesion.

In a study of 24 children from 2 to 14 years of age, half of whom were referred because of psychiatric disturbances and the other half because of suspected deafness, Robier, Lemaire, Garreau, Ployet, Martineau, Delvert, and Reynaud (1983) found that the combined use of ABR and late AEPs enabled them to modify the initial diagnosis of 11 of the 24 children. Absent ABR and late AEPs were generally associated with sensorineural deafness; normal ABR and absent or pathologic late AEPs were associated with autism. The authors concluded that the combined clinical data from ABR and late AEPs were helpful in separating deafness from psychiatric disturbance in difficult-to-test children.

CONCLUSIONS AND SUMMARY

Auditory evoked potentials, particularly ABR, have made a profound contribution to the differential diagnosis of auditory problems in the child or adult too impaired physically or mentally to cooperate in behavioral testing. With inherent advantages of being able to assess cochlear and auditory brainstem function through surface electrodes under sleep or sedation, ABR has been utilized by audiologists and electrophysiologists to investigate both the clinical and neurophysiologic nature of the sensory and cognitive deficits presumed to be common in many subpopulations of the neurologically, mentally, or behaviorally impaired.

ABR does provide a means of identifying hearing impairment in children and adults often poorly served due to limitations of existing test procedures. The implications for audiology are numerous. A means is now available to identify and clinically manage not only the previously undiagnosed hearing impaired child or adult but also those mistakenly thought to be deaf. Properly interpreted, the results of ABR testing with the multiply handicapped can contribute information critical to the differential diagnostic process. Although ABR data may be obtained in an objective manner, the very nature of the multiply handicapped population places a premium on interpretation and the need for caution by a less-than-objective examiner.

Both the audiologist and the electrophysiologist must realize that an abnormal ABR may be due to neurologic dysfunction, not necessarily hearing loss. Absent ABR, abnormal waveform morphology, or prolonged neural conduction times are frequent findings in subpopulations of the neurologically, mentally, or behaviorally impaired. The risk of misinterpretation of ABR results in these patients is particularly high. As an example, it is impossible to determine the extent to which the absence of sound evoked bioelectric activity reflects sensorineural hearing loss, brainstem neuropathology, or both. In patients with suspected or confirmed neurologic dysfunction, and in the absence of behavioral audiologic testing, inferences regarding hearing sensitivity based on an abnormal ABR should be made with caution. Similarly, without contributory audiologic data, caution must be exercised in ascribing ABR abnormalities, such as shortened neural conduction time and steeper wave V intensity-latency functions, solely to auditory brainstem dysfunction.

Given these cautions, the repeatedly confirmed observations of decreased central conduction times in Down's syndrome patients, prolongation of ABR waves in infantile autism, and other ABR evidence of brainstem dysfunction in various subgroups of the multiply handicapped have potentially important implications. If, as several investigators have speculated, there is a relationship between auditory brainstem dysfunction as revealed by ABR and auditory processing problems, an organic basis for some forms of communication and learning disorders may be revealed. It seems certain that the combined use of ABR, MLR, and the late AEP will be increasingly studied in children presenting a variety of behavioral symptoms associated with auditory, language, or learning disorders.

BIBLIOGRAPHY

Arezzo, J., Pickoff, A., & Vaughn, H. G. (1975). The sources and intracerebral distribution of auditory evoked potentials in the alert rhesus monkey. *Brain Research, 90*, 57–73.

Banik, N. L., Davison, A. N., Palo, J., & Savolainen, H. (1975). Biochemical studies of myelin isolated from the brains of patients with Down's syndrome. *Brain, 98*, 213–218.

Benda, C. E. (1969). *Down's syndrome*. New York: Grune & Stratton.

Blegvad, B., Svane-Knudsen, V., & Børre, S. (1984). ABR in patients with congenital/early acquired sensorineural hearing loss, abnormal stapedius reflex thresholds, and speech retardation. *Scandinavian Audiology, 13*, 41–46.

Brooks, D. N., Wooley, H., & Kanjilal, G. C. (1972). Hearing loss and middle ear disorders in patients with Down's syndrome (mongolism). *Journal of Mental Deficiency Research, 16*, 21–29.

Buchwald, J. S., Hinman, C., Norman, R. J., Huang, C. M., & Brown, K. A. (1981). Middle and long-latency auditory evoked potentials recorded from the vertex of normal and chronically lesioned cats. *Brain Research, 205*, 91–109.

Callner, D. A., Dustman, R. E., Madsen, J. A., Schenkenberg, T., & Beck, C. E. (1978). Life span changes in the averaged evoked responses of Down's syndrome and nonretarded persons. *American Journal of Mental Deficiency, 82*, 398–405.

Celesia, G. G. (1976). Organization of auditory cortical areas in man. *Brain, 99*, 403–414.

Coats, A., & Martin, J. (1977). Human auditory nerve action potentials and brainstem evoked responses: Effects of Audiogram shape and lesion location. *Archives of Otolaryngology, 103*, 605.

Cohen, M. M. (1982). Coronal topography of the middle latency auditory evoked potentials in man. *Electroencephalography and Clinical Neurophysiology, 53*, 231–236.

Cohen, M. M., & Rapin, I. (1978). Evoked potential audiometry in neurologically impaired. In R. Naunton & C. Fernandez (Eds.), *Evoked electrical activity in the auditory nervous system*. New York: Academic Press.

Crome, L., Cowie, V., & Slater, E. (1966). A statistical note on cerebellar and brain-stem weight in mongolism. *Journal of Mental Deficiency Research, 10*, 69–72.

Crowley, D. E., Davis, H., & Beagley, H. A. (1975). Survey of the clinical use of electrocochleography. *Annals of Otology, Rhinology, and Laryngology, 84*, 1–11.

Cullen, J. K., Berlin, C. I., Gondra, M. I., & Adams, M. L. (1976). Electrocochleography in children. *Archives of Otolaryngology, 102*, 482–486.

Davis, H. (1976). Principles of electric response audiometry. *Annals of Otology, Rhinology, and Laryngology Supplement, 28*, 1–80.

Davis, H., & Hirsh, S. K. (1979). A slow brainstem response for low-frequency audiometry. *Audiology, 18*, 445–461.

Dustman, R.E., & Callner, A.A. (1979). Cortical evoked responses and response decrement in nonretarded and Down's syndrome individuals. *American Journal of Mental Deficiency*, *83*, 391-397.

Eggermont, J. J., Odenthal, D. W., Schmidt, P. H., & Spoor, A. (1974). Electrocochleography. Basic principles and clinical application. *Acta Otolaryngology Supplement*, *316*, 1-84.

Engel, R. (1971). Early waves of the electroencephalic auditory response in neonates. *Neuropaediatrie*, *3*, 147-154.

Folsom, R. C., Widen, J. E., & Wilson, W. R. (1983). Auditory brain-stem responses in infants with Down's syndrome. *Archives of Otolaryngology*, *109*, 607-610.

Frye-Osier, H. A., Goldstein, R., Hirsch, J. E., & Webster, K. (1982). Early and middle-AER components to clicks as response indices for neonatal hearing screening. *Annals of Otology, Rhinology, and Laryngology*, *91*, 272-276.

Galambos, R., & Hecox, K. (1977). Clinical applications of the brain stem auditory evoked potentials. In J.E. Desmedt (Ed.), *Auditory evoked potentials in man. Progress in clinical neurophysiology* (vol. 2). Basel: S. Karger.

Galbraith, G., Aine, C., Squires, N., & Buchwald, J. (1983). Binaural interaction in auditory brainstem responses of mentally retarded and nonretarded individuals. *American Journal of Mental Deficiency*, *87*, 551-557.

Geisler, C. D., Frishkopt, L. S., & Rosenblith, W. A. (1958). Extracranial responses to acoustic clicks in man. *Science*, *128*, 1210-1211.

Goff, G. D., Matsumiya, Y., Allison, T., & Goff, W. R. (1977). The scalp topography of human somatosensory and auditory evoked potentials. *Electroencephalography and Clinical Neurophysiology*, *42*, 57-76.

Graziani, L. J., Katz, L., Cracco, R. Q., Cracco, J. B., & Weitzman, E. D. (1974). The maturation and interrelationship of EEG patterns and auditory evoked responses in premature infants. *Electroencephalography and Clinical Neuphysiology*, *36*, 367-375.

Harker, I. A., Hosick, E., Voots, R. J., & Mendel, M. (1977). Influence of succinylcholine on middle component auditory evoked potentials. *Archives of Otolaryngology*, *103*, 133-137.

Harris, S., Broms, P., & Mollerstrom, B. (1981). ABR in the mentally retarded child. *Scandinavian Audiology Supplement*, *13*, 149-150.

Hecox, K. E., Cone, B., & Blaw, M. E. (1981). Brainstem auditory evoked response in the diagnosis of pediatric neurologic diseases. *Neurology*, *31*, 832-840.

Hecox, K. E., & Galambos, R. (1974). Brainstem auditory evoked responses in human infants and adults. *Archives of Otolaryngology*, *99*, 30-33.

Hinman, C. L., & Buchwald, J. (1983). Depth evoked potentials and single unit correlates of vertex mid latency auditory evoked responses. *Brain Research*, *264*, 57-67.

Hirsch, H.V., & Spinelli, D.N. (1970). Visual experience modifies disruption of horizontally and vertically oriented receptive fields in cats. *Science*, *168*, 869-871.

Hubel, D. H., & Wiesel, T. N. (1970). The period of susceptibility to physiologic effects of unilateral eye closure in cats. *Journal of Physiology*, *206*, 419-436.

Igarashi, M., Takahashi, M., Alford, B. R., & Johnson, P. E. (1977). Inner ear morphology in Down's syndrome. *Acta Otolaryngology*, *83*, 175-181.

Kaga, K., Hink, R., Shinoda, Y., & Suzuki, J. (1980a). Evidence for a primary cortical origin of a middle latency auditory evoked potential in cats. *Electroencephalography and Clinical Neurophysiology*, *50*, 254-266.

Kaga, K., Marsh, R. R., & Fukuyama, Y. (1982). Auditory brainstem responses in infantile spasms. *International Journal of Pediatric Otorhinolaryngology*, *4*, 57-67.

Kaga, K., Tokoro, Y., Tanaka, Y., & Ushijima, H. (1980b). The progress of adrenoleukodystrophy as revealed by auditory brainstem evoked responses and brainstem histology. *Archives of Otorhinolaryngology*, *228*, 17-27.

Kileny, P., & Berry, D. A. (1983). Selective impairment of late vertex and middle latency auditory evoked responses. In G. Mencher & S. Gerber (Eds.), *The multiply handicapped hearing impaired child*. New York: Grune & Stratton.

Kraus, N., Ozdamar, O., Heydemann, P. T., Stein, L., & Reed, N. (1984). Auditory brainstem responses in hydrocephalic patients. *Electroencephalography and Clinical Neurophysiology, 59*, 310–317.

Kraus, N., Ozdamar, O., Hier, D., & Stein, L. (1982). Auditory middle latency responses (MLRs) in patients with cortical lesions. *Electroencephalography and Clinical Neurophysiology, 54*, 275–287.

Kraus, N., Ozdamar, O., Stein, L., & Reed, N. (1984a). Absent auditory brain stem response: peripheral hearing loss or brain stem dysfunction? *Laryngoscope, 94*, 400–406.

Kraus, N., Reed, N., Smith, D. I., Stein, L., & Cartee, C. (1984b). Middle latency responses in infants and children. International Congress of Audiology Abstracts.

Lenhardt, M. (1981). Childhood central auditory processing disorder with brainstem evoked response verification. *Archives of Otolaryngology, 107*, 623–625.

Lyons, G.D., Berlin, C.I., Lousteau, R.J., Ellis, M.S., & Yarbrough, W.M. (1974). Electrocochleography with retardates. *Laryngoscope, 6*, 990–997.

McRandle, C. C., Smith, M. A., & Goldstein, R. (1974). Early averaged electroencephalic responses to clicks in neonates. *Annals of Otology, Rhinology, and Laryngology, 83*, 695–701.

Mendel, M. I., & Hosick, E. C. (1975). Effects of secobarbital on the early components of the auditory evoked potentials. *Revue de Laryngologie, 96*, 178–184.

Mendelson, T., & Salamy, A. (1981). Maturational effects on the middle components of the averaged electroencephalic response. Journal of Speech and Hearing Research, *46*, 140–144.

Naunton, R. F., & Zerlin, S. S. (1978). Electrocochleography: behavioral threshold comparisons. In R. Naunton & C. Fernandez (Eds.), *Evoked electrical activity in the auditory nervous system*. New York: Academic Press.

Ochs, R., Markand, O. N., & DeMyer, W. E. (1979). Brainstem auditory evoked responses in leukodystrophies. *Neurology, 29*, 1089–1093.

Ornitz, E. M., Brown, M. B., Mason, A., & Putnam, N. H. (1974). Effects of visual input on vestibular nystagmus in autistic children. *Archives of General Psychiatry, 31*, 369–375.

Ozdamar, O., & Kraus, N. (1983). Auditory middle-latency responses in humans. *Audiology, 22*, 34–49.

Ozdamar, O., Kraus, N., & Curry, F. (1982). Auditory brainstem and middle latency responses in a patient with cortical deafness. *Electroencephalography and Clinical Neurophysiology, 53*, 224–230.

Picton, T.W., & Hillyard, S.A. (1974). Human auditory evoked potentials. II. Effects of attention. *Electroencephalography and Clinical Neurophysiology, 36*, 191–199.

Picton, T. W., Hillyard, S. A., Krauz, H. I., & Galambos, R. (1974). Human auditory evoked potentials. I. Evaluation of components. *Electroencephalography and Clinical Neurophysiology, 36*, 179–191.

Rapin, I., & Graziani, L. J. (1967). Auditory-evoked responses in normal, brain damaged, and deaf infants. *Neurology, 17*, 881–894.

Rapin, I., Graziani, L. J., & Lyttle, M. (1969). Summated auditory evoked responses for audiometry: experience in 51 children with congenital rubella. *International Audiology, 8*, 371–376.

Rapin, I., Ruben, R. J., & Lyttle, M. (1970) Diagnosis of hearing loss in infants using auditory evoked responses. *Laryngoscope, 80*, 717–722.

Robier, A., Lemaire, M. C., Garreau, B., Ployet, M. J., Martineau, J., Delvert, J. C., & Reynaud, J. (1983). Auditory brain stem responses and cortical auditory-evoked potentials in difficult-to-test children. *Audiology, 22*, 219–228.

Rosenblum, S. M., Arick, J. R., Krug, D. A., Stubbs, E. G., Young, N. B., & Pelson, R. O. (1980). Auditory brainstem evoked responses in autistic children. *Journal of Autism and Developmental Disorders, 10*, 215–225.

Schafer, E. W., & Peeke, H. V. (1982). Down syndrome individuals fail to habituate cortical evoked potentials. *American Journal of Mental Deficiency, 87*, 332–337.

Schulman-Galambos, C., & Galambos, R. (1975). Brainstem auditory evoked responses in premature infants. *Journal of Speech and Hearing Research, 18*, 456–465.

Skinner, P., & Glattke, T. J. (1977). Electrophysiologic response and audiometry: State of the art. *Journal of Speech and Hearing Disorders, 42*, 179–198.

Skoff, B. F., Mirsky, A. F., & Turner, D. (1980). Prolonged brainstem transmission time in autism. *Psychiatric Research, 2*, 157–166.

Sohmer, H., & Student, M. (1977). Auditory nerve and brain-stem responses in normal, autistic, minimal brain dysfunction, and psychomotor retarded children. *Electroencephalography and Clinical Neurophysiology, 44*, 380–388.

Sohoel, P., Mair, I. W., Everland, H. H., & Laukli, E. (1979). Brainstem-evoked responses. Audiometry in difficult to test patients. *Acta Otolaryngology Supplement, 360*, 56–57.

Squires, N., Aine, C., Buchwald, J., Norman, R., & Galbraith, G. (1980). Auditory brain stem response abnormalities in severely and profoundly retarded adults. *Electroencephalography and Clinical Neurophysiology, 50*, 172–185.

Squires, N., Buchwald, J., Liley, F., & Strecker, J. (1982). Brainstem auditory evoked potential abnormalities in retarded adults. In J. Courjon, F. Maguiere, & M. Revol (Eds.), *Clinical applications of evoked potentials in neurology*. New York: Raven Press.

Stein, L,, Ozdamar, O., & Schnabel, M. (1981). Auditory brainstem responses (ABR) with suspected deaf-blind children. *Ear and Hearing, 2*, 30–40.

Stein, L., Palmer, P., & Weinberg, B. (1982). Characteristics of a young deaf-blind population. *Annals of the Deaf, 127*, 828–837.

Suzuki, T., Hirabayashi, M., & Kobayashi, K. (1983). Auditory middle responses in young children. *British Journal of Audiology, 17*, 5–9.

Suzuki, T., Yasuhito, H., & Horiuchi, K. (1981). Simultaneous recording of early and middle components of auditory electric responses. *Ear and Hearing, 2*, 276–282.

Tanguay, P. E., & Edwards, R. M. (1982). Electrophysiological studies in autism: the whisper of the bang. *Journal of Autism and Developmental Disorders, 12*, 177–184.

Teas, D. C., Kiang, N.Y. (1964). Evoked response from the auditory cortex. *Experimental Neurology, 10*, 91–119.

Vaughn, H. G., & Ritter, W. (1970). The sources of auditory evoked responses recorded from the human scalp. *Electroencephalography and Clinical Neurophysiology, 28*, 360–367.

Werman, S., & Clopton, B. M. (1977). Plasticity of binaural interaction. I. Effect of early auditory deprivation. *Journal of Neurophysiology, 40*, 1266–1274.

Williams, H. L., Tepas, D. I., & Morlock, H. C. (1962). Evoked responses to clicks and electroencephalographic stages of sleep in man. *Science, 183*, 685–686.

Wolf, K. E., & Goldstein, R. (1980). Middle component AERs from neonates to low level tonal stimuli. *Journal of Speech and Hearing Research, 23*, 185–191.

Wood, C. C., & Wolpaw, J. R. (1982). Scalp distribution of human auditory evoked potentials. II. Evidence from overlapping sources and involvement of auditory cortex. *Electroencephalography and Clinical Neurophysiology, 54*, 25–38.

Worthington, D. W., & Peters, J. F. (1980). Quantifiable hearing and no ABR: paradox or error? *Ear and Hearing, 5*, 281–285.

Yellin, A. M., Lodwig, A. K., & Jerison, H. J. (1980). Auditory evoked brain potentials as a function of interstimulus interval in adults with Down's syndrome. *Audiology, 19*, 255–262.

Zerlin, S. S., & Naunton, R. R. (1978). Recording and analysis techniques. In R. Naunton & C. Fernandez (Eds.), *Evoked electrical activity in the auditory nervous system*. New York: Academic Press.

Chapter 19

Auditory Brainstem Response Hearing Aid Applications

Thomas M. Mahoney

INTRODUCTION

Other chapters of this text have explicitly delineated the many aspects of the auditory brainstem response (ABR) phenomena, making available a detailed description of the electrophysiological basis of the response, methods utilized in its generation and recording, and its clinical application to early identification, differential diagnosis, and neurologic function. In reviewing this wealth of information, one can hardly not be impressed by the amount of new knowledge ABR has afforded clinical practitioners and researchers in just over 10 years. Its total contribution to the fields of audiology, neurology, and auditory physiology seems unprecedented by any other single procedure. The topic of this chapter exemplifies even further the versatility of ABR, by taking it beyond investigative and diagnostic utilization, into the field of auditory habilitation.

Need

As pointed out in a recent state-of-the-art hearing aid report (Studebaker & Bess, 1982), considerable controversy continues concerning both the determination of hearing aid candidacy and the best electroacoustic fitting for a specific hearing-impaired individual. Studebaker (1980) reports that progress in hearing aid research during the past 50 years has been painfully slow, and Bryne (1979) noted that although clinicians have been involved in hearing aid selection for more than 30 years, there is little agreement on how the task should be approached. In making these pessimistic statements about contemporary hearing aid evaluations (HAE), these authorities were commenting on clinical procedures for cooperative adults. Unfortunately, we are even less adept in determining the most suitable amplification for nonverbal children or difficult-to-test individuals, who are not able to cooperate for even the simplest conventional test procedures. In the case of hearing-impaired infants, we are in a tenuous position of being able to do the least for the population that could potentially benefit the most from appropriate hearing aid fittings.

It is almost universally accepted that early language intervention is critical to a hearing-impaired child's optimal developmental potential (Edwards, 1968; Lenneberg, 1967; Mencher & Gerber, 1981; Northern & Downs, 1978). However, we are often severely limited in achieving optimal habilitative goals by an inability to provide appropriate pediatric hearing aid prescriptions. To illustrate, Bess and McConnell (1981) noted that hearing aid selection for a very young child is one of the most difficult tasks confronting the audiologist and that present procedures must be considered in developmental stages. Ross and Tomassetti (1980) reported that the basic premise of the initial hearing aid selection for infants is that the recommendations are tentative, and Schwartz and Larson (1977) suggested that there is no single preferred method for the selection of amplification in young children.

The basic problem in fitting infants with hearing aids is that the clinician is faced with making clinical determinations on difficult to obtain and often questionable nonverbal data. Some audiologists continue to practice the art of "prognostic therapy" as their single strategy in this important area. Recommended at a national conference on hearing aid evaluation procedures (ASHA, 1967), this effort involves "continuous monitoring" of the child while various hearing aids or hearing aid adjustments are made. Presumably, this monitoring focuses on observing the child's behavioral reactions under different listening conditions, in hope of making intelligent decisions concerning hearing aid type, electroacoustic settings, ear preference, and earmold modifications. Even the most didactic clinicians would agree that an infant's auditory behavior under amplification must be considered a basic complement to the total evaluation procedure. Most also realize, however, that more rational criteria are needed for this age group, at least to establish competence in selecting the initial instrument to be tried.

Objective Approach

Behavioral methods

Infant developmental levels obviously preclude hearing aid selection based upon speech intelligibility performance. Over a period of years, several methods have evolved that attempt to circumvent this problem by utilizing basic principles of nonverbal behavioral audiometry. These include comparisons between sound-field aided versus unaided conditioned warble tone or narrow-band thresholds and the speech spectrum procedure proposed by Gengel, Pascoe, and Shore (1971). Unfortunately, young children habituate quite rapidly to conditioning protocols required in these techniques, making it difficult to maintain adequate stimulus response control over long HAE sessions. The number of total responses necessitated for HAEs often exceed the recommended limit of approximately 30 stimulus presentations over a 20-min time span (Talbott, Wilson, & Moore, unpublished data; Thompson & Wilson, 1984). Further, in our experience many infants do not condition as well in repeated test sessions, so that final selection data may be compromised even when second or third appointments are scheduled.

Two HAE procedures that more closely fit a rigid definition of objective techniques (i.e., those requiring no active participation) are those utilizing the middle ear acoustic reflex and auditory evoked potentials. These techniques seemingly offer a clinically valid approach to objective HAEs and may, by virtue of their theoretical potential, change the future direction of HAEs for nonverbal and difficult-to-test patients.

Acoustic reflex method

Tonisson (1975) and Rappaport and Tait (1976) were among the first to suggest that acoustic reflex measurements could be used to adjust hearing aid gain to levels resulting in improved speech perception. It has since been recommended as a test to assess frequency-specific real-ear gain and loudness discomfort in preverbal children (Schwartz & Konkle, 1981) and as a method of transferring pathologic input–output functions into the normal range by appropriate amplification (Kiessling, 1980). The major limitation of the acoustic reflex is that it is present in less than half of the children in need of amplification (Kiessling, 1980). Additionally, usefulness of acoustic reflex measurements in this area is limited by the fact that even when they are clearly measurable, they often demonstrate little difference from the normal ear due to the abnormal loudness growth of the pathologic cochlea (Stecker, 1982). Finally, a clear relationship between the middle ear acoustic reflex and loudness discomfort continues to be clouded in controversy.

Evoked potential methods

Using electrophysiological data to assist in hearing aid selection is not a new idea. Rapin and Graziani (1967) were perhaps the first to demonstrate altered evoked auditory potentials under amplification. They reported that when a hearing aid was fitted on an infant whose mother had rubella during pregnancy, it could be adjusted to produce clear cortical evoked potentials, whereas maximum stimulation by the earphone alone resulted in no recognizable waveforms. Spreng (1971) used cortical responses to make hearing aid adjustments by normalizing input–output functions under amplification, and Fritsche, Flach, and Knothe (1978) presented data from over 70 children in whom vertex responses assisted in the selection of appropriate hearing aid fittings.

In light of the generally acknowledged poor reliability of cortically evoked potentials in children, ABR procedures have gained favor in further attempts at electrophysiological HAEs. Hecox, Breuninger, and Krebs (1975) and Mokotoff and Krebs (1976) were among the first to generate ABR responses under amplification from normal and hearing-impaired adults. These early efforts demonstrated the feasibility of the procedure from a technical standpoint and showed favorable correlations between ABR, behavioral audiometry, and hearing aid measures on cooperative patients. While remaining in an admitted preliminary state, later research emerged which reported aided versus unaided ABR data from pathological adult and infant ears (Cox & Metz, 1980; Jacobson, Seitz, Mencher, & Parrott, 1981; Kileny, 1982; Mahoney, Condie, & Snyder, 1980). These studies were optimistic that a valid ABR HAE would eventually be realized for infants, young children, and difficult-to-test populations. Due to the complex nature of the subject, however, a variety of divergent methodologies were proposed, including an ABR wave V latency paradigm (Hecox, 1983), wave V amplitude–intensity (A–I) growth (Kiessling, 1982; 1983) and a combination of ABR latency and amplitude determinations (Stecker, 1982). These efforts are reviewed in detail in the Applications section of this chapter. of this chapter.

TECHNICAL ASPECTS

Basic Considerations

A center already equipped to provide infant ABRs can easily accomplish ABR-assisted HAEs. One major consideration unnecessary in conventional clinical ABR is a sound-isolated environment. When ambient room noise is amplified by a hearing aid under trial, we have found that poor aided ABR waveform morphology often results, complicating waveform interpretation.

In an ABR HAE the stimulus must be presented a specified distance from the hearing aid microphone. Although both loudspeakers and earphones have been used as transducers, most investigators seem to favor the latter. Aside from allowing more precise control over distance and sound pressure, standard earphones help maintain the acoustic qualities of conventional ABR stimuli. Additionally, Mahoney et al. (1980) found that some amplifier–speaker combinations produce considerable click distortion and add as much as 10 dB of energy from 250 to 1000 Hz. Figure 19-1 shows a common desk lamp arm that was modified to hold a standard audiometric earphone for aided ABRs in our facility.

Many infants requiring ABR HAEs are under 1 year of age and do not require sedation. With these patients we instruct parents to impose sleep deprivation, which helps assure a longer and deeper sleep state during the test session. In older children we conventionally recommend the use of 50 mg/kg of 500 mg/5 ml chloral hydrate (Noctec) for sedation. It is necessary that medical coverage be immediately available whenever medication is administered and that all staff who administer sedation be currently certified in cardiopulmonary resuscitation.

Figure 19–1.
Common desk lamp arm modified to hold earphone for sound field ABR. As shown, the arm is also useful in conventional ABR procedures, greatly reducing the chance of the earphone collapsing the ear canal.

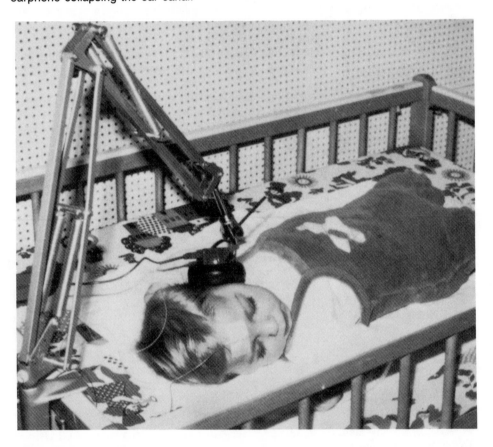

Transducer Distance

The most obvious effect of removing a transducer from the ear and stimulating at a distance is a corresponding increase in ABR waveform latency. The calculated velocity of sound at room temperature (20°C) is about 1 cm per 0.03 ms. When not correcting for additional shift due to reduced sound pressure, Hecox (1983) reported a latency increase of 0.3 ms when placing the earphone 3 cm from the external auditory meatus. Jacobson et al. (1981) recorded a latency shift of 3.51 ms at 1 meter, or 0.6 ms over the expected velocity of sound. They explained the difference as due to variations between earphone and speaker frequency response, resonance characteristics of an occluded and unoccluded auditory canal, and room reverberation.

In our clinic we have chosen to stimulate 8 cm away from the hearing aid microphone, a distance that significantly reduces radiation artifact, and yet allows for adequate stimulus intensity. The 8-cm transducer placement also conveniently amounts to an approximate 0.25-ms distance correction factor, when stimulus intensity is held constant. If we want to compare latency between the field condition and the usual pinna placement, we increase click intensity 20 dB at 8 cm to compensate for loss of sound pressure due to distance. Then, the 0.25 travel time correction factor can be accurately applied. The 20-dB difference was determined by behavioral threshold judgments, wave V latency equalization procedures, and sound pressure level comparisons between a closed 6-cc coupler and the sound-field condition.

Radiation Artifact

Whenever sound is generated by a conversion of electric to acoustic energy, or in the opposite case to a lesser extent, a certain amount of energy is lost in the form of radiant electrical waves. These are sometimes referred to as electrostatic or electromagnetic artifacts, which are described in detail in procedures that require direct electrophysiological monitoring of the cochlea (Vernon & Meikle, 1973). Stimulus artifact has also been the subject of considerable attention in various far-field recordings, including ABR. During ABR the energy that is radiated by high-intensity earphone activation is in relatively close proximity to the active recording site. Consequently, it can be picked up by the surface electrodes and may contaminate the average response for as long as 4 ms poststimulus. Various attempts have been suggested to control this artifact, including alternating the polarity of the stimulus, shielding the transducer, and separating the transducer from the subject (Coates, 1983).

In aided ABR conditions, the addition of an amplifier close to the recording electrodes is cause for increased concern for artifact contamination. In the process of amplification, all hearing aids emit electrical radiation, mainly from their magnetic receivers. The amount may vary according to signal strength, current drain, amplifier type, and the method of shielding used to reduce transient responses. According to Staab (personal communication), there are presently no manufacturing standards for controlling electrical radiation in the hearing aid industry. In our clinic several hearing aids were found to be virtually impossible to evaluate by the ABR procedure, due to excessive radiation artifact (Mahoney et al., 1980). Recently, the use of state-of-the-art ABR equipment and establishment of minimum electrode impedance levels have served to lessen this problem.

Poststimulus radiation from a click-activated hearing aid is shown in Figure 19-2. When such contamination occurs, the clinician should not automatically reject the hearing aid from further consideration, since there is no evidence to suggest that electrical radiation by itself has a detrimental effect on electroacoustic performance.

Signal Processing

The auditory click is the most commonly used ABR stimulus because its abrupt rise time elicits maximal response from primary auditory neurons in the acoustic nerve and brainstem. It is usually generated by a rapid-onset, short-duration electrical impulse sent to a receiver, usually an audiometric earphone, that responds according to its natural resonance. Resulting temporal and spectral properties are determined by the shape of the input signal and transducer response characteristics, with the latter offering the major contribution.

In our discussion of transducer distance we have already noted a significant decrease in click intensity when the earphone is taken off the pinna and positioned 8 cm from the patient's ear. Additional change occurs in the stimulus waveform as shown in Figure 19-3. As evaluated by the Knowles Electronics mannikin for acoustic research (KEMAR), it can be seen that sound-field click stimulation produces a definite bimodal envelope, compared to the positive-polarity waveform generated in a 6-cc coupler. It is significant that alternating-polarity clicks have previously been shown to distort neural response waveforms, especially in patients with high-frequency hearing loss (Coates & Martin, 1977). Of concern is the fact that bimodal waveforms within a single stimulus may have similar effect.

Figure 19-2.
ABR artifact caused by electromagnetic radiation emitted from a high powered hearing aid.

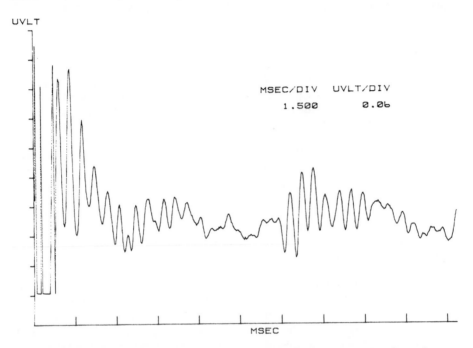

Sound-field stimulation also affects click frequency response. Figure 19-4 shows the average spectrum of 64 clicks delivered through a 6-cc coupler and then through KEMAR with the same TDH 50 earphone held 8 cm away. Intensity was equated between the two conditions. A definite high-frequency emphasis was realized during sound-field KEMAR stimulation, manifested by both the reduction of low-frequency energy and the addition of high-frequency energy at major peaks of 2900 and 4600 Hz. When compared to directly stimulating a one-half inch Bruel & Kjaer microphone 8 cm from the earphone, we see that KEMAR itself adds high-frequency energy to the click, while not altering the low-frequency attenuation introduced by the field condition.

A most intriguing aspect of ABR hearing aid signal processing is the effect amplification may have on the ABR stimulus. In transducing the signal, the amplifying device has a decisive impact on signal amplitude. Less obviously, it also may alter frequency and temporal parameters that can only be detailed through in-depth study. Although hearing aids have recently undergone drastic electronic improvements, harmonic, transient, and intermodulation distortion remains, all of which may impose changes in the ABR stimulus. Additionally, the complex and multiple varieties of compression circuits logically impose certain signal modifications that need to be clarified. Mahoney, et al. (1980) reported that click waveform properties, particularly the important rise-time considerations, were generally preserved under amplification and that other characteristics, such as frequency response settings, compression characteristics, and earmold modifications have a direct influence on KEMAR-processed click stimuli.

It has been suggested that ABR HAEs are limited by the fact that ABR stimuli are necessarily shorter ($<$ 0.01 ms) than the attack time of most compression hearing aids (Kiessling, 1982; Levillain, Garcon, & Le Her, 1979; Stecker, 1982). Because the ABR is dependent upon instant stimulus onset, it is asserted that compression characteristics cannot be evaluated by the ABR procedure. This notion was not verified in KEMAR analysis of various compression instruments.

Figure 19-3.
Waveforms of one auditory click measured through a closed 6 cc coupler (dashed tracing) and 8 cm away from KEMAR (solid tracing). A definite bimodal effect is demonstrated in the sound field KEMAR condition.

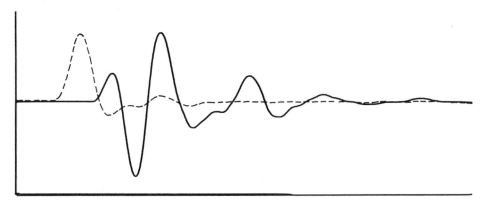

Using a 0.01-ms click at a repetition rate of 21.4/s, Figure 19-5 shows the reduction of click energy imposed by the compression circuit of two hearing aids, one with a measured attack-release time of 5 and 10 ms, respectively, and the other with 1 and 6 ms. These amplitude differences converted to an equivalent of 8 and 15 dB at areas of peak energy. In addition to this evidence, Hecox (1983) has shown that ABR wave V latency may be influenced by adjusting hearing aid compression settings in normal and pathologic ears. In our clinic we have found similar effects on wave V latency and amplitude, suggesting that compression characteristics may in fact be assessed by the ABR HAE technique.

Calibration

Early in this section methods were presented to correct stimulus intensity and wave V latency differences between placement of the stimulus earphone on the pinna and 8 cm removed. It is important to note that even when such corrections are made, inter- and intrasubject latency wave V replication is a little more variable in sound-field conditions, making direct comparison to pinna stimulation somewhat tenuous. Transducer distance, head baffle differences, variations in acoustic absorption, stimulus polarity changes, and phase and spectral differences may all contribute to this problem.

Although there are presently no universal calibration standards for even conventional ABR, an excellent review of several psychoacoustic and electroacoustic methods are offered by Durrant (1983) and Coates (1983).

APPLICATIONS

The primary purpose of this section is to present a summary of the various ABR HAE procedures that have recently emerged in the literature. There is an attempt to synthesize information into several major evaluation strategies, discussing possible advantages and disadvantages when applicable. Because this area is new and complicated by technical variables, it is premature to recommend a specific clinical procedure. However, the prospect of valid ABR

Figure 19–4.
Average spectrum of 64 auditory clicks delivered at equal intensity through a closed 6 cc coupler (solid tracing), 8 cm from KEMAR (dashed tracing), and 8 cm from a Bruel and Kjaer 1 inch field microphone (dash-dot tracing). Note that low frequency click energy is significantly attenuated in the sound field, whereas KEMAR itself enhances peaks at 2900 Hz and 4600 Hz.

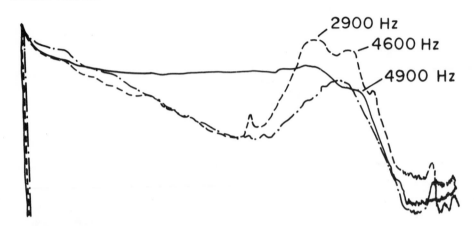

HAEs for preverbal or uncooperative patients is truly exciting. An electrophysiological index of appropriate gain, frequency response, output, and compression dynamics would for the first time instill clinical confidence in fitting this difficult population. In this light, it is hoped that the following discussion will help formulate a reasonable estimate that these amplification characteristics may be validly prescribed by ABR in the near future.

Before proceeding, some basic information is reviewed. First, we know that sound-field ABRs can be produced with reliability. Figure 19-6 shows a rather classic latency–intensity (L-I) function from sound-field stimulation of a normal adult ear. Note that at a repetition rate of 21.4/s, adequate waveform morphology is presented in the sound-field condition. The illustration also depicts the L-I function of the same individual under 30 dB of linear amplification from a hearing aid set on normal frequency response. Clearly, reasonably good ABRs can be generated when the stimulus is transferred through and amplified by a wearable hearing aid. It follows that in individuals who have enough intact hearing to produce a recognizable ABR, hearing aid decisions and adjustments may be determined by the effects they have on the ABR potential. The basic premise underlying this contention is that ABR waveform latency, amplitude, and morphology are directly affected by acoustical parameters of the stimulus. In the pathologic ear these parameters may be altered, via amplification modifications, to produce ABR results that more closely approximate normalcy. Accordingly, hearing aid decisions may be based on objective electrophysiological results.

The various proposed ABR HAEs procedures can be generally categorized into those utilizing wave V threshold, latency, and amplitude. Depending upon the amount of confidence and skill one has with these parameters, clinical application may vary from basic ear selection to precise prescription of hearing aid gain, frequency response, output, and compression characteristics.

ABR Threshold Methods

Early ABR HAE reports illustrated that the technique was feasible on normal hearing and hearing-impaired patients. They showed that unaided ABR sound-field thresholds could be

Figure 19–5.
KEMAR averaged spectrum of 64 auditory clicks amplified through two hearing aids under conditions of compression off (solid tracing) and compression on (dashed tracing). In the top tracing, the aid had an attack-release time of 5 ms and 10 ms, in the bottom the aid had times of 1 and 6 ms. Sound pressure reduction under compression converted to 8 and 15 dB for the two instruments.

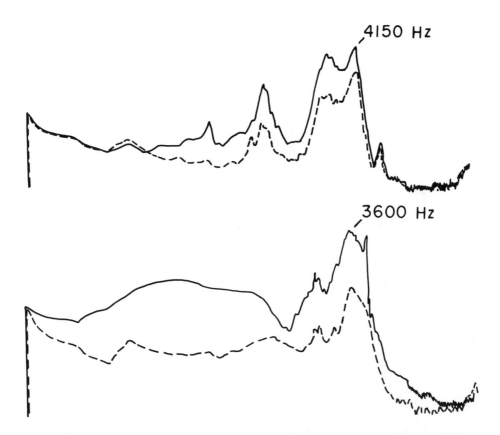

enhanced by the introduction of amplification. Although latency values may have been mentioned for waveform verification, they were not suggested as primary indicators of aided improvement. Amplitude measurements were completely ignored. Mokotoff and Krebs (1976) obtained unaided and aided ABR thresholds, audiometric thresholds, and electroacoustic measures on cooperative adult hearing aid users, and found favorable correlations between these procedures. Mahoney et al., (1980) presented aided versus unaided wave V L–I functions from a number of hearing-impaired infants and young children. Taken from this study, Figure 19-7 shows a series of ABR waveforms from a 2 1/2-year-old boy with suspected high-frequency hearing loss. Note that in the 60-dB HL input sound-field unaided condition there is no recognizable ABR, but when 20 dB of additional gain was afforded by a hearing aid, wave V appeared at 8 ms poststimulus. When stimulus intensity was reduced 10 dB the response disappeared, whereas reintroduction of 30 dB of gain with 60-dB input again produced a wave V at 7.5 ms. In this case ABR offered an electrophysiological index of hearing aid gain in an otherwise difficult-to-test child. The rather large (0.5 ms) L–I shift for only a 10-dB intensity change is attributable to the fact that the waveforms are very near threshold. Jacobson et al. (1981) generated aided sound-field L–I functions from a hearing-impaired adult by first reducing the gain of the instrument and then

Figure 19–6.
ABR sound field latency-intensity functions from a normal adult ear. In the top series the ear was stimulated at a distance of 8 cm from the pinna with a Telex 1470 earphone. In the bottom series the same ear was given 30 dB of linear amplification from a standard frequency response hearing aid.

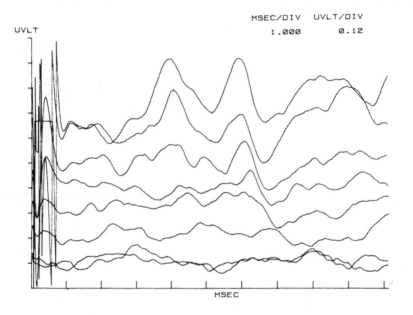

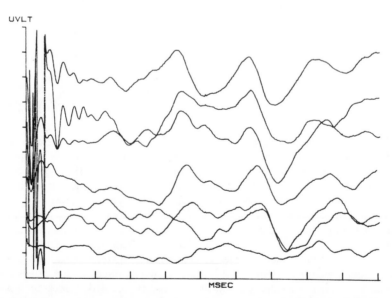

by reducing click stimulus intensity. Improved ABR thresholds were noted under amplification, as were increased wave V latencies during decreased gain and decreased stimulus intensity. In presenting case reports from young and difficult-to-test patients, Kileny (1982) also suggested that aided ABR thresholds could be used to predict the feasibility of amplification and assist in selecting the ear to be amplified.

Pure tone threshold audiometry has been criticized when used as a sole determinant of cochlear function, because data suggest it does not always accurately reflect total hair cell integrity (Pollack & Lipscomb, 1979). Similarly, threshold determinations in both conventional ABR and ABR HAEs offer only limited clinical information, necessitating further measures of suprathreshold auditory function and auditory dynamic range. In traditional adult hearing aid evaluations, threshold information is supplemented by comfort levels, discomfort levels, speech discrimination tests in quiet and in competition, recruitment estimates, frequency information, and hearing aid trials in various listening enviornments. Although aided ABR thresholds provide necessary gain and ouput measures, they alone leave inaccessible the more valuable information concerning dynamic hearing aid function. Consequently, wave V latency and amplitude have undergone serious investigation in ABR HAEs. Because ABR latency and amplitude reflect different physiological processes, which can vary independently or change concurrently (Buchwald, 1983), their combined use has the immediate appeal of offering a dynamic look at suprathreshold hearing aid performance on pathologic ears.

ABR Latency Methods

Several studies (Cox & Metz, 1980; Hecox, 1983) suggest the use of ABR wave V absolute latency and/or L-I slope to predict appropriate hearing aid specifications. The basic premises, although not entirely proven, are that normal wave V latencies require an intact auditory system up to the neural generator, that normal L-I slope suggests normal dynamic loudness function, and that speech intelligibility and ABR latency are correlated. It follows that if a hearing aid can be adjusted in gain, output, and compression characteristics to generate as normal an ABR as possible in a pathologic ear, the procedure has merit as a tool for the evaluation of amplification.

Cox and Metz (1980) presented data from eight hearing aid users who were given standard behavioral tests, aided speech discrimination tests in quiet and in noise, and unaided versus aided click- and tone pip-elicited ABRs. At a sound-field level corresponding to the recommended 50 dB HTL for speech audiometers, a variable hearing aid was adjusted to three different settings. L-I functions were obtained at levels 10 dB above and below comfort, and ABR threshold and latency data were rank-ordered into three hearing loss categories. Speech discrimination results were ranked according to best combined scores for quiet and noise. ABR ranking was determined by hearing aid settings that produced the shortest wave V latencies and lowest wave V thresholds. Although there was some discrepancy between stimuli, hearing aid settings which produced the best speech discrimination scores also generally produced the shortest wave V latencies and vice versa. ABR threshold determinations did not produce consistent results and were not recommended as a practical clinical method. Interestingly, subjects with sloping pure tone configurations produced speech discrimination/ABR correlations that were poorer than the total group, and in the two precipitous audiometric configurations, there was perfect speech discrimination/ABR agreement. An obvious limitation of this study was the small number of subjects in each of the test categories. Also, hearing aid compression settings were not evaluated.

Another ABR HAE latency-based study was presented by Hecox (1983), who asserted that "the most significant contribution of ABR will be in the quantification of suprathreshold auditory function, primarily as it relates to characterizing the dynamic range of the impaired listener" and "the careful quantification of the ABR will ultimately assist in the development of quantitative predictions regarding optimal electroacoustic properties of hearing aids" (p. 51). Adults and infants were first tested by routine ABR procedures. After conventional ABR, an earphone was placed 3 cm away from the hearing aid microphone and aided L-I functions were generated at the preferred hearing aid settings using a click intensity of 40 dB SPL. No

Figure 19–7.
Standard sound field and sound field–aided ABR tracings from a 2½ year old boy with suspected high frequency sensorineural loss. Top tracings show conventional ABR wave V response at 70 dB nHL with a possible threshold wave V at 60 dB nHL. In the 60 dB unaided sound field condition, no wave V is evident, whereas wave V appeared at 8 ms after the stimulus with the addition of 20 dB hearing aid gain. When input was reduced 10 dB in the aided condition, wave V disappeared, whereas increasing the hearing aid gain to 30 dB at the original 60 dB input produced a wave V at 7.5 ms. From Mahoney et al. (1980). Early ABR equipment precluded precise latency measurement.

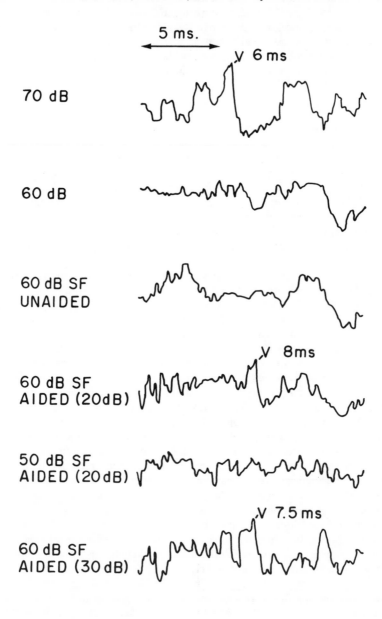

mention ws made on how hearing aids were adjusted on the infant subjects. Unaided and aided ABR responses were compared to determine improvement, which was reflected in absolute latency reduction and L-I slope normalization. A 0.3-ms latency correction for transducer distance was required in the aided condition. Results were reported in categories of satisfactory performance, unsatisfactory performance, recruiting patterns, and central auditory dysfunction. Figure 19-8 illustrates hearing aid performance in a patient using a compression versus a linear hearing aid. Hecox noted that the $400\text{-}\mu s/dB$ L-I slope implies electrophysiological recruitment, suggestive of inner ear pathology. Little L-I slope change was noted from linear amplification, whereas the introduction of compression changed the slope to a near-normal $67\ \mu s/dB$, greatly increasing the patient's effective dynamic range. A more striking example of the effects of compression on aided ABR L-I slope is shown in Figure 19-9. Using a master hearing aid with various compression ratios, a hearing-impaired patient's slope more closely approximated normal when maximum compression was used. Identical wave V latency between the two compression settings at 60 dB signifies the importance of establishing complete L-I functions for each hearing aid characteristic being assessed.

Four primary assertions were made in the Hecox study: (1) the greater the displacement of the L-I function from normal, the larger the gain requirements when L-I is held constant, that is, effective amplification should diminish the discrepancy between normal and pathologic latencies for the frequency region assessed; (2) the steeper the L-I function the more likely that compression will be superior to linear amplification; (3) there is no advantage to amplification that introduces latencies of less than 6 ms for 60 dB HL signals; and (4) amplification is unlikely to improve the communication skills of patients with pure central auditory dysfunction.

It seems inevitable that ABR wave V latency and L-I slope will provide a major role in future ABR HAEs. In our clinic we find it difficult to perform the many repeated L-I series necessary to evaluate various electroacoustic characteristics for each ear in the time allowed by hypnotic sedation. Another practical problem is difficulty in finding exact wave V latencies in the distorted waveform morphologies of some patients. A narrow window such as 10 ms is recommended to accentuate latency differences.

ABR Amplitude Methods

ABR amplitude is thought to be a function of graded postsynaptic potentials, initiated on the dendrites or soma and electronically spread over portions of the postsynaptic cell (Buchwald, 1983). Absolute amplitude has been termed a nebulous parameter in diagnostic ABR procedures and relative amplitude ratios change at an unpredictable maturational rate in infants (Stockard & Stockard, 1983).

In spite of the above facts, amplitude measures have undergone considerable investigation in ABR HAEs, particularly as reported in European literature. Relative intrasubject ABR wave V amplitude growth has been proposed as a direct index of cochlear loudness function (Kiessling, 1982, submitted for publication; Stecker, 1982), offering a valid electrophysiological index of preferred amplification characteristics. Kiessling (1982; submitted for publication) used an unaided ABR projection system, based on normal and pathological amplitude growth, to prescribe appropriate hearing aid gain, compression ratio, and compression onset. Asserting that ABR amplitudes correlate with actual loudness perception, Kiessling suggested that hearing aid settings can be adjusted in accordance with amplitude normalization. Aided ABR functions were not determined because compression instruments were said to have onset time constraints in excess of the stimuli required to generate the ABR. To enhance the procedures' sensitivity, negative wave V amplitude was utilized. This is the amplitude from baseline to wave V's negative trough, which is reported to dominate even at low stimulation levels.

Figure 19-8.
The effect of compression (aid 2) versus linear (aid 1) amplification on the latency-intensity function of a patient with sensorineural impairment. Note that the rather steep latency-intensity slope (420 ɲs/dB) in the unaided and linear aided conditions approximate normalcy (67 ɲs/dB) under compression amplification. Both aids provided sufficient gain to produce a 60 dB wave V at 6 ms. From Hecox, (1983).

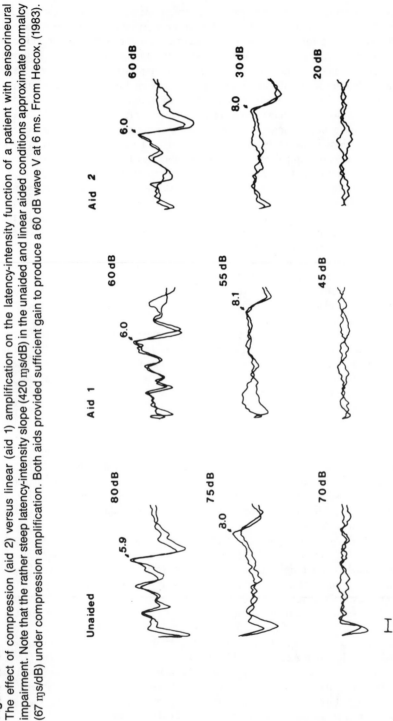

Figure 19–9.
A plot of the latency-intensity function for a sensorineural hearing loss patient in the unaided condition (a) and amplified with aids (b) and (c), which differed in their compression ratios. Note that the slope of the responses obtained with the higher compression ratio more closely approximates normal, although the improvement provided at 60 dB is equivalent for the two devices. From Hecox (1983).

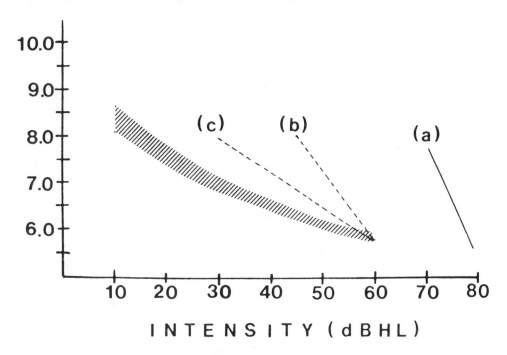

INTENSITY (dBHL)

An unaided amplitude–intensity (A–I) procedure was tested on 29 (Kiessling, 1982) and 59 (Kiessling, submitted for publication) hearing-impaired children. First, normal A–I functions were obtained from normal hearing adults and children, with no significant differences noted once intrasubject variability was reduced by repeated tests. Normal A–I function is displayed with that of a recruiting ear in Figure 19-10. Note that the normal dynamic range of 40 to 80 dB is projected upward to the normal A–I curve. At these points horizontal lines are drawn to the pathological A–I function and then vertically, yielding the dynamic range required for the pathologic ear. Figure 19-11 shows a projection diagram of the data, indicating that a 33-dB gain hearing aid was required with a 0.35 linear compression factor and a 40-dB onset level. Figure 19-12 demonstrates the complete procedure on a child with sensorineural hearing loss. With an ABR wave V threshold at 40 dB, L-I functions of waves I, III, and V are slightly shifted, but interpeak values are within the normal range. However, A–I shows a steep rise in this pathologic ear, suggesting sensorineural loss with recruitment. The resulting projection diagram was used to determine gain, dynamic range, compression type, compression factor, and compression onset level. Importantly, this work indicates that wave V amplitude may be more sensitive than wave V latency as an index of pathologic loudness in sensorineural hearing impairment.

Kiessling (submitted for publication) reported that hearing aid specifications gained by these procedures are in good agreement with those obtained by conventional speech audiometry. An interesting note was that the compression factors recommended by the procedure were

Figure 19-10.
Determining the dynamic range of an ear with pathology by the amplitude-intensity method described by Kiessling (1982). The intensity-amplitude function of negative wave V (V/N₅) in normal ears (top left) is displayed together with a curve from a recruiting ear (bottom right). Normal 40 to 80 dB speech intensity is projected upwards to the normal amplitude curve, then horizontally to the pathologic amplitude curve. The vertical projection from these points gives the output dynamic range of an appropriate hearing aid. (From Kiessling, 1980.)

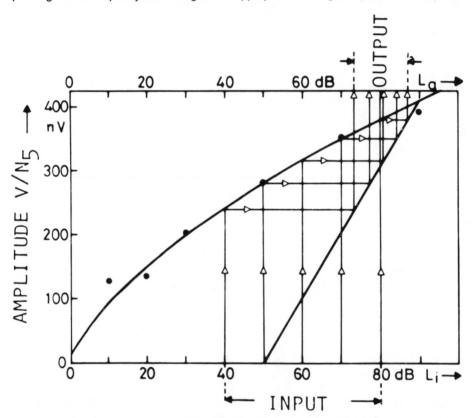

generally greater than those available in commercial hearing aids. Nearly 75% of the 59 subjects required ratios higher than those available in the Federal Republic of Germany.

The A–I projection method has the immediate appeal of not requiring unaided versus aided ABR measurements. This significantly reduces test time and eliminates problems related to the hearing aid transfer of ABR stimuli. To maximally utilize valuable sedated sleep time for testing, Kiessling evaluates A–I data away from clinical sessions using an interactive semiautomatic BASIC computer program, which calculates and displays recommended hearing aid specifications. Although the procedure needs to be replicated by other investigators, with special attention to amplitude variability and intertest reliability, it would seem to offer considerable promise as a clinically feasible, valid ABR HAE procedure.

Combined Approaches and Considerations

At the Utah Department of Health Bureau of Communicative Disorders we have addressed a variety of ABR HAE procedures. The most compelling problem is completing a rather lengthy

Figure 19–11.
Projection diagram derived from intensity-amplitude functions in Figure 19–10, indicating a hearing aid with 33 dB gain, a compression factor of 0.35, and a compression onset of 40 dB. (From Kiessling, 1982.)

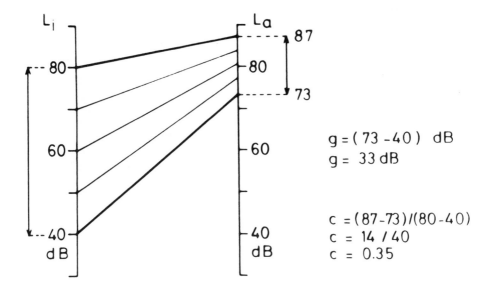

$$g = (73 - 40)\ dB$$
$$g = 33\ dB$$

$$c = (87 - 73)/(80 - 40)$$
$$c = 14 / 40$$
$$c = 0.35$$

test protocol during the typical 1 1/2- to 2-hour sedated sleep time. Because of the need for ongoing investigation in this area and the fact that a totally satisfactory protocol has not yet emerged, we have not committed ourselves to a single test procedure at the time of this writing. Patients scheduled in our clinic for aided ABRs have usually had previous conventional ABR procedures. Severe and profound sensorineural losses that do not generate a conventional ABR under maximum earphone stimulations (99 dB nHL) usually do not generate an aided ABR. Apparently, patients in this category do not have enough high-frequency cochlear integrity, even at extremely high hearing aid gain and output setting. Intense stimulation may also introduce such upward spread of energy that cochlear overload, saturation, or distortion obviates residual mid- and basal-turn electrophysiological generation.

In our aided protocol, we begin click stimulation at 50 dB SPL at the hearing aid microphone, a level accomplished at a 70-dB dial setting on our equipment in a sound-isolated environment. This level was chosen because it approximates the average speech spectrum from 2000 to 4000 Hz (Gengel et al., 1971), the frequency area primarily addressed by the ABR procedure. If no ABR is generated at high hearing aid gain, the input intensity is increased. Our first procedure is to assess gain by rotating the hearing aid volume control to a point where wave V latency stabilizes and its amplitude saturates. At this level we then record L-I slope at various frequency and compression settings to determine the most favorable amplified dynamic range. Due to time constraints we begin at maximum compression settings because they seem to normalize the L-I slope best in most sensorineurally impaired ears, a finding consistent with the A–I data of Kiessling, (submitted for publication). We are often unable to complete the total HAE procedure in one setting and must frequently settle on gain and/or output determinations on the first visit. In such cases, when sensorineural impairment in suspected, the instrument is set near maximum compression until the next appointment. Consequently, we choose hearing aids whose compression variations demonstrate little or no effect on gain.

An interesting clinical observation we often note in the aided condition is an apparent L-I "rollover" effect. Wave V latency decreases with increased amplification to a point of maximal

Figure 19–12.
Complete ABR procedures used by Kiessling (1982) in a sensorineural impairment. ABR V/N_5 values (a) are followed by intensity-latency functions of wave I, III, and V/N_5 plotted against normal (solid lines) (b), intensity-amplitude function of V/N_5 plotted against normal (solid lines) (c), and the resulting projection diagram indicating recommended hearing aid characteristics (d). (From Kiessling, 1982.)

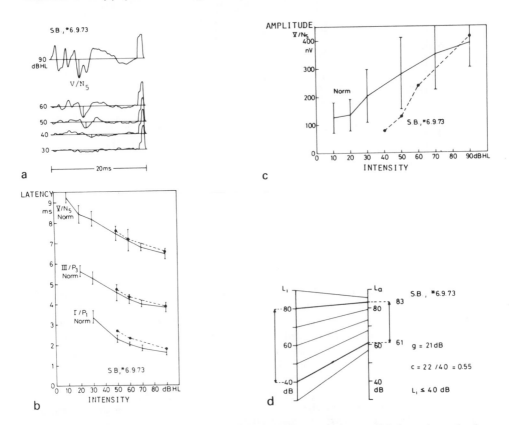

shift, upon which further gain not only stabilizes but increases it to a slightly prolonged value. One possible explanation for this phenomenon is that at output saturation further gain only increases internal distortion, which serves to degrade the stimulus envelope and decrease wave V latency. A second consideration is that we are observing real electrophysiologic degradation. At high intensity the pathologic cochlea's output becomes saturated, whereas further increases produce cochlear overload, reduced neural generation, and prolonged wave V latency. Upward spread of masking may also contribute to this "reverse latency shift," an example of which is illustrated in Figure 19-13.

Stecker (1982) reported on the use of a combination of threshold, latency, and amplitude measurements in ABR HAEs. Aided ABR information determined frequency response and gain, but, similar to the procedure of Kiessling (1982), estimates of compression were made from unaided A–I functions. Frequency response judgements were made by comparing unaided click to 500- and 1000-Hz tone pip-generated ABRs. For example, if wave V click threshold was found to be significantly higher than the 500- or 1000-Hz waveforms, a high-frequency emphasis hearing aid was indicated. (As a point of caution, note that Stecker did not address the possibility that 500- or 1000-Hz tone pip ABRs generated in isolation may not actually

Figure 19–13.
The wave V "reverse latency shift" phenomenon observed in many aided latency-intensity functions. In this case of moderate to severe sensorineural hearing impairment, wave V latency decrease as expected from 7.10 ms at 40 dB nHL to 6.78 ms at 60 dB, but then reverses itself to 7.02 ms at higher input intensity of 90 dB. Hearing aid distortion, cochlear overload, and upward spread of masking are hypothesized as contributing factors.

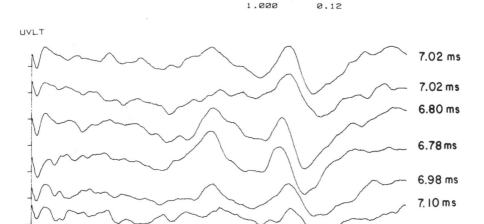

be resolving a similar frequency area of the cochlea.) Hearing aid output was set at a level where further increases did not decrease wave V latency and wave V amplitude saturation. It was pointed out that normal latencies may be approximated in conductive and gently sloping sensorineural losses, but that the distorted waveform morphology of steep sloping sensorineural losses may preclude attempts at normalization.

The many and diverse approaches to ABR HAEs testify to the complex nature of issues within this topic, and the widespread recognition of the need for valid, feasible test protocols in this area. On a more positive note, the rather large amount of ABR HAE investigation suggests good potential for the eminent development of clinical strategies that will enjoy more general application.

LIMITATIONS AND FUTURE DIRECTIONS

Most investigators who have had experience in the ABR hearing aid applications outline various limitations of the procedure. The most controversial is the notion that hearing aids with compression circuits cannot be evaluated because their circuits cannot follow the very fast stimulus rise times necessary to elicit an ABR (Levillain et al., 1979; Kiessling, 1982; Stecker, 1982). As previously discussed, however, it has been demonstrated at our clinic that compression aids may in fact be assessed by the ABR procedure. We have found that amplified click output is significantly reduced by compression, that ABR L-I functions are appropriately affected, and that rather good waveform morphology is maintained under amplification, suggesting adequate stimulus onset. In spite of this information, we must consider that ABR amplitude and latency changes during compression may in fact reflect stimulus duration or associated interstimulus interval modification, rather than actual output compression. For instance, Durrant (1983) has shown that input pulse duration directly influences the sound pressure of clicks generated from a standard earphone. In the present case, it is possible that such influences imposed by the hearing aid circuitry may be mistakenly interpreted as actual compression amplification.

A more universally accepted limitation is the high-frequency emphasis of the ABR HAE procedure. This is in concurrence with Coates and Martin (1977) and Møller and Blegvad (1976), who show that click-generated ABR reflects primarily the frequency range of 1000 to 4000 Hz. In reality this limitation is not overly concerning, since frequencies above 1000 Hz are most important to speech intelligibility and successful hearing aid use. To better assess low-frequency amplification some investigators have recommended the use of tone pips (Cox & Metz, 1980; Stecker, 1982), but, as previously noted, the frequency resolution of the cochlea by these signals in ABR must be interpreted cautiously.

The limited use of ABR in selecting amplification in severe and profound hearing losses was addressed earlier. In the profoundly impaired, an ABR usually cannot be generated even under maximum amplification, rendering the procedure useless. In severe losses there is often insufficient dynamic range to produce adequate L-I or A-I functions. However, we have found that even distorted wave Vs at maximum intensity are of some value, often assisting in determining the ear better suited for amplification or assisting in basic gain and output adjustments. Hecox (1983) reported that in their experience ABR HAEs are rarely productive in losses greater than 75 dB.

Future directions in ABR hearing aid applications present very exciting possibilities. Hecox (1983) described plans to develop a master hearing aid able to transform pathological into normal ABR input–output functions, wherein the properties required to normalize the ABR would be matched by the electroacoustic properties of the amplifier. We can expect that this approach will be dramatically enhanced by the inevitable application of digital processing technology to hearing aids. On-line latency/amplitude data could be fed directly into the hearing aid microprocessor to effect on-line ABR normalization. The hearing aid settings that produce the normal ABR would in turn serve as the basic electrophysiological prescription for amplification.

Finally, future research may well explore the feasibility of middle evoked responses and/or the 40-Hz phenomena in electrophysiological HAEs. These endeavors may yield more frequency-specific information than the ABR approach.

In summary, this chapter has noted the pressing need for valid HAE procedures in infants and difficult-to-test patients and has reviewed various attempts at accomplishing this goal. The major impetus for these efforts lies in the fact that while we are faced with an urgent desire to apply amplification as early as possible, we are cautioned by evidence that overamplification may damage residual hearing (Hawkins, 1982; Rintelmann & Bess, 1977). We have asserted that behavioral HAEs are tedious and difficult to accomplish in infants and that acoustic reflex measurements are of limited use. ABR procedures, in spite of several limitations, may serve to accomplish clinically valid pediatric HAEs through the use of stable and reliable electrophysiological data. They provide a dynamic assessment of suprathreshold auditory function, can be performed on patients displaying diverse levels of development, and are not precluded by middle ear lesions.

In reviewing the favorable results of several emerging ABR HAE strategies, we can conclude that a clinically useful procedure is probably forthcoming in the near future. It is not intended that the reader interpret these techniques as offering a "black-box" approach to infant HAEs. There is enough evidence, however, to encourage their replication and further investigation. The establishment of positive correlations between ABR information and successful hearing aid use and the development of hearing aid technology capable of normalizing pathologic ABR data should expedite the more general utilization of these procedures.

The author thanks Dr. Robert Brey and Dr. Richard Harris of Brigham Young University for their kind assistance and collaboration in the acoustical analysis procedures incorporated in this chapter.

REFERENCES

American Speech and Hearing Association (1967). A conference on hearing aid evaluation procedures. *ASHA Reports No. 2*. Washington DC: American Speech and Hearing Association.

Bess, F. H., & McConnell, F. E. (1981). *Audiology, education, and the hearing impaired child*. St. Louis: Mosby.

Bryne, D. (1979). Hearing aid selection. *Archives of Otolaryngology, 105*, 519–525.

Buchwald, J. S. (1983). Generators. In E. J. Moore (Ed.), *Basis of auditory brain-stem evoked responses*. New York: Grune & Stratton.

Coates, A. C. (1983). Instrumentation. In E. J. Moore (Ed.), *Basis of auditory brain-stem evoked responses*. New York: Grune & Stratton.

Coates, A. C., & Martin, J. L. (1977). Human auditory nerve action potentials and brainstem evoked responses. *Archives of Otolaryngology, 103*, 605–622.

Cox, L. C., & Metz, D. A. (1980). ABER in the prescription of hearing aids. *Hearing Instruments, 31*, 12–15.

Durrant, J. D. (1983). Fundamentals of sound generation. In E. J. Moore (Ed.), *Basis of auditory brain-stem evoked responses*. New York: Grune & Stratton.

Edwards, E. P. (1968). Kindergarten is too late. *Saturday Review, 51*, 60–79.

Fritsche, F., Flach, M., & Knothe, J. (1978). Zu Ergebmissen der Horgerateanpassung Gei Kleinkinderm Mittels ERA. *HNO Praxis 3*, 124.

Gengel, R. W., Pascoe, D., & Shore, I. (1971). A frequency response procedure for evaluating and selecting hearing aids for severely hearing impaired children. *Journal of Speech and Hearing Disorders, 36*, 341–353.

Hawkins, D. B. (1982). Overamplification: A well documented case report. *Journal of Speech and Hearing Disorders, 47*, 376–382.

Hecox, K. E. (1983). Role of auditory brainstem responses in the selection of hearing aids. *Ear and Hearing, 4*, 51–55.

Hecox, K. E., Breuninger, C., & Krebs, D. (1975). Brainstem evoked responses obtained from hearing-aided adults. *Journal of the Acoustical Society of America, 57*, 563.

Jacobson, J., Seitz, M., Mencher, G., & Parrott, V. (1981). Auditory brainstem response: A contribution to infant assessment and management. In G. T. Mencher & S. E. Gerber (Eds.), *Early management of hearing loss*. New York: Grune & Stratton.

Kiessling, J. (1980). Input–output function of the acoustic reflex and objective hearing aid evaluation. *Audiology, 19*, 480–494.

Kiessling, J. (1982). Hearing aid selection by brainstem audiometry. *Scandinavian Audiology, 11*, 269–275.

Kiessling, J. (1983). Clinical experience in hearing aid adjustment by means of BER amplitudes. *Archives of Otorhinolaryngology, 238* (3), 233–240.

Kileny, P. P. (1982). Auditory brainstem responses as indicators of hearing aid performance. *Annals of Otology, 91*, 61–64.

Lenneberg, E. H. (1967). *Biological foundations of language*. New York: Wiley.

Levillain, D., Garcon, F., & Le Her, G. (1979). Apport des potentiels du tronc cerebral dans le controle du gain prothetique. *Revue de Laryngologic, 100*, 739–743.

Mahoney, T., Condie, R., & Snyder, K. (1980). *Hearing aid evaluation by brainstem evoked responses: A feasibility study*. Paper presented at the meeting of the American Speech, Language, and Hearing Association, Detroit, November.

Mencher, G. T., & Gerber, S. E. (1981). *Early management of hearing loss*. New York: Grune & Stratton.

Mokotoff, B., Krebs, D. (1976). *Brainstem auditory-evoked responses with amplification*. Paper presented at the meeting of the Acoustical Society of America, November.

Moller, K., & Blegvad, B. (1976). Brainstem potentials in subjects with sensorineural hearing loss. *Scandinavian Audiology, 5*, 115–127.

Northern, J. L., & Downs, M. P. (1978). *Hearing in children*. Baltimore: Williams & Wilkins.

Pollack, M. C., & Lipscomb, D. M. (1979). Implications of hair-pure tone discrepancies for oto-audiologic practice. *Audiology and Hearing Education 5*, 16–36.

Rapin, I., & Graziani, L. J. (1967). Auditory evoked responses in normal brain damaged and deaf infants. *Neurology, 17*, 881–894.

Rappaport, B. Z., & Tait, C. A. (1976). Acoustic reflex threshold measurement in hearing aid selection. *Archives of Otolaryngology, 102*, 129–132.

Rintelmann, W. F., & Bess, F. H. (1977). High level amplification and potential hearing loss in children. In F. H. Bess (Ed.), *Childhood deafness: Causation, assessment and management*. New York: Grune & Stratton.

Ross, M., Tomassetti, C. (1980). Hearing aid selection for the preverbal hearing-impaired child. In M. Pollack (Ed.), *Amplification for the hearing impaired* (2nd ed.). New York: Grune & Stratton.

Schwartz, D. M., & Konkle, D. F. (1981). Hearing aids for children. In C. D. Bluestone & S. E. Stool (Eds.), *Pediatric otolaryngology*. Philadelphia: Saunders.

Schwartz, D. M., & Larson, V. D. (1977). A comparison of three hearing aid evaluation procedures for young children. *Archives of Otolaryngology, 103*, 401–406.

Spreng, M. (1971). Small computers in evoked response audiometry. *Archives Klinischen Experimentellen Ohren Nasen Kehlkopfheilkunde, 198, 50–63.*

Staab, W. Personal communication, October 20, 1983.

Stecker, M. (1982). Objective hearing aid fitting. *Laryngology, Rhinology and Otology, 61*, 678–682.

Stockard, J. E., & Stockard J. J. (1983). Recording and analyzing. In E. J. Moore (Ed.), *Basis of auditory brain-stem evoked responses*. New York: Grune & Stratton.

Studebaker, G. A. (1980). Fifty years of hearing aid research: An evaluation of progress. *Ear and Hearing, 1*, 57–62.

Studebaker, G. A., & Bess, F. H. (1982). *The Vanderbilt hearing-aid report: State of the art research needs*. Upper Darby, PA: Monographs in Contemporary Audiology.

Talbott, S. A., Wilson, W. R., & Moore, J. M. *Habituation of infant responses to auditory stimuli under two conditions of visual reinforcement*. Unpublished data, 1976.

Thompson, G. & Wilson, W. R. (1984). Clinical application of visual reinforcement audiometry. In T. Mahoney (Ed.), *Early identification of hearing loss in infants. Seminars in Hearing*, Vol 5, part 1, pp. 85–99.

Tonisson, W. (1975). Measuring in-the-ear gain of hearing aids by the acoustic reflex method. *Journal of Speech and Hearing Research, 18*, 17–30.

Vernon, J., & Meikle, M. (1973). Electrophysiology of the cochlea. In R. Thompson & M. Patterson (Eds.), *Recordings of bioelectric activity*. New York: Academic Press.

Chapter 20

Auditory Brainstem Response Testing Strategies

James Jerger
Terrey Oliver
Brad Stach

INTRODUCTION

Ideally, it would be desirable to list a single, universal test procedure applicable to every ABR examination. But differing problems encountered in the clinical situation dictate the need for a variety of testing strategies. One of the most important factors is the specific ABR application; a second is limitation in available testing time; and a third is dependence of results on degree of peripheral hearing loss.

Specific ABR Application

The specific ABR application impacts, to a great extent, on the optimal testing strategy. We can distinguish three fundamental clinical applications of ABR:

1. neonatal screening;
2. evaluation of older infants and young children; and
3. differentiating cochlear from retrocochlear site.

In neonatal screening, the goal is simply to categorize auditory function as either normal or abnormal in order to identify babies in need of subsequent follow-up. The focus is twofold: (1) a gross estimate of overall peripheral sensitivity and (2) a gross estimate of central function. An efficient testing strategy must concentrate on providing data directed to these two fundamental questions in a manner that maximizes the correct identification or "hit" rate, while minimizing the incorrect identification, or "false-alarm" rate.

In the evaluation of older infants and young children, however, the goal is usually more detailed. Here, the typical concern is to obtain as much information as possible about the degree of loss, the nature of the audiometric contour, and the extent of interaural asymmetry.

An effective testing strategy must, therefore, not only estimate overall degree of loss but also provide frequency-specific information about shape of loss, and an estimate of which is the better ear and by how much it differs from the poorer ear.

In differentiating cochlear from retrocochlear disorder, still another goal is pursued. Here, the aim is to explore the exact morphology of the ABR waveform, to document the presence of all component waves, and to measure both absolute and relative latencies of the various component peaks.

Thus, the optimal testing strategy will concentrate on suprathreshold measures designed to enhance all component peaks of the ABR, but especially the early waves upon which accurate estimates of interpeak intervals or "central conduction time" depend.

The differing demands of these three principal applications of ABR have led to specific strategies unique to each application.

Limited Available Testing Time

Limitation of ABR testing time is a factor common to all audiologic evaluation, but is especially prominent in pediatric applications. Since time in the neonatal intensive care unit is always at a premium, the screening of newborn babies must be carried out quickly and efficiently. Similarly, when children in the 1- to 4-year age range are being evaluated under sedation, testing time is effectively limited by the duration of sedative-induced sleep. Even in the case of adults being evaluated for retrocochlear disorder, cost effectiveness dictates the need for rapid and efficient evaluation. Thus, the ubiquitous time constraint has had its own unique impact on ABR testing strategies.

Dependence on Degree of Loss

Finally, degree of hearing loss is a factor affecting all auditory measures, but especially ABR. The extent to which various ABR measures can be effectively interpreted as normal or abnormal depends, to a great extent, on the degree of peripheral sensitivity loss, especially in the critical 1000- to 4000-Hertz (Hz) frequency range. Any effective diagnostic testing strategy must take this critical hearing loss dependence into account.

In the following sections, we list the various testing strategies that have been proposed for each of the three basic clinical applications of ABR, discuss their strengths and weaknesses, and suggest a single recommended test strategy for each ABR application.

NEONATAL SCREENING

Neonatal screening by ABR, first proposed by Galambos (1978), has since been initiated by a number of investigators in a variety of settings. Proposed testing strategies are, however, remarkably uniform. The majority of centers engaged in neonatal screening continue to utilize the test parameters first suggested by Galambos and his associates. They suggested that click presentation levels be 30 and 60 dB nHL, the click rate be 37/s, EEG filters be set to pass a band from 150 to 3000 Hz, 2,048 responses be averaged, and that each ear be tested separately by air conduction only. Only minor variations on this consistent theme have been proposed. In an effort to reduce the false-positive rate, it has been suggested that the 30-dB test level be raised to 35 or 40 dB (Alberti, Hyde, Riko, Corbin, & Abramovich, 1983; Dennis, Sheldon, Toubas, & McCaffee, 1984), that the rate be lowered to 21 (Dennis et al., 1984; Stein, Ozdamar, Kraus, & Paton, 1983) or even 10/s (Jacobson, Seitz, Mencher, & Parrott, 1980), that the EEG passband be lowered to 50 Hz (Thornton, personal communication), and that the number averaged be increased to 4000 (Alberti et al., 1983). In general, however, there is reasonably good agreement on how to carry out the actual screening test procedure.

Most investigators will also agree that the crucial issue confronting neonatal screeners is the high failure rate typically observed when a series of infants is screened in the ICU, and the subsequent apparent resolution of many of the initial failures. Galambos, Hicks, and Wilson (in press) note, for example, that, in their experience, 16% of infants in the neonatal ICU will fail the initial screen, but as many as one-third of these babies will pass a retest administered 6–8 weeks after the initial test.

Most investigators suspect that such apparently resolving loss is due to middle ear disorder on the first test which then resolves before the 6–8 week retest (Cevette, 1984; Finitzo-Hieber, 1982; Hecox, 1984; Stein, 1984), but no one can be sure of the exact numbers involved. Other possibilities that must be entertained, however, include maturation of the ABR response during the first month of life (Hooks & Weber, 1984; Roberts, Davis, Phon, Reichert, Sturtevant, & Marshall, 1982; Starr, Amlie, Martin, and Sanders, 1977) and simple failure of the screening instrument in a certain percentage of cases due to ambient acoustic and electrical noise in the testing environment.

Nevertheless, much of the continuing controversy over the desirability of neonatal screening (Cevette, 1984; Downs, 1982; Jacobson et al., 1980; Roberts et al., 1982) centers on this relatively high false-positive rate. Whether one regards them as the fruit of test flaws, the result of late maturation, or the consequence of subsequently resolving middle ear disease, there is general agreement that such screening failures are undesirable concomitants of the search for significant permanent sensorineural hearing loss. Many feel that unless this false-positive rate can be kept to an acceptable minimum, neonatal screening for hearing loss cannot be cost effective. Others point out, however, that even a relatively high false-positive rate is a small price to pay for the identification of even a small number of children with handicapping hearing loss at so early an age (Northern & Downs, 1974, p. 99).

What may prove to be a useful strategy for minimizing the false-positive rate due to resolving middle ear disorder was first proposed by Weber (1983) and later elaborated by Hooks and Weber (1984). They reasoned that, if conductive hearing loss due to middle ear disease leads to an undesirable screening "fail" then an effective strategy might be to test only by bone conduction (BC). If the click is introduced directly to the infant's skull via a bone-conduction transducer, then the confounding effect of conductive hearing loss would be effectively bypassed. So long as the sensorineural system is intact, the infant should pass the screen in spite of temporary conductive loss.

The presence of a normal ABR response at a BC hearing level (HL) of 30–40 dB would not, of course, ensure normal hearing in both ears. The BC response would reflect only the sensitivity of the better cochlea. Thus, significant interaural asymmetries in sensorineural sensitivity level would be missed by such a procedure. However, if the principal goal of neonatal screening is to identify handicapping hearing loss at the earliest possible age, so that remediation may be introduced according to an optimal schedule, then failure to identify unilateral loss in a child with normal hearing in one ear cannot be regarded as a serious flaw in the strategy.

On the positive side, such a strategy would, in theory at least, virtually eliminate the problem of false-positive results due to resolving middle ear disease in infants.

Although there are some additional problems inherent in the measurement of an ABR by bone conduction (Kavanagh & Beardsley, 1979; Mauldin & Jerger, 1979), and although these problems may be exacerbated in small infants, the proposed BC strategy seems promising and certainly warrants further field evaluation.

Based on the foregoing observations, Table 20-1 summarizes a recommended neonatal ABR screening strategy.

In connection with neonatal screening, it is important to remember that:

(A) The click response only tells you about sensitivity in the 1000- to 4000-Hz region.

(B) The false-positive rate for this test is going to be high, especially if testing by air conduction only.

(C) The "yield" (correct identification of significant permanent sensorineural loss) will depend on the population being screened. Even when screening is confined to high-risk groups, however, the yield may not exceed 1.5–3.5% of infants evaluated (Cox, Hack, & Metz, 1981).

EVALUATION OF OLDER INFANTS AND YOUNG CHILDREN

ABR testing of very young infants can usually be carried out in natural sleep. But in older infants and young children, especially in the 12- to 36-month range, it is usually necessary to sedate or anesthetize the child (Jerger, Hayes, & Jordan, 1980). This usually introduces a time constraint into the clinical evaluation. Depending on the sedative, barbiturate, or anesthetic agent used, the child may be sufficiently immobilized for only a finite period, usually 30–45 min.

Within this time frame, the clinician must explore overall sensitivity, audiometric contour, and interaural asymmetry. A typical strategy in such a situation is to gather all data on one ear, then switch to the other ear and gather similar data. However, there is a very real danger in such a strategy. If the sedation wears off and the child wakes up after one ear has been tested, but before testing can be carried out on the other ear, then the clinician is in the unenviable position of knowing all about the hearing on one ear but of not knowing whether this happens to be the better ear, the poorer ear, or a good representation of both ears. He has no choice but to reschedule the child for another evaluation.

Binaural Strategy

To meet the challenge of this situation, we have evolved, in our own clinical testing of children, an alternative approach called the *binaural strategy*. The essence of the binaural strategy is to initiate testing with the click presented to both ears simultaneously (binaural mode). The clinician then seeks "threshold" in the conventional manner by systematically lowering signal level until the lowest at which the ABR response can be observed is defined. In the binaural strategy, this initial threshold seeking yields the *binaural threshold*, that is, the threshold level for a binaural signal. After this binaural threshold has been defined, the clinician checks for binaural symmetry by testing monaurally in each ear at a level 20 dB above the previously defined binaural threshold. If the two monaural responses are approximately equal, the clinician may safely conclude that sensitivity is about the same in the two ears and testing is complete. If, on the other hand, the two monaural responses are substantially different, then the clinician pursues monaural threshold on the apparently poorer ear. There is no need for further testing of the better ear since, in the case of asymmetry, one may safely conclude that the binaural response is an accurate test of the better ear.

The rationale for the binaural strategy is that, when testing time may be limited and full evaluation curtailed, it is more important to define sensitivity in the better ear, even if one does not know which ear that is, than to obtain detailed information on the right ear but not know what sensitivity is like in the left ear.

If there is only time to complete one threshold run before the child wakes up, then, if that defined threshold is the binaural threshold, one at least knows hearing on the better ear and can plan a reasonably appropriate intervention strategy without further information (e.g., if the binaural threshold is normal, one need not be concerned about the presence of

TABLE 20–1.
Strategy for neonatal ABR screening

Test parameter	Test procedure	
A. Signal: click	A.	Present signal by earphone to each ear separately or by BC transducer on forehead.
B. Polarity: alternating	B.	Present signal at 30–40 dB nHL and 60–70 dB nHL.
C. Rate: 20–30/s	C.	If ABR response at 30–40 dB HL is normal, pass.
D. Level: 30–40 dB nHL; 60–70 dB nHL	D.	If ABR response at 30–40 dB HL is abnormal, raise level to 60–70 dB and retest.
E. Filter passband: 100–3000 Hz	E.	If ABR response at 60–70 dB HL is normal, refer for follow-up exam to investigate possibility of mild–moderate loss.
F. No. averaged: 2048	F.	If ABR response at 60–70 dB HL is abnormal, refer for follow-up exam to investigate possibility of severe–profound loss.

handicapping loss even if there is substantial loss in one ear. Conversely, if the binaural threshold is elevated, one can begin to plan for early appropriate intervention without further information about the status of individual ears. With an experimental binaural hearing aid fitting, for example, one can guarantee optimal stimulation for the ear most likely to benefit from amplification.

In effect, the binaural strategy is based on the following considerations:

(1) There are only two possibilities:

    (a) hearing sensitivity is the same in both ears, or

    (b) hearing sensitivity is different in the two ears.

(2) If sensitivity is the same in both ears, then the binaural threshold is an accurate representation of either ear and there is no need for further, ear-specific, testing.

(3) If sensitivity is different in each ear, then the binaural threshold is an accurate representation of the better ear, and one need explore further only the poorer ear.

(4) If one knows the sensitivity level of a child's better ear, one can initiate a useful and meaningful intervention strategy without further, ear-specific information if such information is not easily obtainable.

Clearly, the validity of the binaural strategy rests squarely on the assertion that the binaural threshold always reflects sensitivity of the better ear. It is possible, however, that the ABR response could be normal in each ear separately, but abnormal to binaural stimulation. We know of no such reports in the world's literature. On the contrary, it has been repeatedly observed (Blegvad, 1975; Gerull & Mrowinski, 1984) that at equivalent SLs the binaural response is always at least as large as, and usually larger than, either monaural response. Suppose, however, that a child has brainstem disease affecting the ABR response. Could this invalidate the binaural strategy by predicting loss when sensitivity was in fact normal in both ears? If the effect on ABR were unilateral, then the binaural response would be normal and prediction of normal sensitivity in at least one ear would continue to hold, and an erroneous prediction of significant peripheral hearing loss would not occur. If the brainstem disease affected the ABR response bilaterally, then the binaural ABR response would, in all likelihood, be abnormal and might lead to the erroneous prediction of significant peripheral hearing loss. But it would be in this respect, no different from the two abnormal monaural responses, each of which would also erroneously predict significant peripheral loss. Thus, the use of the binaural strategy in no way increases the likelihood of this kind of error.

Frequency Specificity

While the binaural click threshold yields a satisfactory estimate of sensitivity in the 1000- to 4000-Hz region of the audiogram, it fails to provide crucial information on audiometric contour. A click threshold in the region of 70 dB HL, for example, is consistent with either a flat loss at 70 dB HL across the frequency range or a steeply sloping contour with normal sensitivity at 500 Hz, but with a contour sharply dropping to 60–80 dB at 2000 and 4000 Hz.

Audiologists do not need to be reminded that intervention strategies would, ideally, be quite different in these two cases. Thus, frequency-specific information about audiometric contour, especially in the 500-Hz region, is highly desirable in the evaluation of infants and children.

Since the click response does not provide such information, it is necessary to employ more frequency-specific test signals. But here one encounters an inevitable interaction between frequency specificity of the test signal and quality of the ABR response (Davis, Hirsh, Popelka, & Formby, 1984). In general, the more energy is confined to a narrow, low-frequency region, the poorer is the "early" evoked response (Klein & Teas, 1978) and, consequently, the less satisfactory is its value as a threshold predictor. At the present time (June, 1984), two approaches to this problem have evolved a loyal coterie of followers. Both approaches advocate similar signals, 2–1–2 tone pips (i.e., tone pips with two-cycle rise, one cycle at maximum amplitude, and a two-cycle fall [Davis et al., 1984]). The two approaches differ, however, in their fundamental approach to the measurement problem. One approach, the SN-10 response (Davis & Hirsh, 1976; Suzuki, Hirai, & Horiuchi, 1977), employs a 20-ms epoch and seeks a surface-negative, evoked response to the tone pip in the latency range from 10–14 ms. The second approach, the 40-Hz event-related potential (ERP) (Galambos, Makeig, & Talmachoff, 1981), also referred to as the high-rate driven response (HRDR), employs a 50- to 100-ms window and seeks an essentially sinusoidal driven steady state response to tone pips presented at a rate of approximately 40 pips/s. This HRDR is thought to be a special case of the well-known middle latency potential (Pa at 20–30 ms) in response to tone pips delivered at relatively slower rates (1–10 pips/s).

Each of these two approaches has characteristic advantages and disadvantages. The SN-10 response is presumably less influenced by state variables (stage of sleep, effects of sedation, etc.) than the relatively longer latency HRDR (but see Klein, 1983), but it tends to be difficult to see at low levels of low-frequency tone pips and the accuracy of its predictions has been questioned (Hayes & Jerger, 1982). The HRDR, on the other hand, tends to be well-defined even at very low signal levels. It seems to work as well, or even better, at low frequencies as at high frequencies. The middle latency response, in general, however, may be more liable to the fluctuating effects of state variables (Brown & Shallop, 1982; Shallop & Osterhammel, 1983). In particular, amplitude declines substantially in sleep (Mendel & Goldstein, 1971) and under sedation. Recent studies of the HRDR by fast-Fourier transform (FFT) techniques, however, show considerable promise of refining this technique from the standpoint of its clinical feasibility (Galambos & Makeig, 1982).

In general, the use of either clicks or tone pips presented either binaurally or monaurally follows traditional methodology for threshold prediction. One systematically varies signal intensity, seeking the evoked response threshold, that is, the lowest level of the signal producing a recognizable and repeatable electrophysiological response. In the case of click-elicited ABRs, this approach has been generally quite successful. In the case of tone pip-elicited responses, however, especially those based on responses in the middle latency range, this traditional method of defining threshold may not be optimal. There is some evidence that more valid threshold estimation may be obtained by eschewing the search for poorly repeatable responses to very low SL signals and extrapolating amplitude versus intensity functions downward to the signal level corresponding to zero amplitude, or to the amplitude of the baseline noise floor of a "no sound" run. Another promising approach is the extraction of amplitude and phase components of the 40-Hz component of the HRDR by FFT analysis.

While these new analytic methods are still in the exploratory stage, there can be no doubt that useful information about audiometric contour can be derived from tone-pip responses (Brown & Shallop, 1982; Davis et al., 1984; Hawes & Greenberg, 1981; Shallop & Osterhammel, 1983). Some form of the response to tone pips should be an integral part of the ABR examination of all infants and young children.

Based on the foregoing observations, Table 20-2 presents a strategy for the evaluation of older infants and young children.

In the use of this strategy, it is important to remember that:

(A) If the sensitivity of the better ear is known, one is in a good position to intervene appropriately.

(B) Click thresholds do not tell all one needs to know about shape of audiogram. Knowledge of sensitivity at 500 Hz is very important for appropriate intervention.

DIFFERENTIATING COCHLEAR FROM RETROCOCHLEAR SITE

The diagnostic value of the ABR depends, to a great extent, on the identification of component waves, evaluation of waveform morphology, and the accurate measurement of both absolute and interwave latencies. The optimization of these various measures requires careful consideration of six specific parameters of the test situation:

1. Test level
2. Test mode
3. Click rate
4. Click polarity
5. Filter passband
6. Interpretive strategy

In the following sections each of these factors is considered in turn.

Test Level

Best results are achieved when the signal intensity is sufficient to elicit a well-defined waveform including, at minimum, identifiable waves I, III, and V. In the ear with normal hearing, this usually requires an intensity level of at least 60 dB nHL. Thus, diagnostic ABR testing is best carried out at relatively high signal levels, usually in the range of 60–80 dB nHL. However, there is some hazard in setting the intensity level too high. Hecox (1983), for example, has pointed out that amplitude relations among component waves, especially the I/V amplitude ratio, may be distorted at very high signal levels (80–100 dB). These considerations suggest that the optimal

TABLE 20-2.
Strategy for ABR testing of infants and children

Test parameter	Test procedure
A. Signals: clicks and 500-Hz tone pips (2-1-2)	Click Phase
	A. Use binaural strategy to define binaural click threshold.
B. Polarity: alternating	B. Test monaurally at binaural threshold +20 dB.
C. Rate: ABR; 10–20/s SN-10; 10–20/s HRDR; 40/s	C. If monaural responses are not equivalent, seek threshold of poorer ear.
D. Level: varied to seek threshold	D. If monaural responses are equivalent, move to tone-pip phase.
E. Filter passband: ABR; 100–3000 Hz SN-10; 30–3000 Hz HRDR; 5–1000 Hz	Tone-Pip Phase
F. No. averaged: ABR; 2048 SN-10; 2048 HRDR; 1024	A. Use monaural strategy to define 500 Hz tone-pip threshold (either SN-10 or HRDR) on each ear.

signal level would be just about 70 dB nHL (or approximately 100 dB peSPL). And, indeed, many laboratories use 70 dB as the standard signal level for diagnostic ABR testing.

If all patients we test had normal peripheral hearing, there would be no need for further discussion of appropriate test levels. But, unfortunately, a substantial number of patients for whom ABR is a useful diagnostic test have some degree of peripheral hearing loss (Hayes, 1980), especially in the high-frequency region of the audiogram so important for mediation of the click response. If there is even moderate high-frequency loss, however, the 70 dB nHL test level may no longer be sufficient to elicit an ideal ABR waveform. If the sensation level of the test signal is not sufficient, then all component waves may not be identifiable, especially the important landmark, wave I. One's first inclination might be to raise the test level by an amount equal to the sensitivity loss in the critical high-frequency region (1–4 kHz); in other words, to maintain a constant 70-dB sensation level. Anyone familiar with the suprathreshold characteristics of the ear with cochlear impairment, however, already knows that this approach will not work. Because of suprathreshold distortions in such ears (e.g., "loudness recruitment"), such an approach would be neither desirable nor practical. If the loss in the 1–4 kHz region were 40 dB, for example, the constant 70-dB sensation level would be achieved at 110 dB nHL. However, this level would almost certainly be extremely unpleasant for the patient with cochlear loss and, as noted above, might distort interwave amplitude relationships. Fortunately, such a high level is not necessary to observe the optimal waveform obtainable from this ear. In fact, a level of 80–90 dB nHL would probably be sufficient to observe the best waveform that the ear is capable of producing. But, even at this optimal level, the response may not show a wave I response as well defined as one expects to see in the response from a normal ear. As the degree of high-frequency hearing loss increases, all of the early waves (I, II, and III), but especially wave I, become increasingly difficult to identify (Hecox & Galambos, 1974). From the standpoint of test strategy, then, the problem is to find the test level that has the best probability of yielding identifiable early waves but that remains within the range of intensities acceptable to the patient. A useful strategy, therefore, is to first examine the pure tone audiometric thresholds in the 1–4 kHz region. If the average of the three thresholds at 1000, 2000, and 4000 Hz (pure tone threshold average; PTA 2) falls in the 0–19 dB range, then it is probably safe to use a standard test level of 70 dB nHL. If the PTA 2 is in the range from 20–39 dB, however, raise the level to 80 dB nHL. For PTA 2 in the range from 40 to 59 dB, raise the test level to 90 dB nHL and for PTA 2 in the range from 60 to 79 dB, raise the test level to 100 dB nHL. For PTA 2 greater than 79 dB, it may be desirable to raise the level an additional 5 dB to 105 dB nHL, although many commercial ABR systems are not capable of delivering such high signal levels.

Test Mode

In diagnostic evaluation, it is customary to test only in the monaural mode. Since the binaural ABR reflects only the response from the better ear, it is a more efficient use of time to test the two ears separately and compare the two monaural responses for symmetry. It should be noted, however, that Dobie and Berlin (1979) have proposed a procedure for comparing the binaural response with the sum of the two monaural responses in order to derive a difference measure thought to be sensitive to certain forms of central disorder. Apart from this unique application, however, common diagnostic evaluation typically proceeds by testing the two ears separately and examining each monaural response for normalcy of waveform, absolute and interwave latencies, and amplitude ratios. Diagnostically significant abnormalities take the form of degraded morphology, absence of component waves, delayed absolute or interwave latencies or both, and abnormal amplitude ratios (Hecox, Cone, & Blaw, 1981; Starr & Achor, 1975; Starr & Hamilton, 1976; Stockard & Rossiter, 1977).

Click Rate

Click rate is an important variable in diagnostic evaluation (Gerling & Finitzo-Hieber, 1983; Hecox, 1983). It is usually desirable to set the click rate low enough to ensure observation of all component waves. Commonly a rate in the vicinity of 10–20 clicks/s is appropriate for this task. At this point, the examiner evaluates the response carefully. If the morphology is relatively good, all essential component waves can be observed, and latencies seem reasonably normal, then it may be desirable to stress the mechanism by retesting at a higher click rate (Pratt, Ben-David, Peled, Podoshin, & Scharf, 1981). Some investigators will routinely raise the click rate to 70 clicks/s and retest. Other investigators may take the time to generate an entire rate function by retesting at rates of 40, 60, and 80 clicks/s, or even at smaller intervals. It is sometimes the case that responses looking reasonably normal at click rates of 10–20/s will show some pathologic degradation at high click rates, suggesting retrocochlear disorder (Shanon, Gold, & Himmelfarb, 1981; Zöllner & Eibach, 1981).

If the morphologic characteristics of the response to clicks at 10–20/s are decidedly abnormal, then the appropriate strategy is to decrease the click rate in order to probe for a more well-defined response. In the case of high-frequency peripheral hearing loss, for example, wave I may not be indentifiable at a click rate of 20/s but may appear if the click rate is lowered to 10 or 5/s. The strategy for varying click rate, therefore, should be to increase the rate when the response at the standard rate looks good and to decrease rate when the response at the standard rate looks bad. There is, however, one important exception to this simple algorithm. It has been observed that, in some patients with demyelinating disease, the response to clicks at a relatively fast rate (50–70/s) may actually be better formed than the response to clicks at the standard slower rate (10–20/s). This observation argues for a flexible strategy in which probing at high click rates becomes a relatively standard test condition.

Click Polarity

Click polarity, in diagnostic ABR evaluation, is still a matter of some dispute. Arguments have been made in support of condensation (C) only, rarefaction (R) only, and alternation of polarity. Perhaps the most persuasive data bearing on this issue have been provided by Salt (1982). Using an ear canal probe–microphone technique, this investigator showed that what begins electrically as a condensation click actually turns out to be an acoustic condensation in the real ear canal in only about 60% of subjects. In the remaining 40%, the acoustic properties of the ear canal actually reverse the polarity at the ear drum. In this circumstance, the best strategy would appear to be use of alternating clicks in order to maintain signal constancy from patient to patient. In some patients with steeply sloping high-frequency sensorineural loss, however, there may be marked differences in responses to C and R clicks (Borg & Löfqvist, 1981, 1982) arguing for testing both responses separately as well as in the alternating condition.

Filter Passband

Filter passband is another issue that has been hotly debated over the years. Early in the history of ABR testing, some investigators advocated a narrow band from 300–3000 Hz in order to minimize low-frequency artifact from the ongoing EEG. Other investigators, however, felt that a good deal of useful information lay in the region from 50 to 300 Hz and should not be discarded. A reasonable compromise between these two positions now seems to have been achieved with a fairly universally accepted passband from 100 to 3000 Hz.

Interpretive Strategy

Over the years, several strategies have been proposed for evaluating the diagnostic significance of ABR waveforms. The various proposed indices of abnormality include

(1) absolute latency of wave V
(2) wave V interaural difference
(3) I–V interwave interval
(4) interaural difference in I–V interwave intervals
(5) I/V amplitude ratio
(6) interaural difference in I/V amplitude ratios
(7) selective loss of late waves
(8) grossly degraded waveform morphology

The last two indices, selective loss of late waves and grossly degraded waveform morphology, while less objective than the first six, tend to be fairly obvious and dramatic when they do occur. But abnormality in the various latency and amplitude measures is not always so obvious and dramatic. In some early cases of acoustic tumor, for example, waveform morphology may be very good on both ears, the abnormality on the tumor ear being confined to a 0.4–0.5 ms interaural difference in the I–V interpeak interval. In these latter cases, there has been some disagreement as to the best strategy for taking normal variability into account in diagnostic evaluation. The conventional notion of defining normal limits as a band, plus or minus two standard deviations, around the normal mean is compelling but fails to deal with three important related issues:

(1) Is the underlying distribution truly normal or even symmetric?

(2) Is 5% actually the appropriate risk of alpha error in the typical diagnostic evaluation?

(3) How should one weigh abnormalities revealed by the various indices? Are some abnormalities more significant than others?

We have fairly good evidence on the first question. Stockard, Stockard, and Coen (1983) and Klein and Teas (1978) have shown that indices like absolute and interwave intervals are indeed normally and symmetrically distributed and with remarkably constant standard deviations. It is not, therefore, unreasonable to define normal variability as a range of values encompassing a given number of standard deviations around the arithmetic mean.

Not so straightforward, however, is the tacit adoption of a 5% alpha error level by adopting the two-standard deviation (more appropriately 1.96 SD) boundary. In so doing we are, in effect, saying that we are willing to be wrong on 5% of the occasions that we identify an ABR measure as abnormal. Is this acceptable? Is the value of a correct identification sufficient to justify a 5% false alarm rate? A strong argument can be made for an affirmative answer to such a question. In fact, one could argue that an even higher alpha error is desirable. If, goes the argument, one purpose of the ABR test is to act as a screen to identify patients with potentially life-threatening diseases (e.g., intra- or extraaxial brain tumors) and the consequence of an abnormal finding is simply further testing, perhaps by sophisticated radiographic or other scanning technique to confirm the presence of a lesion, then a relatively high alpha error level is tolerable. The value of correct identification, especially to the patient, is high, and the cost of a false alarm is no more than the cost and inconvenience of further testing. In this circumstance, one could argue for an alpha level of 10 or even 20%. There is, indeed, nothing magical about the 5% level of confidence in this example. Yet, 5% limits are so ingrained in our thinking that it would be very difficult to find acceptance for higher levels of alpha error.

However, a more sophisticated approach to the problem of selecting an appropriate confidence level would be to base such selection on a careful analysis of relative costs and values associated with the various possible correct and incorrect outcomes rather than on appeal to tradition.

We still lack sufficient data to assign relative weights to the various indices of abnormality. Many investigators would readily rank order at least some of the indices, placing least weight on amplitude ratios (see, however, Musiek, Kibbe, Rackliff, & Weider, 1984), somewhat more weight on absolute latencies, and even more weight on interwave intervals. And, one could probably find strong support for weighting interaural differences higher than ear-specific measures. We still do not have enough data, however, to tell us exactly how much these various weights should be in a quantitative sense. The issue is further complicated by the fact that all possible indices are not always available for each patient. The most valuable indices, those based on interwave intervals, for example, cannot be computed if wave I is not identifiable, a circumstance that arises often when there is substantial high-frequency hearing loss in the ear under test.

Based on the foregoing observations, Table 20-4 presents a strategy for diagnostic evaluation. In the use of this strategy it is important to remember the following points:

A. Do not lose sight of the forest for the trees. Before dwelling on the fine grain of tenths of milliseconds of interwave intervals, it is well to ask the basic questions:

1. Is the ABR waveform morphology obviously abnormal?
2. Is the ABR abnormality consistent with the configuration of the audiogram?
3. Can an ABR interaural difference be explained by the audiometric interaural difference?

In a fairly large share of patients with retrocochlear disorder, answers to these fundamental questions are straightforward and obviate the necessity for anguishing over the precise identification of component waves or the exact measurements of either absolute or relative latencies.

B. When in doubt, slow up. There is nothing magical about a click rate of 20/s. It is simply a compromise between the desire for a well-defined waveform and the desire to keep testing time to a minimum. If anything about the ABR response to a relatively fast rate like 20/s looks suspicious, your best strategy is to retest at a slower rate (10/s or even 5/s) in order to achieve better waveform definition, especially of wave I.

CONCLUSION

We have attempted to present relatively specific test strategies for the three fundamental clinical applications of ABR. Inevitably, in such an ambitious undertaking, there must be some compromise to resolve the range of approaches taken by different investigators. Throughout the chapter, therefore, we have attempted to reflect not only those aspects of testing where consistency is the rule, but also those aspects where opinion is still divergent.

Are we advocating, herein, the standardization of ABR testing? Decidedly not! Our sole purpose in presenting these specific test strategies is to distill the wide range of experiences of various investigators into a set of procedures in which the clinician may have confidence. But we do not advocate that any of these recommendations become fixed and immutable. Instead, we recommend continued flexibility in our approach to the test situation and a continuing willingness to modify our approach as new evidence warrants such change.

TABLE 20-4.
Strategy for diagnostic ABR evaluation

Test parameter	Test procedure
A. Signal: click	Evaluate: Examine waveforms for adequacy of morphology and presence of all component waves. If these criteria are met, compute the following six indices:
B. Polarity: alternating and/or condensations and rarefactions separately	1. Absolute latency of wave V on each ear (2)
	2. Interaural difference in wave V latencies (1)
C. Rate: adjustable 1. Begin at 20/s 2. Follow with 70/s 3. If neither rate yields a satisfactory waveform, slow rate to 10 or 5/s	3. I–V Interwave interval on each ear (2)
	4. Interaural difference in I–V interwave intervals (1)
D. Test level: adjust according to PTA2	Categorize results as either normal, questionable, or abnormal according to the interpretive algorithm given above.
PTA2 (dB) Test level (dB nHL) 0–19 70 20–39 80 40–59 90 60–79 100 ≥80 105	
E. Filter passband: 100–3000 Hz	
F. No. averaged: 2048	

REFERENCES

Alberti, P. W., Hyde, M. L., Riko, K., Corbin, H., & Abramovich, S. (1983). An evaluation of BERA for hearing screening in high-risk neonates. *Laryngoscope, 93*, 1115-1121.

Blegvad, B. (1975). Binaural summation of surface-recorded electrocochleographic responses. *Scandinavian Audiology, 4*, 233-238.

Borg, E., & Löfqvist, L. (1981). Auditory brainstem response (ABR) to rarefaction and condensation clicks in normal and steep high-frequency hearing loss. *Scandinavian Audiology, 10* (Supplement 13), 99-101.

Borg, E., & Löfqvist, L. (1982). Auditory brainstem response (ABR) to rarefaction and condensation clicks in normal and abnormal ears. *Scandinavian Audiology, 11*, 227-235.

Brown, D. D., & Shallop, J. K. (1982, fall). A clinically useful 500 Hz evoked response. *Nicolet Potentials, 1*, 9-12.

Cevette, M. J. (1984). Auditory brainstem response testing in the intensive care unit. *Seminars in Hearing, 5*, 57-69.

Cox, C., Hack, M., & Metz, D. (1981). Brainstem-evoked response audiometry: Normative data from the preterm infant. *Audiology, 20*, 53-64.

Davis, H., & Hirsh, S. K. (1976). The audiometric utility of brain stem responses to low-frequency sounds. *Audiology, 15*, 181-195.

Davis, H., Hirsh, S. K., Popelka, G. R., & Formby, C. (1984). Frequency selectivity and thresholds of brief stimuli suitable for electric response audiometry. *Audiology, 23*, 59-74.

Dennis, J. M., Sheldon, R., Toubas, P., & McCaffee, M. A. (1984). Identification of hearing loss in the neonatal intensive care unit population. *The American Journal of Otology, 5*, 201-205.

Dobie, R. A., & Berlin, C. I. (1979). Binaural interaction in brainstem-evoked responses. *Archives of Otolaryngology, 105*, 391-398.

Downs, D. W. (1982). Auditory brainstem response testing in the neonatal intensive care unit: A cautious response. *ASHA, 24*, 1009-1015.

Finitzo-Hieber, T. (1982). Auditory brainstem response: Its place in infant audiological evaluations. *Seminars in Speech, Language and Hearing, 3*, 76-87.

Galambos, R. (1978). Use of the auditory brainstem response (ABR) in infant hearing testing. In S. E. Gerber & G. T. Mencher (Eds.), *Early diagnosis of hearing loss*. New York: Grune & Stratton.

Galambos, R., Hicks, G. E., & Wilson, M. J. (in press). The auditory brainstem response reliably predicts hearing loss in graduates of a tertiary intensive care nursery. *Ear & Hearing*.

Galambos, R., & Makeig, S. (1982). *Electric response audiometry: Improving threshold estimates*. Paper presented at the Annual Convention of the American Speech-Language-Hearing Association, Toronto, November.

Galambos, R., Makeig, S., & Talmachoff, P. J. (1981). A 40-Hz auditory potential recorded from the human scalp. *Proceedings of National Academy of Science USA, 78*, 2643-2647.

Gerling, I. J., & Finitzo-Hieber, T. (1983). Auditory brainstem response with high stimulus rates in normal and patient populations. *Annals of Otology, Rhinology and Laryngology, 92*, 119-123.

Gerull, G., & Mrowinski, D. (1984). Brain stem potentials evoked by binaural click stimuli with differences in interaural time and intensity. *Audiology, 23*, 265-276.

Hawes, M. D., & Greenberg, H. J. (1981). Slow brain stem responses (SN10) to tone pips in normally hearing newborns and adults. *Audiology, 20*, 113-122.

Hayes, D. (1980). Effect of degree of hearing loss on diagnostic audiometric tests. *American Journal of Otology, 2*, 91-96.

Hayes, D., & Jerger, J. (1982). Auditory brainstem response (ABR) to tone-pips: Results in normal and hearing-impaired subjects. *Scandinavian Audiology, 11*, 133-142.

Hecox, K. E. (1983, spring). Brainstem auditory evoked responses: Technical factors Part I. *Nicolet Potentials*, 2, 19–22; 24.

Hecox, K. E. (1984, spring). Auditory evoked response: Audiologic applications Part II. *Nicolet Potentials*, 3, 39–41; 47.

Hecox, K. E., Cone, B., & Blaw, M. E. (1981). Brainstem auditory evoked response in the diagnosis of pediatric neurologic diseases. *Neurology*, 31, 832–840.

Hecox, K., & Galambos, R. (1974). Brain stem auditory evoked responses in human infants and adults. *Archives of Otolaryngology*, 99, 30–33.

Hooks, R. G., & Weber, B. A. (1984). Auditory brain stem responses of premature infants to bone-conducted stimuli: A feasibility study. *Ear and Hearing*, 5, 42–46.

Jacobson, J. T., Seitz, M. R., Mencher, G. T., & Parrott, V. (1980). Auditory brainstem response: A contribution to infant assessment and management. In G. T. Mencher & S. E. Gerber (Eds.), *Early management of hearing loss*. New York: Grune & Stratton.

Jerger, J., Hayes, D., & Jordan, C. (1980). Clinical experience with auditory brainstem response audiometry in pediatric assessment. *Ear and Hearing*, 1, 19–25.

Kavanagh, K. T., & Beardsley, J. V. (1979). Brain stem auditory evoked response. *Annals of Otology, Rhinology and Laryngology*, 88 (Supplement 58), 1–28.

Klein, A. J. (1983). Properties of the brain-stem response slow-wave component: I. Latency, amplitude, and threshold measurement. *Archives of Otolaryngology*, 109, 6–12.

Klein, A. J., & Teas, D. C. (1978). Acoustically dependent latency shifts of BSER (wave V) in man. *Journal of the Acoustical Society of America*, 63, 1887–1895.

Mauldin, L., & Jerger, J. (1979). Auditory brain stem evoked responses to bone-conducted signals. *Archives of Otolaryngology*, 105, 656–661.

Mendel, M. I., & Goldstein, R. (1971). Early components of the averaged electroencephalic response to constant level clicks during all-night sleep. *Journal of Speech and Hearing Research*, 14, 829–840.

Musiek, F. E., Kibbe, K., Rackliffe, L., & Weider, D. J. (1984). The auditory brain stem response I–V amplitude ratio in normal, cochlear, and retrocochlear ears. *Ear and Hearing*, 5, 52–55.

Northern, J. L., & Downs, M. P. (1974). *Hearing in children*. Baltimore: Williams & Wilkins.

Pratt, H., Ben-David, Y., Peled, R., Podoshin, L., & Scharf, B. (1981). Auditory brain stem evoked potentials: Clinical promise of increasing stimulus rate. *Electroencephalography and Clinical Neurophysiology*, 51, 80–90.

Roberts, J. L., Davis, H., Phon, G. L., Reichert, T. J., Sturtevant, E. M., & Marshall, R. E. (1982). Auditory brainstem responses in preterm neonates: Maturation and follow-up. *The Journal of Pediatrics*, 101, 257–263.

Salt, A. (1982). *Presentation on ear canal probe microphone measurements of click polarity*. Paper presented at the 1st International Conference on Standards for Auditory Brainstem Response Measurement, Laguna Beach, CA, February.

Schulman-Galambos, C., & Galambos, R. (1979). Brainstem evoked response audiometry in newborn hearing screening. *Archives of Otolaryngology*, 105, 86–90.

Shallop, J. K., & Osterhammel, P. A. (1983). A comparative study of measurements of SN-10 and the 40/sec middle latency responses in newborns. *Scandinavian Audiology*, 12, 91–95.

Shanon, E., Gold, S., & Himmelfarb, M. (1981). Assessment of functional integrity of brain stem auditory pathways by stimulus stress. *Audiology*, 20, 65–71.

Starr, A., & Achor, L. J. (1975). Auditory brainstem responses in neurological disease. *Archives of Neurology*, 32, 761–768.

Starr, A., Amlie, R. N., Martin, W. H., & Sanders, S. (1977). Development of auditory function in newborn infants revealed by auditory brainstem potentials. *Pediatrics*, 60, 831–839.

Starr, A., & Hamilton, A. E. (1976). Correlation between confirmed sites of neurological lesions and abnormalities of far-field auditory brainstem responses, *Electroencephalography and Clinical Neurophysiology*, 41, 595–608.

Stein, L. K. (1984). Evaluating the efficiency of auditory brainstem response as a neonatal hearing screening test. *Seminars in Hearing, 5,* 71–77.

Stein, L. K., Ozdamar, O., Kraus, N., & Paton, J. (1983). Follow-up of infants screened by auditory brainstem response in the neonatal intensive care unit, *103,* 447–453.

Stockard, J., & Rossiter, V. (1977). Clinical and pathologic correlates of brainstem auditory response abnormalities. *Neurology, 27,* 316–325.

Stockard, J. E., Stockard, J. J., & Coen, R. W. (1983). Auditory brainstem response variability in infants. *Ear and Hearing, 4,* 11–23.

Suzuki, T., Hirai, Y., & Horiuchi, K. (1977). Auditory brainstem responses to pure-tone stimuli. *Scandinavian Audiology, 6,* 51–56.

Thornton, A. Personal communication, May, 1984.

Weber, B. A. (1983). Masking and bone conduction testing in brainstem response audiometry. *Seminars in Hearing, 4,* 343–352.

Zollner, C., & Eibach, H. (1981). Can the differential diagnosis cochlear–retrocochlear disorder be improved using the brainstem potentials with changing stimulus repetition rates? *HNO, 29,* 240–245.

Chapter 21

Special Case Studies

INTRODUCTION

John T. Jacobson, Ph.D.
Department of Communicative Disorders
University of Mississippi
University, Mississippi

The auditory brainstem response is not a panacea; it was never developed with the intent of gaining such stature. The ABR has only been classified as such by those who do not fully understand or appreciate its limitations. The ABR is most useful when recognized in its proper perspective; that is, as an electrophysiological measure of the discharge pattern of a group of neural elements generated from the acoustic nerve and brainstem pathway in response to an auditory stimulus. The ABR is not a test of hearing acuity in the true sense of auditory perception. It does, however, provide an objective insight into the integrity of the peripheral and central auditory mechanism as far as the level of the pons and caudal regions of the midbrain.

It follows, then, that the ABR should not be expected to be definitive in every case study. The use of the ABR in clinical practice will never replace the traditional audiological evaluation. The ABR was not designed to usurp but to supplement the existing test battery, offering an added dimension in objective testing. Pure tone and immittance audiometry will remain the cornerstones of audiological assessment. The ABR must be looked upon as a test procedure that is applied in conjunction with, not independent of, other test protocols. In addition to psychophysical measures, this dependency also includes the support of other electrophysiological procedures, such as the middle latency and slow vertex responses. The ABR is best suited to be a supplement to conventional testing, where it can fully complement other audiological procedures.

To date, there remain a number of unanswered questions that concern ABR test strategy. Although not vital to ABR function, their resolution will assist in the overall logistics of the test measure. For example, When is it appropriate to request an ABR test evaluation? Where does the ABR fit in terms of test sequence? Does the ABR provide sufficient information to differentiate pathology or measure the degree of hearing loss based on a transient stimuli? Should ABR testing be limited to the difficult-to-test population; if not, when is the test considered cost-effective? From experience, we have learned that any test "in vogue" will be requested regardless of its efficiency (e.g., tuning fork tests and other traditional site-of-lesion test protocols). What justifies use? For instance, is the ABR a necessary procedure in the case of a young child who offers reliable behavioral and immittance measures? Too often there is a tendency to reject the conventional test battery, which may provide all the necessary information for an accurate diagnosis. A conservative approach taken by this author suggests that except for the unwilling or incapable patient, for whom the ABR or other objective procedures may present themselves as the tests of choice in auditory or neurological evaluation, the ABR should be integrated into the auditory assessment only after other psychophysical procedures have failed to provide conclusive evidence or when further confirmation is dictated. In this manner, optimum use of time, cost, energy, and expertise is appropriately weighted in the overall diagnosis.

With these concepts in mind, the purpose of this final chapter is to provide the reader with a series of documented case studies in which several important clinical ABR issues are addressed. Not only is this chapter the culmination of this text, but it also reflects the sum and substance of the preceding five Sections. Throughout, there has been a concerted effort to systematically review the brainstem response from a practical viewpoint. Thus, a major goal of this book has been to synthesize the various aspects of the ABR into a concise, usable, and up-to-date literary source. In an attempt to convey the many practical and technical variables discussed herein, the following series of case studies have been selected. These illustrations are, of course, not inclusive, but do offer a representative example of ABR application.

In order to draw from diverse sources of experience, I invited colleagues to submit unusual case findings they thought would be of interest. Each contributor was instructed only to provide an authentic case study that utilized the ABR in some aspect of auditory or neurological diagnosis and that the example should demonstrate the advantages or limitations, or both, of the electrophysiological procedure. Although each study describes a unique aspect of the ABR, the cases also exemplify the importance of the test battery approach. When used in conjunction with other audiological, neurological, and radiological evidence, the ABR may prove to be the most powerful diagnostic prognosticator used today in clinical auditory diagnosis.

Neonatal Intraventricular Hemorrhage

Michael J. Cevette, M.S.,
and
Tracy Karp, R.N., M.S.
Speech-Language-Hearing Center,
Primary Children's Medical Center,
Salt Lake City, Utah

This case study describes the electrophysiological status of a premature neonate's preoperative and postoperative ventricular decompression. Auditory brainstem responses (ABR) were used to monitor the condition of a 32 week adjusted gestational age female infant who was born with a birth weight of 1800 grams. The early neonatal history was significant for birth asphyxia, seizures, developmental hyaline membrane disease, and *Escherichia coli* sepsis with pneumonia. The neonatal course was further complicated by the development of multiple pneumothoraces, respiratory failure, and the need for aggressive mechanical ventilation. On the tenth day of life a severe cardiopulmonary deterioration occurred, resulting in a grade IV (intraventricular and parenchymal) hemorrhage. Secondary to the hemorrhage, progressive noncommunicating hydrocephalus developed by the thirtieth day of life. In addition, prior to and following the hydrocephalus, the infant suffered from brief periods of severe hypercarbia and secondary respiratory acidosis.

Owing to the infant's instability and the elevated cerebrospinal fluid protein values, a ventricular reservoir was placed to allow for ventricular decompression. At 40 weeks PCA, a series of ABR recordings were conducted before and after ventricular tapping via the ventricular reservoir. The amount of cerebrospinal fluid removed measured 30 ml over a 10 minute period. Brainstem responses were recorded on a clinical averager using 85 dB nHL positive polarity clicks at a rate of 13/s. A minimum of 2000 responses were averaged for each run employing a 15 ms time window.

Since ABR evaluations occurred before and after the draining of the cerebrospinal fluid and within 30 minutes of the baseline test, any significant influence due to maturation or transient peripheral auditory abnormality was eliminated. The pretap and posttap ABR results are presented in Figure 21-1 (A, B). The wave I latency responses remain stable and repeatable for both conditions at 1.86 ms, suggesting a normal peripheral measure. In comparison, the wave V latency decreased from 7.26 to 6.78 ms. The 0.48 ms difference in interwave intervals offers a significant improvement in neural conduction time. These observations measured by ABR suggest the possible related physiological changes of decompression and intracranial pressure and show the prognostic value of electrophysiological procedure in neurological monitoring.

Interestingly, further ABR testing at 41 weeks PCA revealed normal ABR responses; however, at 47 weeks, ABRs once again showed abnormal central pathology, suggesting a change in the infant's status.

Figure 21–1.

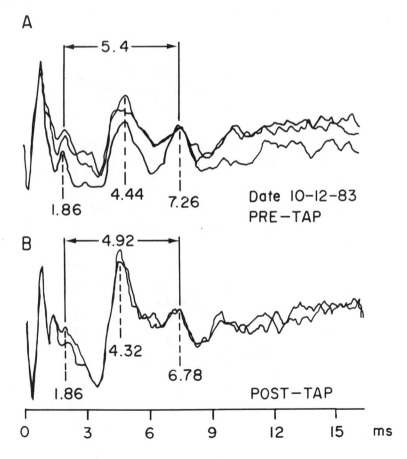

ABR and the Language Delay

L. Clarke Cox, Ph.D.
Department of Speech and Hearing,
Cleveland State University,
Cleveland, Ohio

The client was referred for ABR testing at 4½ years of age due to inconsistencies in behavioral audiometric and language data. The mother reported normal language development until the birth of a sibling when the child was 14 months of age, at which time the client's "speech" development appeared to slow.

Initial audiometric data at 2 years of age revealed elevated speech awareness thresholds and normal acoustic immittance data. Further testing at a second clinic at 2½ and 3 years of age revealed speech thresholds of approximately 40 dB HTL under phones and in soundfield. Responses to bone conduction speech stimuli were at 10 dB HTL. Pure tone thresholds, at 70 dB HTL, were not consistent with speech thresholds. Acoustic immittance data were normal bilaterally.

Figure 21–2.

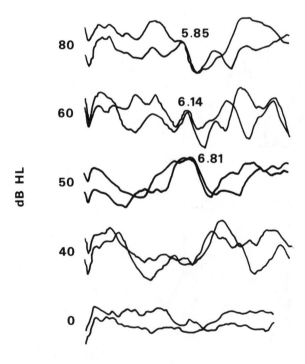

A language evaluation completed at 3 years of age noted delays in language and what appeared to be heavy reliance on lip-reading. The mother reported fluctuation in the client's response to speech and environmental sounds. The client also on occasion complained of ear pain. With the attending ENT physician noting the possibility of eustachian tube dysfunction, the diagnosis of a fluctuating hearing loss was made.

Subsequent testing at 4 years of age produced pure tone and speech thresholds at 25 to 30 dB HTL, while immittance data were normal. The problems of fluctuating hearing loss and language delays were still reported by the mother and speech therapist. Approximately two

Figure 21-3.

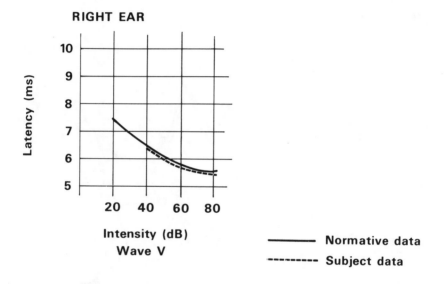

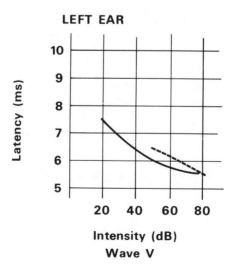

months later, at another clinic, negative middle ear pressure of -150 mm H_2O was noted. At the insistence of the parents, PE tubes were inserted at 4.3 years of age. Follow-up testing noted no change in hearing sensitivity, and the parents reported no change in responsiveness to speech. At that point, questions regarding possible central auditory or functional problems precipitated the referral for ABR.

Initial ABR testing produced what appeared to be normal data from the right ear. Some wave V prolongation and absence of response at lower intensities consistent with a mild cochlear hearing loss was seen in the left ear (Fig. 21-2). The latency-intensity function of 40, 60, and

Figure 21–4.

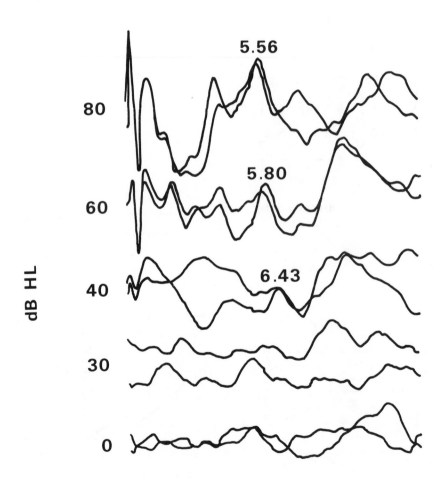

RIGHT EAR

80dB HL in the right ear was normal, with no indication of deviation from normal function (Fig. 21-3).

In analyzing the ABR data in conjunction with the behavioral data and apparent language delay, a mild unilateral hearing loss was not adequate to explain the language data. Further ABR testing could not be completed, however, owing to the client's level of activity.

ABR testing was repeated approximately 30 days later, while the client was sedated. The data obtained below 40dB HL in the right ear was surprising and revealing. Although no deviation from latency-intensity norms was seen above 40dB HL, responses below were absent (Fig. 21-4). In neonates, a response at 40dB HL and an absent response at 30dB HL is not unusual. In a 4½ year old sedated, child, it is highly unusual; this is the only such case seen by the writer. These results were interpreted as the presence of a mild cochlear hearing loss in the right ear. Coupled with a mild to possibly moderate cochlear loss in the left ear, a mild loss in the right ear could contribute to if not account for the language delay and current auditory behavior seen. The ABR results also were in good agreement with the most recent pure tone and speech data.

In view of the results, a mild gain hearing aid fit to the left ear was recommended. A marked improvement to speech and other environmental sounds was noted with the hearing aid. With regard to any changes in language, however, the jury is still out.

Cytomegalovirus

Katherine Pike Gerkin, M.A., and Jerry L. Northern, Ph.D.
Audiology Division,
University of Colorado Health Sciences Center,
Denver, Colorado

Cytomegalovirus (CMV) is one of the more common congenital and perinatal viral infections. In its more severe form it can cause a global central nervous system infection with multiple sequelae to the infant. Infants may shed CMV in their urine yet appear asymptomatic. Reports of sensorineural hearing loss in both symptomatic and asymptomatic cases of CMV have been reported (Pass, Stagno, Myers, & Alford, 1980; Reynolds, Stagno, Stubbs, Dahle, Livingston, Saxon, & Alford, 1974). The pattern and degree of the sensorineural loss varies greatly, and evidence suggests the CMV may cause progressive hearing loss.

Three case studies of infants diagnosed shortly after birth as having cytomegalovirus are presented here.

Case 1. A 5 month old child was referred for audiometric testing and ABR evaluation because of CMV diagnosis. Behavioral audiometric testing suggested normal hearing with startle responses by air conduction to moderately loud stimuli and behavioral responses at lower intensity levels of 45 to 50 dB HL. The ABR results revealed auditory responses at 95 and 80 dB nHL with somewhat prolonged interwave intervals. No ABR response was obtained at 65 dB nHL.

Owing to the inconsistency between the behavioral audiometric responses and the ABR, the child was rescheduled and tested again two months later. During the second testing session, the ABR revealed no response bilaterally at the maximum intensity limits of the equipment. Sound field behavioral auditory responses were observed only to low frequency stimuli at 85 to 90 dB, leading to a diagnosis of profound bilateral sensorineural hearing loss.

Case 2. This client is an 8 month old infant of 33 weeks' gestation with a birth weight of 1360 grams. The infant had a difficult four month hospital course before going home with her parents. She was readmitted at five months of age because of a dusky skin appearance and poor feeding habits. At this time viral cultures were conducted and CMV was discovered in the urine. Negative CMV cultures had been noted previously during the neonatal hospital course.

This child was referred for behavioral hearing testing at 5 months of age, at which time air conduction auditory thresholds were indicated to be approximately 40 dB HL. Tympanograms were immobile and middle ear fluid was observed otoscopically. This child was difficult to follow routinely because her mother subsequently died from complications of a renal transplant, and the infant was placed in the care of various foster parents.

An ABR evaluation, conducted at 9 months of age, demonstrated questionable wave V responses at 80 dB in the left ear. No ABR responses could be replicated at lower intensity levels. Owing to activity level, the right ear could not be evaluated. Behavioral audiometry at 16 months of age confirmed a moderate bilateral sensorineural hearing loss.

Case 3. This 3 month old infant, of 37 weeks' gestation and birth weight of 1600 grams, had a stormy neonatal course and was ultimately diagnosed as having congenital CMV. The behavioral audiometric evaluation showed no behavioral responses to high frequency or broadband stimuli presented at 90 dB. ABR results were absent bilaterally at the intensity limits of the equipment, supporting a diagnosis of profound bilateral sensorineural hearing loss. Although this case did not present with the inconsistencies between behavioral audiometry and ABR noted in the first two cases, there is little doubt that the profound sensorineural hearing loss often accompanies congenital CMV infection.

These three children were fitted with hearing aids and placed in appropriate habilitation programs. Unfortunately, although their hearing losses were identified early, their progress in speech and language development has been poor. This may be related to the extensive central nervous system damage that often accompanies congenital CMV infection.

These cases illustrate several important points: (1) a child's hearing loss would have been missed if behavioral testing alone had been used; (2) hearing sensitivity may have been underestimated if ABR testing had been used independently of other measures. Our results indicate cases of rapid deterioration of hearing sensitivity as a result of CMV infection, suggesting the need for serial audiometrics, including the ABR.

REFERENCES

Pass, R.F., Stagno, S., Myers, G.J., & Alford, C.A. (1980). Outcome of symptomatic congenital cytomegalovirus infection: Results of long-term longitudinal follow-up. *Pediatrics, 66,* 758–762.

Reynolds, D.W., Stagno, S., Stubbs, K.G., Dahle, A.J., Livingston, M.M., Saxon, S.S., & Alford, C.A. (1974). Inapparent congenital cytomegalovirus infection with elevated cord IgM levels. *New England Journal of Medicine, 290,* 6.

Acoustic Tumor

Martyn L. Hyde, Ph.D.
Silverman Hearing Research Laboratory,
Mount Sinai Hospital,
Toronto, Ontario, Canada

The patient is a male, aged 43 years, who first presented in 1981 with right-sided hearing difficulty, tinnitus, and episodic dizziness. ENT examination was unremarkable. Audiologic testing revealed bilateral sloping sensorineural hearing loss, mild on the left and moderate to severe on the right. SRTs were 10 dB and 40 dB, respectively; on the right, the maximum PB score was 68%, with rollover. Electronystagmography revealed substantial caloric depression on the right.

ABR examination with 85 dB nHL, 20/s alternating polarity click stimuli showed normal response on the left, and only a delayed wave V on the right; the interaural wave V latency difference was 0.6 ms, which was corrected to 0.3 ms by subtracting 0.15 ms per 10 dB of pure tone loss above 55 dB at 4000 Hz. The ABR results were thought to be consistent with cochlear dysfunction. As a further check, endomeatal electrocochleography was performed to enhance wave I on the right side. This was successful, and the interpeak latency difference from I to V was 4.1 ms, similar to that observed for the left side. This reinforced the impression that the lesion was cochlear in nature.

The physician's judgment was that further investigation was warranted. A CT scan with positive contrast showed a subtle area of increased density adjacent to the right internal auditory canal. An additional scan three weeks later confirmed the presence of a small, well-defined lesion, which was considered unlikely to be an acoustic tumor because of its lack of relationship to the petrous bone and the internal auditory canal. Cerebral angiography showed normal posterior fossa vasculature. A repeat ABR investigation gave identical results to those obtained previously.

Surgical exploration failed to reveal a tumor, but a loop of blood vessels was found to be pressing on the seventh and eighth nerves. This was mobilized away from the nerves. The CT abnormality was attributed to a redundant posterior-inferior cerebellar artery.

Two months after surgery, some improvement has occurred in the patient's symptoms, but there has been intermittent recurrence of tinnitus and dizziness; the audiologic findings are essentially unchanged.

This case study illustrates various elements of ABR investigation. The basic ABR yielded delayed wave V and no wave I on the suspected side, which is a common pattern. The uncorrected ILD V was abnormal, but it is essential to correct ILDs to avoid many false-positive diagnostic errors due to cochlear hearing loss. The corrected ILD was just within normal limits; we consider 0.4 ms to be an appropriate diagnostic criterion. Of course, the inference is graded in the borderline region. ECochG was a useful adjunct test to clarify wave I and enable the interpeak latency to be measured.

Because the sensitivity of the ABR to acoustic tumors is very good, the electrophysiologic results suggested that there was no such tumor; this was correct. Because acoustic tumor is the most common retrocochlear pathology and cochlear disease is by far the most common alternative diagnosis, the inference that cochlear disease was present was reasonable. The investigation could easily have stopped at that point, and in most cases the pathology would indeed be solely cochlear. In retrospect, the continuation to invasive radiologic studies was opportune. The high-quality scan interpretation, having shown a lesion which was probably not an acoustic tumor, radically reduced the diagnostic value of the "cochlear" ABR pattern; this is so because the ABR is less sensitive to cerebellopontine angle lesions other than acoustic tumor.

The vascular abnormality mimicked several audiologic features of retrocochlear disease, yet did not produce the ABR pattern typical of acoustic tumor. Whether such patterns arise by direct disruption of neural synchrony or by suppression of discharge in high frequency neurons located primarily on the exterior of the acoustic nerve, it is interesting that they did not occur in this case. One possibility is that the vascular anomaly induced cochlear degeneration, which differed somehow from tumor action on the nerve or on the cochlear blood supply.

Neurofibromatosis

John T. Jacobson, Ph.D.,
Department of Communicative Disorders,
University of Mississippi,
University, Mississippi,
and Robin C. Morehouse, M.S.,
Dalhousie University and Nova Scotia Hearing and Speech Clinic,
Halifax, Nova Scotia, Canada

This case study describes a 27 year old female with von Recklinghausen neurofibromatosis who presented with bilateral acoustic neuromas. Prior to audiologic intervention, the patient underwent a craniotomy for the removal of a right temporal and right occipital meningioma. As part of neurologic follow-up, audiologic services were requested. Initial testing showed an unusual peak-trough pure tone configuration with SRTs of 25 and 30 dB HL for the right and left ears, respectively. Immittance audiometry and other site-of -lesion tests were normal. Based on previous history and unique audiometric function, the patient was scheduled for ABR. A 70 dB SL click stimulus was presented monaurally at a rate of 10/s using a vertical montage and a bandpass of 150 to 3000 Hz. Response tracings (Fig. 21-5A) revealed binaural abnormality with greater severity in the right ear. Absolute latencies for the right ear showed prolonged waves III and V and an I–V interwave interval (IWI) of 5.16 ms. The left ear IWI was marginally delayed (4.40 ms). Interestingly, the V/I amplitude ratio was less than 1.0 in both ears. Based on ABR results, a computed tomographic (CT) scanning was ordered, with no evidence of abnormality. No further action was taken.

The patient returned six months later for audiologic evaluation complaining of dizziness and reduced auditory sensitivity. Test results showed a moderate bilateral high frequency sensorineural hearing loss; acoustic reflexes were present but elevated; and reflex was decayed bilaterally at 500 and 1000 Hz. A PIPB produced a positive rollover function. Using a similar protocol to that described previously, ABR revealed a worsening picture (Fig. 21-5B). The I–V IWI increased to 5.6 ms for the right ear and 5.32 ms for the left. Amplitude ratios had decreased to less than 0.5 bilaterally. Prolonged IWIs coupled with reduced amplitude ratio values offered a positive picture of neurologic abnormality. The results of a second CT scan were negative.

Based on continued patient distress, a third ABR was requested by the attending neurologist. At this point, ABR results (Fig. 21-5C) showed a well-defined wave I peak with no identifiable later waves for the right ear and a dramatically reduced wave I amplitude with essentially absent responses thereafter in the left ear. A CT scan with enhancement (air contrast) revealed bilateral acoustic neuromas with greater mass on the right side and evidence of a meningoma posterior to the right-sided tumor.

On admission to surgery, neurologic examination showed right fifth nerve palsy and rapidly deteriorating hearing. Using a right posterior fossa approach, a massive 4 × 4 × 3 cm meningoma was encountered and partially removed; following this, subtotal removal of an

Figure 21-5.

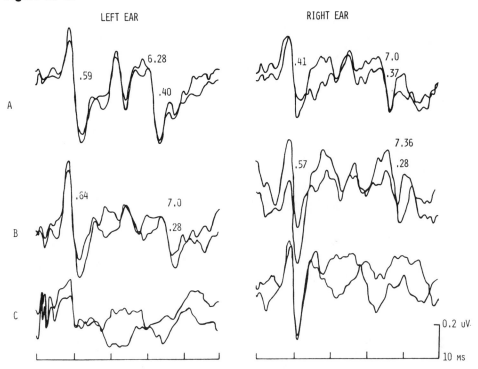

acoustic neuroma was completed with intraoperative ABR monitoring. In an attempt to preserve hearing, the intracanalicular portion of the tumor was not removed. ABR showed stability of hearing in the right ear but postoperative evaluation showed a substantial decrease in auditory sensitivity. A second surgical intervention was scheduled for removal of an acoustic neuroma on the left. A CT scan on the cervical area and expansion of the spinal cord suggested the appearance of a small intramedullary glioma. Unfortunately, during surgery, the patient developed complete left lung collapse that could not be resolved, the operation was terminated. Another operation is presently under consideration. This case illustrates a number of important issues: (1) the sensitivity of ABR in the early detection of acoustic neuroma in the absence of radiologic evidence; (2) the importance of longitudinal data collection to substantiate diagnostic prognostication; and (3) the quantification of latency (prolonged I-V interwave intervals) and amplitude (V/I ratio) values, which were used to identify a neurologic abnormality.

Frequency Specificity

Paul Kileny, Ph.D., and Roger Lundberg, M.S.
Department of Audiology,
Glenrose Hospital
Edmonton, Alberta, Canada

A six year old girl was referred for an audiologic evaluation after she had failed a school hearing screening. Speech and language development have been normal and neither the parents

Figure 21–6.

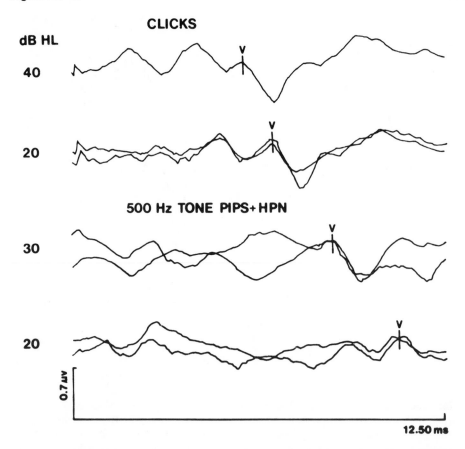

nor the patient had noted the presence of hearing difficulties. There was no family history of hearing impairment on the father's side; however, the mother was known to have had a mid-frequency bilateral mild to moderate sensory hearing loss since childhood. The patient's responses during behavioral audiometry were inconsistent. Tympanometry and acoustic reflex testing indicated normal middle ear function bilaterally with normal contralateral acoustic reflex thresholds bilaterally for all activating frequencies. Owing to the inconsistent results obtained during initial behavioral audiometry, the patient was rescheduled for ABR testing. Brainstem responses were elicited by unfiltered broad band clicks and 500 Hz tone pips embedded in continuous high pass filtered white noise, as described elsewhere (Kileny, 1981).

Figure 21-6 illustrates the auditory brainstem responses obtained following right ear stimulation. The responses obtained following left ear stimulation were identical to those obtained from the right. Well-defined responses to both broad band clicks and 500 Hz tone pips were obtained at 20 dB HL. Based on these results, the absence of any apparent hearing problems and the normal acoustic reflex thresholds normal bilateral hearing sensitivity was presumed. Still, because we never really obtained reliable behavioral audiometric thresholds, behavioral audiometry was repeated eight months later. Figure 21-7 is the audiogram obtained on that date. The accuracy and the reliability of our patient's responses were considered to be good at that time. The pure tone audiogram indicates normal hearing sensitivity at 500 Hz and below and at 4000 Hz and above. There is, however, a moderate hearing loss in the mid-frequencies.

Figure 21–7.

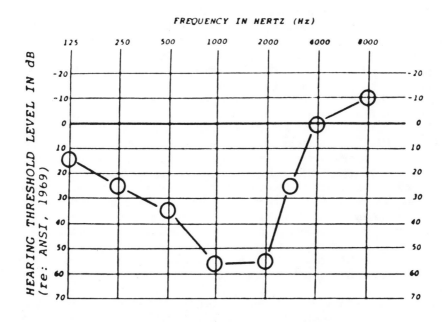

Thus, utilizing 500 Hz tone pips and broad band clicks we accurately predicted normal hearing sensitivity in the high frequency and low frequency regions. The slope of wave V latency-intensity function for clicks was 34 μs/dB, which is considered to be within the normal range. The reason we missed diagnosing a hearing loss in the mid-frequency region was that we did not use 1000 Hz tone pips as well. Based on click and 500 Hz tone pip results, we assumed normal hearing across frequencies. This case underlines the necessity of measuring auditory brainstem response thresholds at mid-frequencies in addition to low frequencies and clicks that coincide with thresholds in the 2000-4000 Hz region (Kileny, 1981).

REFERENCE

Kileny, P. (1981). The frequency specificity of tone-pip evoked auditory brain stem responses. *Ear and Hearing, 2,* 270–275.

Detection of Multiple Level Auditory Pathway Abnormality with Audiometry and Evoked Potentials

George E. Lynn, Ph.D., and Saleem A. Tahir, M.D.
Departments of Audiology and Neurology,
Wayne State University School of Medicine, and
Holden Laboratory of Clinical Neurophysiology,
Harper-Grace Hospital, Detroit, Michigan

This 27 year old, left-handed woman was seen for audiometric and evoked potential tests as part of the diagnostic studies and subsequent follow-up for brain tumor. Her history included otitis media and purulent meningitis at 9 months of age. At 2½ years she developed generalized seizures and was treated with anticonvulsants. At 23 years she had sudden onset of tremors of the right hand and was admitted to the hospital. A neurologic examination revealed the left pupil was larger in diameter (4 mm) than the right (3 mm) and both reacted to light; right central facial palsy; exaggerated tendon reflexes; increased tone in the right upper and lower extremities; equivocal right Babinski sign; and dysmetria of the right upper extremity. CT scans revealed an isodense area in the insular region of the right hemisphere with mass effect, shift of the third ventricle to the left, and effacement of the frontal horn of the right lateral ventricle. The diagnosis of an infiltrating neoplasm of the right insula was made. The positive clinical findings on the right side were considered to reflect pressure effects of the tumor on the left side of the midbrain and left corticopontine and corticospinal pathways. Surgery was not considered owing to the location of the mass, and the patient was treated with steroids, chemotherapy, and radiotherapy. In time, the tremor of the right hand disappeared and the increased tone and exaggerated tendon reflexes returned to normal.

At age 26, the patient was readmitted to the hospital for reevaluation. The neurologic examination revealed the following symptoms: weakness and paresthesia of the left upper and lower extremities, right supraorbital pain, and poor memory. Abnormal signs included increased tone, decreased strength, incoordination of extremities, and exaggerated tendon reflexes all on the left side. A left-sided Babinski response was present. These clinical signs indicated right cerebral hemisphere abnormality. Repeat CT scans (Fig. 21-8A) obtained before and during admission revealed no change in the appearance of the lateral, third and fourth ventricles. However, a definite abnormality was now seen consisting of calcifications occupying the central region of the pons (arrow) and an isodense mass (dots) and associated lucency (arrows) involving the right temporal and parietal lobes. She was again treated with steroids and chemotherapy and discharged with a further course of radiotherapy and chemotherapy as an outpatient.

Audiometric and evoked potential studies obtained during this hospitalization (Fig. 21-8B to D) revealed the following abnormal features: (1) a mild, predominantly high frequency conductive hearing loss in the right ear, (2) decreased middle ear compliance bilaterally with abnormal acoustic reflexes (not shown), (3) reduced ABR amplitudes for waves I, II, and III on the right side (80 dB HL) with increased absolute latencies, but with increased ABR amplitudes on the right side at 90 dB HL, 4) abnormally prolonged ($>$3.0 standard deviations) I–III and I–V interpeak latencies bilaterally compared with female norms, and (5) absent MLR components Pa and Pb recorded from the right temporoparietal region during left ear stimulation, with recognizable Pa and Pb components in the left hemisphere recordings.

The audiometric and evoked potential findings indicated (1) bilateral middle ear dysfunction with slightly greater involvement on the right side, (2) a caudal pontine abnormality involving auditory pathways projecting from both ears, and (3) an abnormality involving the auditory system of the right hemisphere.

One year later, at age 27, this patient was readmitted to the hospital because of significant changes in behavior and psychiatric disorder. A repeat neurologic examination revealed further deterioration in the clinical picture. Repeat CT scans (Fig. 21-9A) continued to show calcifications in the central region of the pons (arrow) and an isodense abnormality pushing on the right lateral ventricle (dots). The previously observed lucency in the right temporal and parietal lobes had partially resolved.

Repeat audiometric and evoked potential studies (Fig 21-9B to D) revealed (1) increased conductive hearing loss on the right side with no change on the left, (2) no change in the impedance measures, (3) significantly reduced ABR amplitudes at 90 dB HL on the right side compared to the first study, (4) abnormally prolonged ABR interpeak latencies bilaterally, and (5) identifiable MLR Pa and Pb components recorded from the right hemisphere, which were absent on the first study. Results continued to demonstrate the middle ear and caudal pontine

Figure 21-8.

Test results at age 26 years. CT (A) shows calcifications in the central pons (arrow) and an isodense mass (dots) with associated lucency (arrows) in the right temporoparietal region. Audiogram and impedance tests (B) and prolonged ABR (C) wave I latency with reduced amplitude indicate conductive involvement. Prolonged ABR I–III and I–V interval latencies indicate pontine level abnormality. Absent MLR (D) Pa component from the right hemisphere indicates a right temporoparietal abnormality. MR = muscle response.

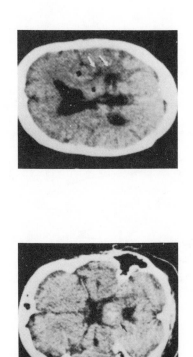

A - CT

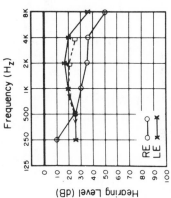

B - Audiometry

Illustration continued on following page.

Fig. 21–8 (continued). See legend on preceding page.

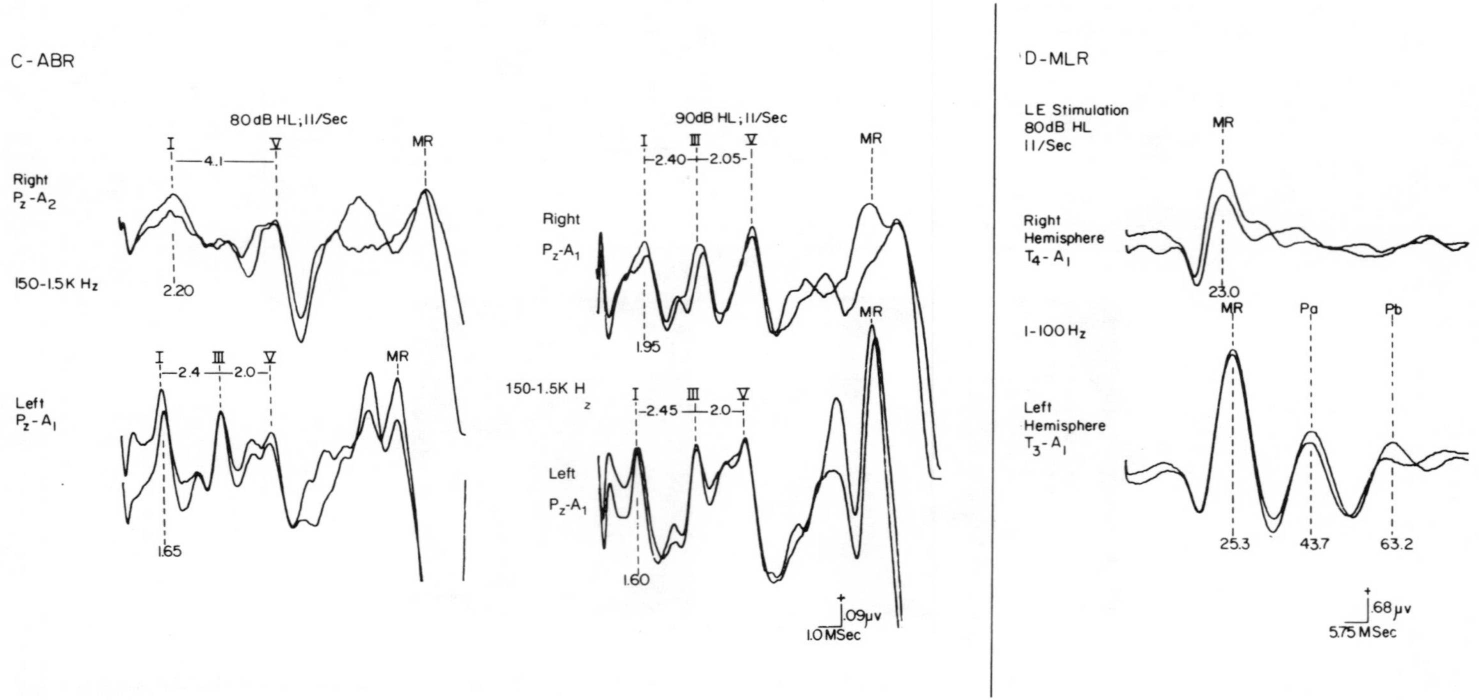
C-ABR
80dB HL; 11/Sec
I
4.1
V
MR
Right
Pz-A2
2.20
150-1.5K Hz
I
2.4
III
2.0
V
MR
Left
Pz-A1
1.65
90dB HL; 11/Sec
I
III
V
2.40
2.05
MR
Right
Pz-A1
1.95
150-1.5K Hz
I
III
V
2.45
2.0
MR
Left
Pz-A1
1.60
+ .09μv
1.0 MSec
D-MLR
LE Stimulation
80dB HL
11/Sec
MR
Right
Hemisphere
T4-A1
23.0
1-100 Hz
MR
Pa
Pb
Left
Hemisphere
T3-A1
25.3
43.7
63.2
+ .68μv
5.75 MSec

Figure 21-9.
Repeat test results at age 27 years. CT (A) shows no change in the pontine calcifications (arrow) or right hemisphere isodense mass (dots) and partial resolution of the right hemisphere lucency. Audiogram (B) shows increased right conductive hearing loss but no change in the tympanogram. ABR (C) reveals prolonged wave I latency, reduced amplitudes, and prolonged I–III and I–V interval latencies consistent with the conductive hearing loss and the pontine abnormality. MLR (D) tracings show a return of the right hemisphere Pa component following partial resolution of the right temporoparietal lucency shown on the CT. MR = muscle response.

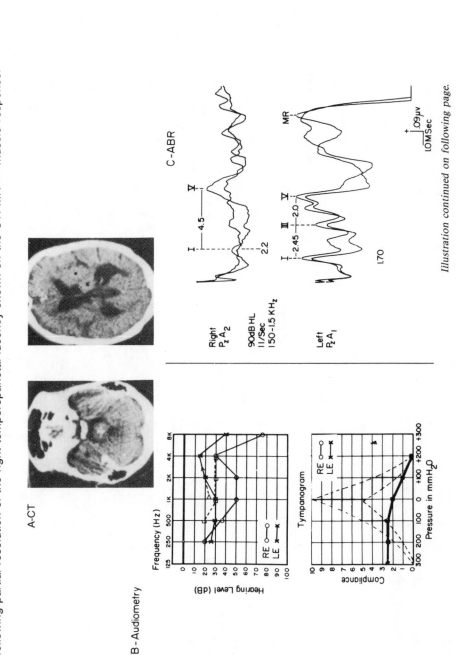

Illustration continued on following page.

Fig. 21-9 (continued). See legend on preceding page.

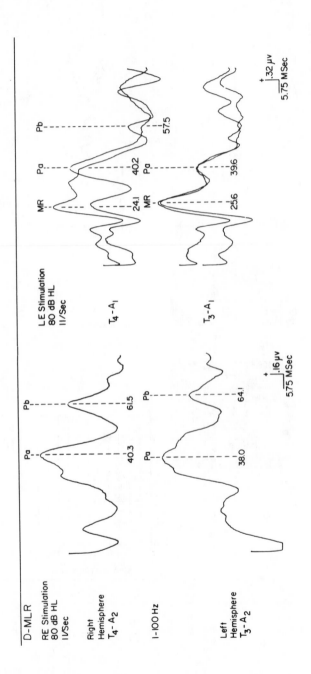

abnormalities. However, at this time there was no MLR evidence of the right hemisphere abnormality, which was clearly present one year earlier.

COMMENT

This case serves as a good example of the role of evoked potentials in diagnosing neurologic problems—that is, the detection and localization of lesions affecting function of the auditory system. Furthermore, when standard and special audiometric procedures are used in conjunction with ABR and MLR, the functional integrity of the entire auditory system may be evaluated from the periphery to the auditory cortex. This is illustrated very well in this case in which the audiometric and evoked potential data correlate well with the clinical and radiologic abnormalities detected during the course of the patient's illness. Even though the reasons for the middle ear and brainstem abnormalities were obscure, the tests nevertheless were sensitive to the effects of the lesions and differentiated the level of the abnormalities. It is also clear from this case that these tests may be useful in monitoring the course of a patient's illness, as shown here by the return of the Pa component of the right hemisphere MLR, which possibly reflects the resolution of the lucency associated with the right temporoparietal lobe mass shown on the CT scan. Finally, it is important to emphasize again that these tests are sensitive to the effects of lesions and serve the important roles of detection, localization, and monitoring of abnormalities to the auditory system.

Acoustic Nerve Microvascular Decompression

Margareta B. Møller, M.D., Ph.D., and Aage R. Møller, Ph.D.
Division of Audiology and
Department of Neurological Surgery,
University of Pittsburgh
Pittsburgh, Pennsylvania

The patient is a 39 year old white male who two years prior to admittance experienced a progressive loss of hearing in his left ear together with constant tinnitus and dizziness. His main problem was dizziness, nausea, and vomiting. He had been seen by two otologists and diagnosed as having Meniere's disease. (However, nothing in the patient's case history indicated Meniere's syndrome. He had no fluctuation in his hearing and no attacks of vertigo, although he was constantly dizzy). The patient mentioned that he often had to stop his truck due to nausea and go out and lie down beside the truck, often vomiting. The patient was seen at the Division of Audiology, Eye and Ear Hospital, in January, 1983. Upon examination tympanic membranes were normal bilaterally. Hearing tests on January 13 showed a flat sensorineural hearing loss of 80 dB in his left ear. He had normal hearing up to 3000 Hz on his right ear and an 80 dB loss at 4000 Hz, most likely caused by noise exposure. Speech discrimination scores were 100 percent in his right ear, and 16 percent in his left ear. Auditory brainstem responses (ABR) showed a normal pattern on the right ear, but the left ear had a delay of wave II, an absence of wave III, and a very small amplitude of wave V (Fig. 21-10). Vestibular testing revealed a peripheral vestibular lesion with a reduced response to caloric stimulation on the left ear. He had elevated acoustic reflex thresholds elicited from the left ear, 105 dB at 500, 1000 and 2000 Hz, indicating an auditory nerve lesion. When elicited from the right ear, the acoustic reflex thresholds were elevated at 1000 and 2000 Hz.

Figure 21–10.

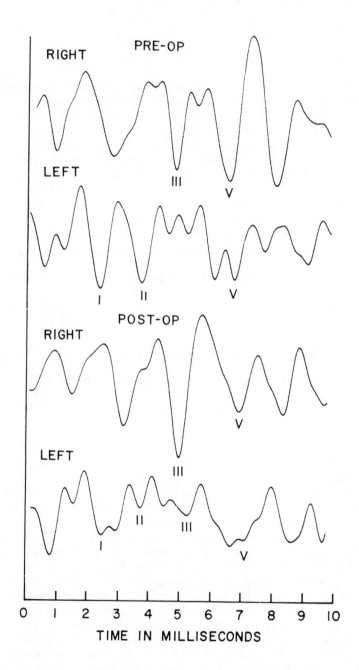

Illustration continued on following page.

Figure 21–10 (continued).

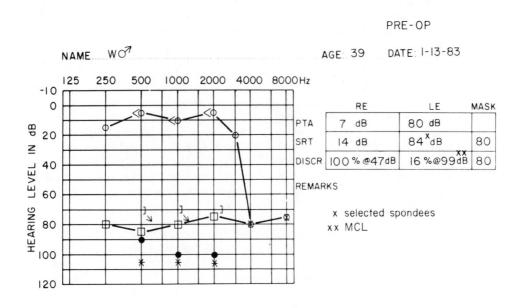

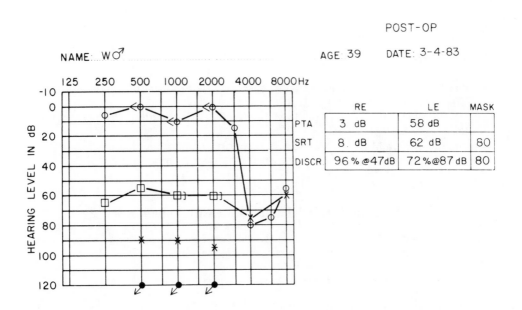

As was shown in Chapter 2, intracranial recordings from the auditory nerve showed that both waves I and II were generated by the auditory nerve (distal and proximal part), and a prolonged latency of wave II and a poorly defined wave III were an indication of a proximal auditory nerve lesion. The changes in the ABR pattern obtained in the left ear of this patient thus indicate involvement of the proximal part of the nerve. The absence of wave III indicates loss of synchrony of firings in the cochlear nucleus, which then results in a poor response of more central nuclei.

The patient was operated upon on January 14, 1983, using the technique described by Jannetta (1977, 1981) and a microvascular decompression of the eighth nerve was done (Jannetta, Møller, & Møller, 1984). It was found that a vessel was compressing the root entry zone of the eighth nerve. During the operation, recordings were made from the auditory nerve, which indicated prolonged latencies of intracranial auditory nerve potentials. After the operation the patient's dizziness improved immediately and his tinnitus gradually improved within two to three weeks. During the postoperative period to February 19, 1983, the patient had a few slight dizzy spells, and he heard an occasional weak humming noise. Upon testing on March 4, 1983, his hearing threshold had improved—a flat loss of 60 dB was present and his speech discrimination was 72 percent on the left ear, compared with 16 percent preoperatively. His acoustic middle ear reflexes on the left ear were normal.

In this case one important objective test result was that the ABR showed clearly that there was an involvement of the auditory nerve and that this involvement was localized to the intracranial portion of the eighth nerve. This finding was confirmed during the operation, when it was found that a blood vessel was pressing on the eighth cranial nerve. This blood vessel was removed from the nerve and an implant of soft Teflon felt was placed between the vessel and the nerve using the technique described for treatment of hemifacial spasm (Jannetta, 1977, 1981). The subsequent clinical finding that the patient's symptoms of dizziness and tinnitus disappeared further supports the diagnosis. In addition, the fact that his speech discrimination score increased further (from 16 to 70 percent) shows that he had an involvement of the auditory nerve and that the technique of microvascular decompression is an efficient treatment of this disorder.

REFERENCES

Jannetta, P.J. (1977). Etiology and definitive microsurgical treatment of hemifacial spasm. *Journal of Neurosurgery, 47,* 321–328.

Jannetta, P.J. (1981). Hemifacial spasm. In M. Samii & P.J. Jannetta (Eds.), *The cranial nerves.* New York: Springer-Verlag.

Jannetta, P.J., Møller, M.B., and Møller, A.R. (in press). Disabling positional vertigo (DPV).

A "Frank's Run" Latency-Intensity Function

Terence W. Picton, M.D., Ph.D., and David R. Stapells, Ph.D.
Human Neurosciences Research Unit,
University of Ottawa,
Ottawa, Ontario, Canada

This case illustrates an unusual latency-intensity function for the click-evoked auditory brainstem response. The patient was an 11 year old girl with a sensorineural hearing loss. Her auditory brainstem responses to broadband clicks are shown in Figure 21-11A. The clicks were presented at a rate of 39/s and the ABRs were recorded from vertex to ipsilateral mastoid using a filter bandpass of 25 to 3000 Hz. Averaging was carried out over 2000 trials after artifact rejection at $\pm 20 \mu$V limits, and replicate averages were obtained at each intensity. The waveforms are plotted such that negativity at the vertex is upward. At high intensities there is a clear wave V (filled triangle), which increases in latency from 5.6 to 6.5 ms as the intensity is decreased from 80 to 60 dB nHL. At 60 dB a second positive wave with a peak latency of 11.0 ms occurs in the waveform. Below 60 dB this second positive wave becomes the dominant component

Figure 21–11. "Frank's Run" latency-intensity function. *A,* Auditory brainstem responses to broad-band clicks. *B,* Latency-intensity function for wave V to clicks. *C,* Pure tone audiogram. *D,* Derived narrow-band auditory brainstem responses at 500 Hz and 2000 Hz.

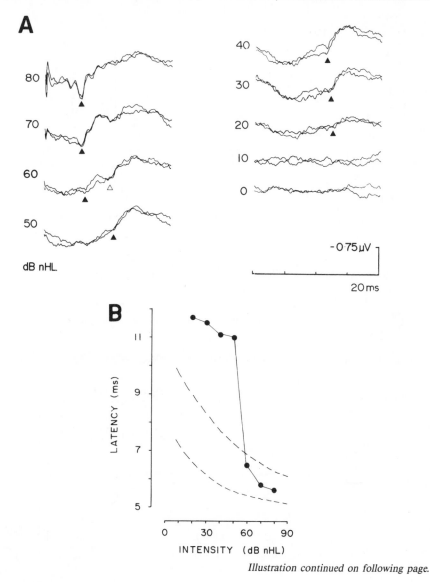

Illustration continued on following page.

Figure 21–11 (continued). See legend on preceding page.

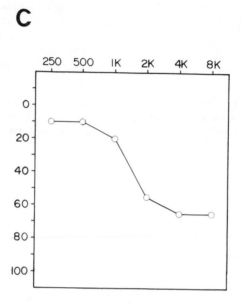

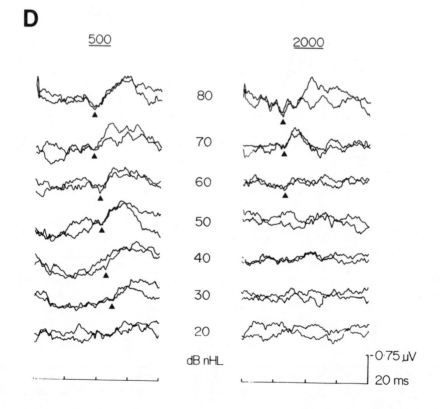

of the response and increases in latency from 11.0 to 11.7 ms as the intensity decreases from 50 to 20 dB. The latency-intensity function, plotted in Figure 21-11B, shows normal latencies at high intensity (the dashed lines represent the $\pm 2SD$ limits) and a sudden change in latency between 60 and 50 dB. This latency-intensity function was morphologically similar to the patient's conventional pure tone audiogram, shown in Figure 21-11C.

This audiogram suggested a possible explanation for the unusual latency-intensity function. The patient has normal thresholds at frequencies of 1000 Hz and lower. At 2000 to 8000 Hz the thresholds are between 55 and 65 dB. We hypothesized that there was a double wave V, with one component originating through the low frequency region of the cochlea and another component through the high frequency region. At high intensities the broadband click would activate all regions of the cochlea. The high frequency regions are more easily synchronized than the low frequency regions and would evoke a large, sharp wave V. This would occur at the normal latency for wave V, since in the normal hearing subject the 2000 to 4000 Hz region of the cochlea is the source of the measured wave V (again because of the synchronizability of discharge from this region). The neural response from the low frequency region of the cochlea would have a later latency because of the traveling-wave delay in the cochlea. Furthermore, it would be less synchronized and would evoke a broad rather than sharp wave V from the brainstem. Much of this could be obscured by the vertex-negative V′ following the wave V elicited through the high frequency region. At 60 dB, which is only just above the threshold at 2000 Hz, the wave V from the 500 to 1000 Hz region would become recognizable. Below 60 dB only the low frequency wave V would be visible.

This hypothesis could be tested by examining the derived responses obtained using high pass noise masking. Auditory brainstem responses were recorded using the same protocols but in the presence of masking noise having high pass cut-offs of 4000, 2000, 1000, and 500 Hz, and sequentially subtracting the responses to obtain the narrow band–derived responses. The derived responses at 500 Hz and 2000 Hz are plotted in Figure 21-11D. The replicability of these recordings is somewhat less than that of the unmasked clicks, for two reasons: first, the subtraction process effectively increases the unaveraged background electrical noise by a factor of 1.4; second, the acoustic noise tends to make the subject more tense and thereby results in higher levels of muscle activity in the recordings. Despite the noisiness of the recordings, a sharp wave V can be recorded in the 2000 Hz response with a peak latency increasing from 6.0 to 6.5 ms from 80 to 60 dB and a broader wave V can be identified in the 500 Hz response increasing in latency from 9.0 to 12.0 ms from 80 to 30 dB. It can easily be seen how the response to the broad band click could be made by combining the responses from the high threshold 2000 Hz region of the cochlea and the responses from the normal threshold 500 Hz region.

"Frank's Run" is a cross-country ski trail in the hills just north of Ottawa. It is characterized by sudden steep slopes, much like this patient's latency-intensity function and pure tone audiogram. The following comments derive from the dangers inherent in examining a patient with an audiogram that changes levels as rapidly as does this ski trail. First, it is important to realize that there may occasionally be two wave V peaks in an ABR. Second, it is essential to use a sweep of longer than 10 ms when recording ABRs in any patient. A sweep of 10 ms would not have allowed the recognition of the delayed wave V to the click stimulus at intensities of below 60 dB. Third, it is always important to record responses at two different subthreshold levels before deciding on an elevated ABR threshold. Because there may be overlapping waves generated at different latencies, it is possible for these to cancel each other out at one particular intensity. This might have happened to the click evoked response at 60 dB if there were not an underlying 40 Hz response recorded. At this intensity the two components of wave V overlap and are not easily distinguishable. Fourth, the interpretation of latency-intensity functions for the click evoked wave V can be very complex. It is probably better to evolve some frequency-specific ABR protocol than to attempt the construction of an audiogram from the latency-intensity function of responses that are not frequency-specific.

The Contralateral Effect of a Large CPA Tumor

Daniel M. Schwartz, Ph.D.
Division of Hearing and Speech Sciences
Vanderbilt University School of Medicine
and Kristine Olson, M.A.,
Speech and Hearing Center,
Hospital of the University of Pennsylvania,
Philadelphia, Pennsylvania

This 22 year old male college student came to the Speech and Hearing Center at the Hospital of the University of Pennsylvania with a chief complaint of hearing loss accompanied by an occasional sensation of pounding in the right ear, which he had experienced during the past eight months. The remaining case history was unremarkable for the presence of tinnitus, numbness, feeling of fullness, vertigo, or visual disturbance.

Figure 21-12A displays the pure tone test results for the right and left ears, respectively. Left ear findings showed essentially normal hearing sensitivity with the exception of a slight conductive component at 250 Hz. A three point performance-intensity function for monosyllabic words indicated excellent word recognition across intensities, with no evidence of rollover at 90 dB HL. Acoustic immittance results showed a tympanogram characterized by a normal shape, normal amplitude, and negative peak pressure point at -180 mm H_2O with no change in peak pressure following Valsalva maneuver. When sound was presented to the left ear the crossed acoustic reflex was elicited at normal reflex hearing and sensation levels, whereas the uncrossed reflex was observed at normal reflex sound pressure levels at all test frequencies. Pure tone results for the right ear suggested a moderate-to-moderately severe sensorineural type hearing loss. Monosyllabic word recognition was severely depressed (8 percent) at 95 dB HL. Acoustic immittance results revealed a normal tympanogram. When sound was presented to the right ear, both the crossed and uncrossed acoustic reflexes were absent, consistent with a diagonal pattern. Because a unilateral sensorineural hearing loss, disproportionately reduced word recognition at high intensity levels and a diagonal acoustic reflex pattern all support an eighth nerve site, auditory brainstem responses were recorded to click stimuli using a vertex-to-earlobe electrode montage.

The results, displayed in Figure 21-12B, showed right ear responses characterized by a wave I at a normal amplitude and latency, a wave II at normal amplitude but slightly delayed latency, and an absence of all subsequent wavelets. Auditory brainstem responses for the left ear showed excellent morphology for waves I, II, and III, all of which had normal absolute latencies and amplitudes; thereafter, there tended to be a marked delay between waves IV and V such that wave V latency and its associated I–V interpeak latency were abnormally prolonged at 75, 85, and 95 dB nHL. Moreover, this latency abnormality tended to persist as stimulus click rate was increased from 11.1/s to 81.1/s.

When these data were viewed with the other auditory test findings, the resulting interpretation was that a large extra-axial neoplasm was present on the right that was compressing the brainstem as evidenced by the left-sided (contralateral) effects shown on the ABR.

Subsequent contrast-enhanced computed tomographic (CT) and nuclear magnetic resonance (NMR) scans demonstrated an enormous tumor mass occupying the anterior portion of the cerebellopontine angle with marked displacement of the brainstem to the left side, which was later partially resected by suboccipital craniectomy.

This case points to the importance of recording the ABR even in the presence of complete sensorineural hearing loss on the suspected side, since large CPA tumors often will compress the brainstem to the point of affecting the contralateral ABR.

Figure 21–12.

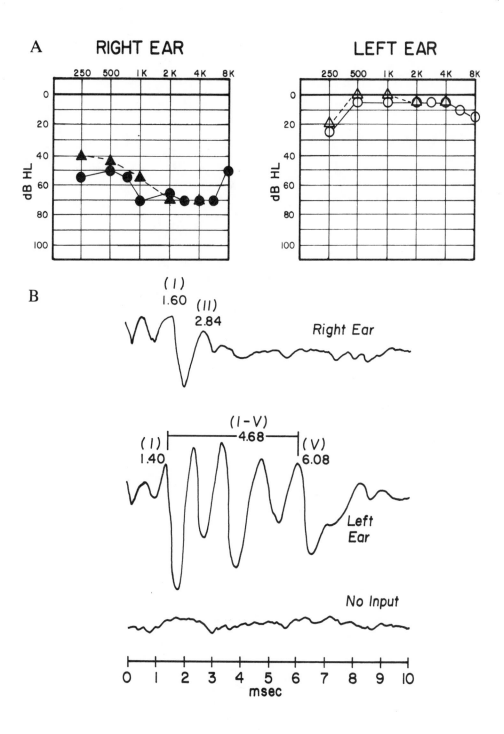

Author Index

Bennett, M., 13, 16, 243, 270
Ben-Yitzhak, E., 153
Bergamasco, B., 226, 231
Berger, H., 4
Berlin, C., 119, 125, 160, 306, 338, 379
Berman, S., 301
Berry, D. A., 344
Berry, G. A., 91, 255
Bes, A., 229
Bess, F. H., 349, 368
Bhargava, V. K., 240
Bickford, R. G., 205, 240, 255
Bjorkman, G., 181, 183, 184, 186, 187,
    188, 189
Blaauw-van Dishoeck, M., 255
Blair, R. L., 110
Blanks, J., 270
Blaw, M. E., 226, 287, 288, 298, 299, 342,
    379
Bledsoe, S. W., 256
Blegvad, B., 86, 255, 306, 342, 368, 375
Bleich, N., 153
Bluestone, C., 118, 125
Bobbin, R. P., 91, 239, 263
Boezeman, E., 119
Bohne, B., 182
Bonikowski, F., 190, 204
Borbely, A. A., 239
Bordley, J. E., 5
Borg, E., 75, 11, 118, 380
Børre, S., 342
Bosatra, A., 223
Bostock, H., 220
Boston, J. R., 71, 72, 243, 260, 306
Bouman, M. A., 51
Bowman, R., 51
Bowman, T., 90
Braakman, R., 255
Brackman, D., 9
Brackmann, D. E., 110, 137, 157, 158,
    159, 181, 183, 184, 185, 186, 187,
    289
Branch, C., 237, 238
Brattson, A., 118, 119
Braun, C., 50
Brazier, M. A. B., 237, 239
Bremer, D., 311
Bresnaw, M. J., 288
Breuninger, C., 351

Brewer, C. C., 255
Brinkman, R. D., 165, 305
Britt, R. H., 13, 255, 263
Broms, P., 341, 342
Bronshvag, M., 297, 298
Brooks, D. N., 338
Brooks, E. B., 225, 276, 287
Broughton, R. J., 237, 238
Brown, C. K., 126
Brown, D. D., 376, 377
Brown, K. A., 126, 205, 343
Brown, M. B., 340
Brown, R. M., 4
Bruce, D. A., 255, 263
Brugge, J. F., 182
Brunberg, J. A., 245
Brune, M. J., 222
Bryne, D., 349
Buchwald, J., 13, 28, 204, 205, 339, 343,
    359, 361
Buda, F. B., 88, 300, 318
Burkard, R., 148, 153, 160, 167, 169, 298,
    299, 302, 305, 306, 307, 310
Bustion, P. F., 270
Bzoch, K., 126

C

Cacace, A. T., 71, 72
Calder, C., 225
Callner, A. A., 340
Campbell, K. B., 50, 139, 150, 303, 304
Campbell, K. R., 76
Cann, J., 54, 75
Cant, B. R., 255
Cantrell, R. W., 72, 75, 76, 86
Cao, M., 297
Capon, A., 255, 256
Carlin, J., 256
Carasso, R., 224, 231
Carhart, R., 222
Cartee, C., 342
Casey, D., 119
Celesia, G. G., 237, 238, 343, 372
Cevette, M. J., 373
Chaplin, E. R., 310
Charachon, R., 182

Jaggi, J., 263
Jahrsdoerfer, R., 255, 269, 271
Jannetta, P. J., 13, 14, 16, 17, 19, 20, 22, 23, 24, 26, 29, 184, 188, 243, 244, 245, 270, 410
Jasper, H. H., 84
Javel, E., 51, 91, 240
Jennett, B., 255, 257
Jerger, J. J., 83, 89, 90, 110, 119, 137, 150, 185, 186, 187, 223, 287, 311, 373, 374, 376
Jerger, S., 9, 119
Jerison, H. J., 340
Jewett, D. I., 203
Jewett, D. L., 5, 8, 65, 69, 71, 75, 255, 297
Jones, T. A., 205
Johnson, J. H., 184
Johnson, K. P., 222
Johnson, M. J., 8, 87, 103, 299, 300, 302, 303, 307
Johnson, P. E., 338
Johnson, S., 117
Jordan, C., 374
Josey, A., 9, 184, 289

K

Kaga, K., 189, 226, 241, 245, 248, 272, 287, 307, 310, 341, 342, 343
Kanjilal, G. C., 338
Kapteyn, T., 119
Karnahl, Th., 75, 226
Karnaze, D. S., 255
Karp, H. R., 204, 206
Katinski, S., 261
Katz, L., 343
Katz, R. B., 277
Kaufman, I., 118
Kaufman, L., 300, 306, 307, 310
Kavanagh, K. T., 373
Keith, R. W., 223, 226, 270
Kennedy, I., 256
Kerley, S. M., 307
Kevanishvili, Z., 71, 75
Kiang, N. Y. S., 149, 182, 239, 299, 303, 308, 343
Kibbe, K., 67, 184, 185, 188, 189, 190, 382

Kibler, R. F., 221
Kidder, H. R., 165
Kiessling, J., 350, 351, 354, 361, 363, 364, 365, 366, 367
Kileny, P., 167, 170, 240, 241, 245, 259, 307, 319, 321, 344, 351, 358, 400, 401
Kinarti, R., 67
Kinney, S., 189
Kirikae, I., 90
Kitazumi, E., 287
Kjaer, M., 231, 300
Klass, D. W., 256
Klauber, M. R., 255
Klee, M. R., 241
Klein, A. J., 163, 165, 167, 376, 381
Klein, J., 125
Kleinberg, F., 309
Klem, G., 272
Kline, D. G., 184
Klug, N., 255, 270
Knickerbocker, G. G., 5
Knothe, J., 351
Knott, J., 54, 75
Kobayashi, K., 343
Koblin, D. D., 238
Kodama, K., 287
Kodera, K., 139, 150, 153, 165, 305, 307
Kondo, C., 245
Konishi, M., 311
Konishi, T., 240
Konkle, D. F., 350
Korein, J., 272
Kraus, H. I., 237, 338, 343
Kraus, N., 237, 319, 321, 342, 343, 372
Krauz, H. J., 6
Krebs, D., 351, 357
Krug, D. A., 340, 341
Krumholz, A., 75, 319, 321, 328
Kuba, T., 190, 204
Kubik, C., 219
Kupperman, G. L., 71
Kurkland, L. T., 221
Kurmin, K., 319, 321
Kylen, P., 118, 119

L

Lacomme, Y., 16, 229
Lader, M., 239

Maurer, K., 225, 231
Maurizi, M., 90, 189
May, J. G., 91, 239
May, J. T., 263
Mazzoni, A., 182
McAlpine, D., 221, 223
McCabe, B. F., 241
McCaffee, M. A., 319, 321, 372
McCandless, G. A., 90
McCarthy, C. S., 255
McClelland, R., 300
McConnell, F. E., 349
McCracken, G., 126
McCrae, R., 300
McCullough, D. W., 239, 255
McCutcheon, M. J., 80, 81, 303
McDermott, J. C., 125
McDonald, J. M., 167
McGee, J., 91, 240
McGee, T., 184, 187
McGee, T. J., 111, 113, 114, 116, 125, 126
McKay, A. R., 255
McKean, C. M., 88, 116, 125, 126, 240,
    297, 298, 299, 300, 318
McKhann, G. M., 222
McPherson, D., 270, 306, 307, 308
McRandle, C. C., 343
Meder, R. N., 245
Meikle, M., 353
Mencher, G. T., 83, 87, 297, 298, 318,
    321, 349, 351, 352, 357, 372, 373
Mendel, M. I., 71, 240, 343
Mendel, M. L., 376
Mendelson, T., 116, 125, 126, 298, 299,
    300, 307, 310, 343
Merino-Canas, A., 256
Merrill, R. E., 288
Metz, D. A., 87, 299, 300, 301, 307, 309,
    310, 311, 318, 351, 359, 368, 374
Michalewski, H. J., 90
Miller, J. D., 254, 255, 256
Minderhoud, J. M., 255
Mirsky, A. F., 341
Miyazaki, H., 184, 292
Mjoen, S., 255, 307, 319
Mo, A., 303
Mokotoff, B., 226, 351, 357
Møller, A. R., 13, 14, 15, 16, 17, 19, 20,
    21, 22, 23, 24, 26, 29, 183, 184, 186,

188, 243, 270, 410
Møller, K., 306, 368
Møller, M. B., 13, 16, 29, 183, 184, 186,
    188, 243, 256, 270, 410
Mollerstrom, B., 307, 341, 342
Molner, C. E., 4
Monstrey, Y., 255
Montandon, P., 297
Moody, R. A., 270
Moore, D. R., 311
Moore, E. J., 5, 153, 307
Moore, J. K., 28
Moore, J. M., 350
Moore, R. Y., 28
Morehouse, C. R., 8, 87, 103, 299, 300,
    302, 303, 307, 321
Morest, K., 182
Morgan, A., 307, 310
Morgan, S. H., 255, 262, 271
Mori, K., 184, 239
Morlock, H. C., 338
Morra, B., 83
Moruzzi, G., 239
Mouney, D. F., 91, 240
Moushegian, G., 5, 148
Mrowinski, D., 375
Mueller, R. J., 184, 185, 190, 231, 271
Mundy, M. R., 111
Murray, B. M., 91
Murray, T. J., 220, 221, 223
Musiek, F. E., 9, 67, 184, 185, 186, 188,
    189, 190, 231, 271, 382
Myers, G. J., 395
Myokai, K., 241, 245, 248

N

Nagao, S., 255, 270
Nager, G. T., 5, 226
Narayan, R. K., 256
Naunton, R. F., 338
Neame, J. H., 239
Nelson, B. J., 222
Nemoto, S., 21, 278
Nencioni, C., 186
Newlon, P. G., 255, 256
Nichimoto, H., 255
Nielsen, B. L., 256

Y

Z

Subject Index*

*Page numbers in italics refer to illustrations or tables.